# Gastroenterology

*Guest Editors*

JAMES WINGER, MD
AARON MICHELFELDER, MD

# PRIMARY CARE:
# CLINICS IN OFFICE PRACTICE

www.primarycare.theclinics.com

*Consulting Editor*
JOEL J. HEIDELBAUGH, MD

September 2011 • Volume 38 • Number 3

SAUNDERS an imprint of ELSEVIER, Inc.

**W.B. SAUNDERS COMPANY**
*A Division of Elsevier Inc.*

1600 John F. Kennedy Boulevard, Suite 1800 ● Philadelphia, PA 19103-2899

http://www.theclinics.com

**PRIMARY CARE: CLINICS IN OFFICE PRACTICE Volume 38, Number 3**
**September 2011 ISSN 0095-4543, ISBN-13: 978-1-4557-1188-8**

Editor: Yonah Korngold

*Primary Care: Clinics in Office Practice* (ISSN: 0095–4543) is published quarterly by Elsevier Inc., 360 Park Avenue South, New York, NY 10010-1710. Months of issue are March, June, September, and December. Periodicals postage paid at New York, NY and additional mailing offices. Subscription prices are $203.00 per year (US individuals), $336.00 (US institutions), $101.00 (US students), $248.00 (Canadian individuals), $395.00 (Canadian institutions), $159.00 (Canadian students), $309.00 (international individuals), $395.00 (international institutions), and $159.00 (international students). Foreign air speed delivery is included in all *Clinics* subscription prices. All prices are subject to change without notice. POSTMASTER: Send address changes to *Primary Care: Clinics in Office Practice*, Elsevier Periodicals Customer Service, 11830 Westline Industrial Drive, St. Louis, MO 63146. Customer Service Health Sciences Division, Subscription Customer Service, 3251 Riverport Lane, Maryland Heights, MO 63043. **Customer Service: 1-800-654-2452 (U.S. and Canada); 314-447-8871 (outside U.S. and Canada). Fax: 314-447-8029. E-mail: journalscustomerservice-usa@elsevier.com (for print support); journalsonlinesupport-usa@elsevier.com (for online support).**

*Reprints.* For copies of 100 or more, of articles in this publication, please contact the Commercial Reprints Department, Elsevier Inc., 360 Park Avenue South, New York, NY 10010-1710. Tel. (212) 633-3812; Fax: (212) 482-1935; E-mail: reprints@elsevier.com.

*Primary Care: Clinics in Office Practice* is covered in *MEDLINE/PubMed (Index Medicus)* and *EMBASE/ Excerpta Medica, Current Contents/Clinical Medicine,* and *ISI/BIOMED.*

Printed and bound by CPI Group (UK) Ltd, Croydon, CR0 4YY

Transferred to Digital Print 2011

# Contributors

## CONSULTING EDITOR

### JOEL J. HEIDELBAUGH, MD
Clinical Assistant Professor and Clerkship Director, Department of Family Medicine; Clinical Assistant Professor, Department of Urology, University of Michigan Medical School, Ann Arbor, Michigan

## GUEST EDITORS

### JAMES WINGER, MD, CAQ
Primary Care Sports Medicine, Assistant Professor of Family Medicine, Department of Family Medicine, Loyola Stritch School of Medicine, Maywood, Illinois

### AARON MICHELFELDER, MD, FAAFP, FAAMA
Vice-Chair and Associate Professor of Family Medicine and Bioethics and Health Policy, Department of Family Medicine, Loyola Stritch School of Medicine, Maywood, Illinois

## AUTHORS

### JOHN AFFRONTI, MS, MD
Professor of Medicine, Division of Gastroenterology, Hepatology and Nutrition, Stritch School of Medicine, Loyola University of Chicago, Maywood, Illinois

### JOSEPH AHN, MD, MS, FACG
Assistant Professor of Medicine, Medical Director, Liver Transplantation, Loyola University Medical Center, Maywood, Illinois

### MANJULA CHERUKURI, MD
Assistant Professor, Department of Family and Community Medicine, University of Texas Southwestern Medical Center at Dallas, Dallas, Texas

### HOONBAE JEON, MD, FACS
Associate Professor of Surgery, Director, Liver Transplant and Hepatobiliary Surgery, Transplant Surgery Fellowship Program, Division of Transplant (MC958), Department of Surgery, University of Illinois at Chicago, Chicago, Illinois

### DONGSHENG JIANG, MD
Assistant Professor of Family Medicine, Family and Community Medicine, Hershey Medical College; Penn State University, State College, Pennsylvania

### MANJULA JULKA, MD
Associate Residency Director, Department of Family and Community Medicine, University of Texas Southwestern Medical Center at Dallas, Dallas, Texas

**RAHELE LAMEH, MD**
Assistant Professor, Department of Family and Community Medicine, University of Texas Southwestern Medical Center at Dallas, Dallas, Texas

**BRODI LYNCH, MD**
Resident Physician, Family Medicine Residency Program, St Luke's Hospital, University of Toledo, Maumee, Ohio

**JOHN MABEE, PhD, PA-C**
Assistant Professor of Clinical Family Medicine, Department of Family Medicine, University of Southern California, Los Angeles; Principal Faculty and Course Director-Pathophysiology, KSOM-USC Primary Care Physician Assistant Program, Alhambra, California

**MICHAEL A. MALONE, MD**
Assistant Professor and Associate Medical Director, Department of Family Medicine, Penn State College of Medicine, Hershey, Pennsylvania

**REBECCA L. MCCLARREN, MD**
Assistant Professor of Family Medicine, Family Medicine Residency Program, St Luke's Hospital, University of Toledo, Maumee, Ohio

**AARON MICHELFELDER, MD, FAAFP, FAAMA**
Vice-Chair and Associate Professor, Department of Family Medicine and Bioethics and Health Policy, Stritch School of Medicine, Loyola University Chicago, Maywood, Illinois

**WADIE I. NAJM, MD, MSED**
Clinical Professor, Department of Family Medicine and Geriatrics, Susan Samueli Center of Integrative Medicine, University of California, Irvine, Orange, California

**NEELIMA NYAYAPATI, MD**
Resident Physician, Family Medicine Residency Program, St Luke's Hospital, University of Toledo, Maumee, Ohio

**AMIMI S. OSAYANDE, MD**
Assistant Professor of Family Medicine, Department of Family and Community Medicine, University of Texas, Southwestern Medical Center, Dallas, Texas

**ZAFREEN SIDDIQUI, MD**
Assistant Professor of Family Medicine, Director of Maternity Care; Fellow High Risk Obstetrics for Family and Community Medicine, University of Texas Southwestern Medical Center, Dallas, Texas

**AUGUSTINE J. SOHN, MD, MPH**
Assistant Professor, Clinical Family Medicine, College of Medicine, University of Illinois at Chicago, Chicago, Illinois

**KASHYAP TRIVEDI, MD**
Staff Gastroenterologist, Hertz and Associates in Gastroenterology, Los Alamitos, California

**ANNE WALSH, MMSc, PA-C**
Instructor of Clinical Family Medicine, Department of Family Medicine, University of Southern California, Los Angeles; Interim Director, KSOM-USC Primary Care Physician Assistant Program, Alhambra; Senior Physician Assistant, Hertz and Associates in Gastroenterology, Los Alamitos, California

**JAMES WINGER, MD, CAQ**
Primary Care Sports Medicine, Assistant Professor, Department of Family Medicine, Stritch School of Medicine, Loyola University Chicago, Maywood, Illinois

# Contents

> Peptic ulcer disease (PUD) is due mostly to the widespread use of low-dose aspirin and nonsteroidal anti-inflammator drugs. It occurs mostly in older patients and those with comorbidities. Pain awakening the patient from sleep between 12 and 3 a.m. affects two-thirds of duodenal ulcer patients and one-third of gastric ulcer patients. Older adults (>80 years old) with PUD often do not present with abdominal pain; instead, epigastric pain, nausea and vomiting are among their most common presenting symptoms.

> Malabsorption syndrome encompasses numerous clinical entities that result in chronic diarrhea, abdominal distention, and failure to thrive. These disorders may be congenital or acquired and include cystic fibrosis and Shwachman-Diamond syndrome; the rare congenital lactase deficiency; glucose-galactose malabsorption; sucrase-isomaltase deficiency; adult-type hypolactasia leading to acquired lactose intolerance. The pathology may be due to impairment in absorption or digestion of nutrients resulting in Nutritional deficiency, gastrointestinal symptoms, and extra gastrointestinal symptoms. Treatment is aimed at correcting the deficiencies and symptoms to improve quality of life. Common disorders of malabsorption celiac disease, pernicious anemia, and lactase deficiency are discussed in this article.

> Crohn disease and ulcerative colitis are the most common forms of inflammatory bowel disease (IBD) likely to be encountered in primary care. Patient-centered care is essential for positive outcomes, and should include long-term continuity with an empathetic primary care provider who can provide skillful coordination of the requisite multidisciplinary approach. Early suspicion of the diagnosis and referral to expert gastroenterologists for confirmation and medical management is essential. Coordinating interdisciplinary consultations, including colorectal surgeons, radiologists, stoma therapists, psychologists, and rheumatologists, in combination with comprehensive patient education, is key to decreasing overall morbidity, mortality, and health care costs associated with IBD.

Better understanding about treatment is the key for primary care providers to provide better care for this group of patients. This review focuses on the treatment of the most common causes of chronic liver disease, including hepatitis B, hepatitis C, alcoholic cirrhosis, nonalcoholic fatty liver disease, and hemochromatosis.

Chronic rejection of liver graft is an insidious process. Major immunosuppression medications such as tacrolimus, cyclosporin, and sirolimus have dose-related toxicity and narrow therapeutic windows. Certain drugs can affect metabolism of calcineurin inhibitors. Primary care physicians should be vigilant for any unusual opportunistic infection in liver transplant recipients. The quality of life of liver transplant recipients is an important aspect of care by primary care physicians. Alcohol relapse and possibility of depression in liver transplant recipients should be a continuous concern for primary care physicians. This article provides a guideline for the care of liver transplant recipients.

The evaluation, management, and follow-up of patients with chronic pancreatitis (CP) can be simple, but it can also be complex, so having a good referral network of subspecialists experienced in this field is essential. Identifying the cause of CP requires a systematic review of the many potential causes when the cause is not obvious. The identification of patients with autoimmune CP is particularly important because treatment with steroids may be effective. Alterations in pain or other symptoms in patients with CP should not be attributed to worsening disease before evaluations for complications including malignancy are done.

Infectious diarrhea is both a local and a global concern. Illnesses can range from mild inconveniences to life-threatening epidemics. Although diarrhea can be caused by a vast array of pathogens, the cornerstone of prevention is provision of a safe food and water supply, application of basic hygiene principles, and the development and administration of vaccines. The cornerstone of treatment is rehydration. Selection of specific antimicrobial therapy should be based on disease presentation and epidemiologic factors.

**VISIT THE CLINICS ONLINE!**

Access your subscription at:
**www.theclinics.com**

# Foreword

# The Burden of Digestive Diseases

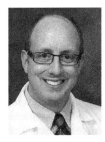

Joel J. Heidelbaugh, MD
  *Consulting Editor*

Digestive, liver, and pancreatic diseases result in greater than 100 million outpatient visits and 13 million hospitalizations annually at a cost of $141.8 billion.[1] A report published in 2009 by the National Institute of Diabetes and Digestive and Kidney Diseases highlighted the 10 most costly digestive diseases in the United States in both direct and indirect costs:

1. Digestive cancers: $24.1 billion
    a. $9.5 billion cost of colorectal cancer
    b. $4.3 billion cost for pancreatic cancer
2. Liver disease: $13.1 billion
3. Gastroesophageal reflux disease (GERD): $12.6 billion
4. Gallstones: $6.2 billion
5. Abdominal wall hernia: $6.1 billion
6. Diverticular disease: $4.0 billion
7. Pancreatitis: $3.7 billion
8. Viral hepatitis (A, B, C): $3.3 billion
9. Peptic ulcer disease: $3.1 billion
10. Appendicitis: $2.6 billion.

It's very easy to be intimidated by these statistics relative to expenditures, as well as seemingly increasing incidences of most of these disorders. As obesity becomes more prevalent, its association with acute and chronic gastrointestinal disorders becomes a greater burden on primary care, gastroenterology, and society.

While cancer screening remains a salient point of primary care, evidence-based guidelines exist for colorectal cancer screening, yet there are no acceptable provisions for pancreatic cancer screening. Deaths related to digestive diseases gradually declined between 1979 and 2004 (236 million cases), largely attributable to a decrease

Prim Care Clin Office Pract 38 (2011) xi–xii
doi:10.1016/j.pop.2011.06.002
0095-4543/11/$ – see front matter © 2011 Elsevier Inc. All rights reserved.

**primarycare.theclinics.com**

in colorectal cancer mortality due to increased screening rates through primary care. Chronic liver disease and cirrhosis ranks twelfth in mortality with an age-adjusted mortality rate of 9.2%.[2] The incidences of alcoholic cirrhosis, viral hepatitis (especially hepatitis C), and non-alcoholic fatty liver disease are all increasing. As we see more and more cases of liver disease, the primary care clinician will be required to know more about identification, etiology, and how to coordinate the complex care of the liver transplant patient.

Upper gastrointestinal disorders, including GERD and peptic ulcer disease, continue to be significant sources of distress for our patients, comprising the majority of referrals to gastroenterologists for management and endoscopic evaluation. Pharmaceutical costs of anti-secretory therapy (mainly proton pump inhibitors) exceeds $1.6 billion annually, plus the costs of over-the-counter medications.[3]

This volume of *Primary Care: Clinics in Office Practice* spans an enormous range of gastrointestinal disorders that affect our patients. Dedicated articles to common diseases of the upper and lower segments, solid organs, and relationship to obesity and transplantation offer up-to-date reviews of guidelines and pertinent trials.

I sincerely thank Drs Winger and Michelfelder, as well as their dedicated authors, for compiling an evidence-based and practical collection of reviews on common topics in gastroenterology. This volume will serve primary care clinicians well in their daily practices, providing the necessary statistics, diagnostic algorithms, and treatment plans to help minimize the burden of such chronic gastrointestinal diseases.

Joel J. Heidelbaugh, MD
Departments of Family Medicine and Urology
University of Michigan Medical School
Ann Arbor, MI
Ypsilanti Health Center
200 Arnet Street, Suite 200
Ypsilanti, MI 48198, USA

E-mail address:
jheidel@umich.edu

## REFERENCES

1. Everhart JE, editor. The burden of digestive diseases in the United States. US Department of Health and Human Services, Public Health Service, National Institutes of Health, National Institute of Diabetes and Digestive and Kidney Diseases. Washington, DC: US Government Printing Office; 2008. NIH Publication No. 09–6443.
2. Kochanek KD, Xu J, Murphy S, et al. National Vital Statistics Report. Deaths: Preliminary Data for 2009;59(4). March 16, 2011.
3. Pharmacy Facts and Figures. Drug Topics [Web site]. Available at: http://drugtopics.modernmedicine.com/drugtopics/data/articlestandard//drugtopics/252010/674961/article.pdf. Accessed on June 11, 2011.

# Preface

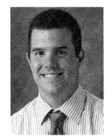 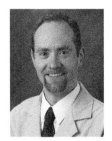

James Winger, MD, CAQ     Aaron Michelfelder, MD
*Guest Editors*

Primary care providers play an important role in the treatment of common gastroenterological disorders. This issue of *Clinics in Office Practice* examines that role in further detail. In the coming decades, our aging population will likely see rises in the prevalence of colorectal cancer, inflammatory bowel disease, *H pylori* infection, and associated gastric ulcers. The ability of primary care providers to efficiently and appropriately care for patients with myriad concerns will be paramount as our health care system undergoes its inevitable changes.

This issue of *Clinics in Office Practice* is dedicated to gastroenterology that may be encountered and treated in a primary care office. Certain articles of this issue deal with specific symptoms, such as jaundice, and their appropriate evaluation. Others address particular gastroenterological disorders and diseases themselves, such as conditions of malabsorption and inflammatory bowel disease. Conditions that may be of increasing importance to primary care providers, such as the primary care of the hepatic transplant recipient, will also be considered.

It has been a pleasure to play a role in producing this issue of *Clinics in Office Practice*. To the reader, we hope this issue serves as a useful tool in providing efficient care to your patients, as well as increasing knowledge of important conditions. To the authors who tolerated our constant reminders, subtle and not so, regarding content and deadlines, thank you for the excellent products you have produced.

James Winger, MD, CAQ
Aaron Michelfelder, MD

Department of Family Medicine
Loyola Stritch School of Medicine
2160 South First Avenue
Building 54, Room 260
Maywood, IL 60153, USA

E-mail addresses:
jwinger@lumc.edu (J. Winger)
amichel@lumc.edu (A. Michelfelder)

Prim Care Clin Office Pract 38 (2011) xiii
doi:10.1016/j.pop.2011.05.010
0095-4543/11/$ – see front matter © 2011 Elsevier Inc. All rights reserved.

# Peptic Ulcer Disease

Wadie I. Najm, MD, MSED

**KEYWORDS**

• Gastric ulcers • Duodenal ulcers • *Helicobacter pylori*

Peptic ulcer can be defined as mucosal lesions that penetrate the muscularis mucosae layer and form a cavity surrounded by acute and chronic inflammation. Gastric ulcers are located in the stomach, often along the lesser curvature in the transition zone from corpus to antrum mucosae. Duodenal ulcers are located in the duodenal bulb.

## EPIDEMIOLOGY

Peptic ulcer disease (PUD) tends to have a chronic remitting course with imperfect correlation between symptoms and the presence of an ulcer. This leads to a limitation in the ability to accurately document its incidence and prevalence. To do so would require technically difficult, expensive population-based endoscopic surveys. The only published study that has taken this approach reported a 4.1% prevalence of PUD (2% gastric ulcers and 2.1% duodenal ulcers).[1]

In the United States, approximately 8.4% of subjects in the National Health Interview Survey (NHIS) between 1997 and 2003 reported a history of PUD.[2] Another study of patients in the United States, between 1997 and 2007, reported that the annual incidence, based mainly on physician diagnoses, was 0.10% to 0.19%, while the incidence based on hospitalization was 0.03% to 0.17%.[3]

The prevalence of PUD reached a peak early in the 20th century but decreased during more recent decades.[3] The continued occurrence of PUD is due, at least in part, to the widespread use of low-dose aspirin (ASA) and nonsteroidal anti-inflammatory drugs (NSAIDs) especially in Western countries, older patients and those with comorbidities. The decreasing prevalence of peptic ulcers is also thought to result both from the reduction of a formerly large pool of patients with recurrent ulcer disease treated for *Helicobacter pylori* and from the decreasing prevalence of *H pylori* infection in the population.[4] The latter is related to several factors, such as improved hygiene and living conditions, decreased family sizes, and the use of antimicrobial therapy.

A similar trend was also noted in 6 European countries between 1921 and 2004, where the risk of dying from PUD increased among consecutive generation born

No funding support was provided for this review. The author declares no conflict of interest.
Department of Family Medicine & Geriatrics, Susan Samueli Center of Integrative Medicine, University of California, Irvine, 101 The City Drive, Building 200, #512, Orange, CA 92868, USA
*E-mail address:* winajm@uci.edu

during the second half of the 19th century until shortly before the turn of the century and decreased in all subsequent generations.[5]

Another factor that plays a role is the duration of institutionalization. The incidence of PUD and gastric cancer in institutionalized adults, who have intellectual disabilities and developmental disabilities (IDDD), is twofold to threefold higher than the general population. This is due to the high prevalence of H pylori infection and oral–oral transmissions in these patients.[6] Oral H pylori infection might not be eradicated with treatment.

Despite the changes in overall incidence, the prevalence of hospitalization from PUD and its complications did not significantly change between 1996 and 2005.[7] Better management of H pylori did not decrease the prevalence of hospitalization secondary to PUD, but decreased episodes of rebleeding and recurrence rates. Similar trends were also reported in European studies.[8] However, a retrospective study from Scotland did show a slight decrease in the admissions rate of PUD among young patients between 1982 and 2002, while an increased incidence of duodenal ulcer bleeding (both sexes), and an increased incidence of gastric ulcer bleeding (in men) was noted in older patients.[9]

### Risk Factors

The major risk factors for PUD are attributed to H pylori infection and NSAID or ASA use.[10] Causes of non-H- pylori non-NSAID ulcers are the use of antiplatelet agents, stress, Helicobacter heilmanii, cytomegalovirus infections, Behcet disease, Zollinger Ellison syndrome, Crohn disease, and cirrhosis with portal hypertension. Other risk factors include older age and ethnicity (**Table 1**).

H pylori, a gram-negative spiral bacteria, is transmitted via fecal–oral, oral–oral, iatrogenic or from mother-to-child routes. Risk factors for H pylori infection show geographic variation, with birth in developing countries and lower socioeconomic status being highly prevalent.[10] Although a causal relationship with PUD is generally accepted, it is estimated that H pylori-positive subjects have a 10% to 20% lifetime

| Table 1 Etiology and risk factors for peptic ulcer disease | |
|---|---|
| **Risk Factor** | **Odds Ratio** |
| Nonsteroidal anti-inflammatory drugs | 3.7 |
| Helicobacter pylori | 3.3 |
| Chronic obstructive pulmonary disease | 2.34 |
| Chronic renal insufficiency | 2.29 |
| Current tobacco use | 1.99 |
| Former tobacco use | 1.55 |
| Three or more doctor visits in a year | 1.49 |
| Coronary heart disease | 1.46 |
| Former alcohol use | 1.29 |
| African Americans | 1.20 |
| Obesity | 1.18 |
| Diabetes | 1.13 |

Data from Garrow D, Delegge MH. Risk factors for gastrointestinal ulcer disease in the US population. Dig Dis Sci 2010;55(1):66–72; and Kurata JH, Nogawa AN. Meta-analysis of risk factors for peptic ulcer. Nonsteroidal antiinflammatory drugs, Helicobacter pylori, and smoking. J Clin Gastroenterol 1997;24(1):2–17.

risk of developing PUD.[4] This suggests possible, yet unknown, cofactors responsible for ulcer formation.

Among the US population, a higher rate of infection is reported in older adults, African Americans, and Hispanics. Interestingly, Mexican Americans had a lower rate of PUD despite a high prevalence of *H pylori*. This discrepancy has been attributed to the higher intake of fiber (vegetables, fruits, and beans) compared with other groups.[2] The prevalence of *H pylori*-negative PUD remains high in countries with high *H pylori*, even after excluding factors such as Crohn disease or NSAID use. A high rate of PUD recurrence is noted even after eradication of *H pylori* infection. These findings suggest that *H pylori* could be a cause of resistance to ulcer healing or its chronicity.[10,11]

In western countries, NSAIDs, less commonly cyclooxygenase inhibitors (COX) and ASA, are the most common causes of PUD.[12] The risk of NSAID-related ulcers is lower in women than men. Factors that increase the risk of PUD with NSAIDs are: a history of ulcer(s), older age, alcohol consumption, *H pylori* infection, and concurrent use of medications such as ASA, clopidogrel, selective serotonin reuptake inhibitors (SSRIs), oral vitamin K antagonists, and glucocorticoids. The risk of ulcer formation is increased seventeenfold when NSAID users are infected with *H pylori*. Contrary to common beliefs, gastrointestinal (GI) mucosal injury caused by NSAIDs and ASA is related to the systemic rather than local toxicity.[12] Use of glucocorticoids alone does not seem to increase risk of ulcer formation.

The incidence of PUD among NSAID users is higher than non-NSAID users, and it is also noted to increase in a linear fashion with each age group. Among older adults, almost 1 of 4 (18%–23%) NSAID users develop PUD.[13] A higher incidence of PUD is reported with the use of COX-1 rather than COX-2 inhibitors. Controlled trials with COX-2 inhibitors have demonstrated a lower risk of PUD and its complications.[14,15] A recent large study, comparing etoricoxib with diclofenac confirmed this the reduction in upper GI events with COX-2, but noted that it was limited only to uncomplicated events and not to serious complicated events.[16] The concurrent use of NSAIDs or COX-2 inhibitors with ASA significantly increased the incidence of PUD compared with using aspirin alone; gastric ulcers (GUs) were twice as common as duodenal ulcers (DUs).[17]

### Clinical Manifestation

A history of night time awakening or episodic epigastric pain relieved following food intake are the most specific clinical findings of PUD.[18]

Typical symptoms of PUD (80%–90% of patients) include episodic gnawing, dull, burning (dyspepsia) epigastric pain. The pain is often localized and occurs when the stomach is empty, 2–5 hours after meals, or at night. Pain is relieved with food, antacids or antisecretory agents.[19] The natural history and clinical presentation of PUD differ in individual populations. Asymptomatic ulcers are common among the elderly (29.4%–35%)[20] and in certain parts of the world where two-thirds of patients are reported to be asymptomatic.[21] Dyspeptic symptoms may be influenced by intrinsic and extrinsic factors such as high body mass index (BMI) due to high plasma levels of endorphins, drinking at least 200 mL of tea daily due to the blocking of adenosine receptors by theophylline, and ulcer size less than 1 cm.

Pain awakening the patient from sleep between 12 and 3 a.m. affects two-thirds of DU patients and one-third of gastric ulcer patients; therefore it is a key symptom of DUs. However, it is also seen in one-third of patients with nonulcer dyspepsia. Substantial vomiting and weight loss suggest gastric outlet obstruction or gastric malignancy. In a meta-analysis, 46% of patients had reflux symptoms, probably due to concomitant reflux disease including heartburn and acid regurgitation.[19] Less common features of PUD are indigestion, belching, vomiting associated with gastric or pyloric stenosis, loss of appetite, intolerance of fatty foods, anemia caused by GI blood loss, and a positive family history. Weight loss precipitated by fear of food intake is also characteristic of gastric ulcers.[22]

Inflammatory ulcers can produce significant constitutional symptoms such as weight loss, cachexia, malnutrition, and chronic abdominal pain. This constellation may mislead the clinician to suspect malignancy as the most likely diagnosis. Abdominal pain, mostly in the epigastric area, sometimes the left upper quadrant, or radiation into the back, is the most common presenting symptom of giant DUs. The pain of these ulcers has been described as more persistent than classically for small ulcers, and is it not relieved by food or antacids. Most giant DUs present with hemorrhage that may manifest as melena, hematochezia, hematemesis, or a combination of these.

Abdominal pain is more prevalent among younger patients than older patients, while the opposite has been found for bleeding.[19] One-third of patients with PUD present with bleeding as an initial symptom, and almost one-third of patients presenting with bleeding peptic ulcer have no history of pain.

Older patients with PUD are less likely to have symptoms, and this may place them at higher risk of having a serious complication of PUD such as perforation or GI bleeding. The most common symptoms of PUD among aged patients (>80 years old.) are epigastric pain (74%), nausea (23%), and vomiting (20%).[19] Among elderly patients, perforation may present with mild pain or or no pain.[23] Among pregnant women, ulcer symptoms may remain mild. Symptoms my manifest as postprandial or nocturnal vomiting that worsens during the third trimester.[18]

Physical examination findings can have low predictive value; however, they are central for identifying ulcer complications. Patients with PUD may experience several potential complications. The three most common complications are GI bleeding, perforation, and gastric outlet obstruction.

### GI Bleeding

Approximately 80% to 85% of upper GI bleeding stops spontaneously, and supportive therapy only is required. The prevalence of bleeding complications has increased during the past decades, particularly in subjects 65 years of age or older.[24] Patients with a bleeding PUD can be asymptomatic or may present with hematemesis, coffee ground emesis, melena, tachycardia, or shock. Subjects with a large initial bleed, continued or recurrent bleeding, or severe comorbid illnesses have the greatest risk of death. Up to 15% of peptic ulcers bleed, and affected patients have an overall mortality rate of 10%. Recent studies have pointed that most PUD bleeding patients died of nonulcer bleeding-related causes (80%).[25,26] Multiorgan failure (24%), pulmonary conditions (24%), and terminal malignancy (34%) were the most common reasons of nonulcer bleeding. Nasogastric aspiration is usually confirmatory of the upper GI bleeding. Urgent upper GI endoscopy is important to detect the cause of bleeding and to start appropriate therapy. When shock is present, aggressive resuscitation and blood transfusion should be initiated.

Endoscopic treatment remains the first-line therapeutic modality in the management of bleeding PUD, even in those with massive bleeding.[27] Adding a high-dose proton pump inhibitor (PPI) infusion after the initial endoscopic hemostasis can alleviate the discomfort of patients undergoing second-look endoscopy.[28] Scheduling a second endoscopy and adjunctive high-dose PPI infusion are important strategies for preventing ulcer rebleeding after the primary endoscopic hemostasis.

Predictors for bleeding following endoscopy are active bleeding, comorbid illness, hemodynamic instability, large ulcer size (>1cm), posterior DU, and lesser gastric curve ulcer.[29] Large ulcers (>2 cm) and hypotension at rebleeding are independent factors predicting failure of endoscopic retreatment. Surgery remains a definite indication and the best treatment method in cases where endoscopy or interventional radiology fails to stop bleeding.[30]

### Perforation

Lifetime prevalence of perforation in patients with PUD is approximately 5%. The most important factors leading to perforation are the use of NSAIDs and the presence of *H pylori* infection.[31] Symptoms of perforation vary based on the location of the ulcer. Posterior perforation often presents with bleeding, while perforation at other sites can present with a sudden onset of severe, sharp abdominal pain. Pain is often generalized, and occasionally it can present as a severe epigastric pain. Abdominal examination findings often identify generalized tenderness, guarding, rigidity, and rebound tenderness. Patients may also present with signs and symptoms of septic shock, such as tachycardia, hypotension, lethargy, anuria, and cyanosis. Caution should be used with older adults and immunocompromised or diabetic patients, as indicators of shock may be absent.

Perforated DU is a surgical and medical emergency. Simple surgical closures, intensive medical treatment, *H pylori* eradication, and NSAID withdrawal have been reported to result in very low recurrence rates. Recurrence rates following *H pylori* eradication are lower than for patients treated with PPIs alone.[32] Patients with perforated DU who are appropriate candidates for proximal gastric vagotomy in addition to omental patch closure and antibiotic therapy do well; however, the true benefit of proximal gastric vagotomy over omental patch closure with antibiotic therapy is yet to be demonstrated. Similar outcomes in morbidity and mortality have been reported for both laparoscopic and open surgery.[33] Laparoscopic surgery was associated with shorter hospital stay and recovery time and less need for analgesics. Risk factors that increase mortality following perforation are severe comorbidity, shock on admission, and delayed presentation for more than 24hours.[34]

One study reported that elective ulcer-definitive surgery may be considered for the uninfected patients who have already received appropriate medical therapy.[35] The authors recommended that in uncomplicated cases, medical treatment could be initiated and work-up to rule out Zollinger-Ellison syndrome should be started before surgery is scheduled.

### Gastric Outlet Obstruction

Gastric outlet obstruction is more commonly due to malignancy than PUD. Patients experiencing gastric outlet obstruction present with nausea, vomiting, bloating, indigestion, epigastric pain, and weight loss. Diagnosis can be made with an upper GI radiography; however, endoscopy has the advantage of being diagnostic and can rule out possible malignancy. Malignant obstruction is reported in 66% of patients.[36] Dehydration and electrolyte imbalance occur as a result of the nausea and vomiting. Treatment should include rehydration, correction of electrolyte imbalance, and relief of obstructive symptoms with nasogastric suction. Peptic ulcer-induced gastric outlet obstruction can be treated safely with endoscopic balloon dilation. About 65% of patients sustain symptom relief, but many require more than 1 dilation session. Data about the effectiveness of balloon dilatation are controversial. A retrospective study reported that 92% of patients with gastric outlet obstruction due to PUD required surgery within 3 years.[37] Another study, however, reported that 70% of patients remained asymptomatic after 2.5 years.[38] Outcomes may be improved with effective ulcer therapy with acid reduction and eradication of *H pylori*.[39] Surgery is associated with significant morbidity and mortality and should be reserved for endoscopic treatment failures. Surgical palliation for malignant disease has poor results and high rates of morbidity and mortality.

### Diagnosis

Uncomplicated PUD can be suspected based on the presence of typical clinical symptoms such as dyspepsia, epigastric burning pain, nocturnal pain, and pain relief with food or antacids. A careful history and physical examination may assist in evaluating the extensive different differential diagnosis (**Table 2**). Several additional tests are helpful in confirming the diagnosis, confirming or excluding PUD complications, and in narrowing the differential diagnosis. Definitive diagnosis is made by direct visualization of the ulcer via radiography (upper GI barium swallow, double contrast) or upper GI endoscopy (EGD). Referral to EGD should be considered in all patients 50 years of age or older, with persistent symptoms, anorexia, weight loss, vomiting, and in the presence of signs of GI bleeding.

The presence of *H pylori* should be confirmed in all patients suspected of PUD. Four tests are commonly used:

Blood antibody test (enzyme-linked immunosorbent assay [ELISA]). This test detects exposure to *H pylori* but cannot be used to confirm successful treatment.

| Table 2 Differential diagnosis of peptic ulcer disease | | |
|---|---|---|
| **Condition** | **Test(s)** | **Findings** |
| Gastritis | Upper gastrointestinal endoscopy | Gastric inflammation |
| Gastroesophageal reflux disease | Symptoms | Dyspepsia worse with eating and upon lying down |
| Gastroparesis | History | History of diabetes |
| Cholelithiasis | Examination Abdominal ultrasound | Right upper quadrant tenderness Gallstones |
| Pancreatitis | Amylase/lipase | Elevated |
| Gastric cancer | Upper gastrointestinal endoscopy Abdominal CT scan | Biopsy |
| Abdominal aortic aneurysm | Abdominal ultrasound Abdominal CT scan | Size of aorta |
| Hepatitis | Liver function tests | Elevated |
| Myocardial ischemia | Cardiac enzymes Electrocardiogram | Elevated $CPK_{MB}$ Elevated troponin ST segment changes Deep symmetric T wave inversion |
| Mesenteric ischemia | Symptoms Abdominal CT | Pain after meals Mesenteric edema; bowel dilatation; bowel wall thickening; intramural gas; mesenteric stranding |

*Abbreviation:* $CPK_{MB}$, creatine phosphokinase-MB.

Urea breath test. This test is aadequate for screening and for confirming cure following treatment. The use of PPIs within 2 weeks of testing can interfere with the results.

Stool antigen test. This test is adequate for screening and for confirming cure following treatment;

Stomach biopsy. This test is considered the gold standard. It is adequate for screening and for confirming cure. Results depend on the number of biopsies and the experience of the pathologist.

### Treatment

Treatment of PUD consists of healing the ulcer and prevention of complications. All plans should include appropriate management of PUD risk factors. Patients should be advised to discontinue smoking; additionally, they should be offered stress management programs and counseled to avoid NSAIDs, aspirin, and alcohol abuse.

Management of patients with PUD requires detection and eradication of H pylori infection and the administration of antisecretory therapy, preferably PPIs, for a minimum of 4 weeks (see **Table 3** for additional drugs used for PUD). If patients recover after the first course of treatment, they should be observed. If symptoms persist, antisecretory therapy with PPIs or histamine receptor (H2) blockers should be continued for an additional 4 to 8 weeks, and repeat EGD should be considered. Patients also should be re-evaluated for H pylori infection. Economic modeling suggests that Cox-1 NSAIDs plus H2 blockers or Cox-1 NSAIDs plus PPIs are the most cost-effective strategies for avoiding endoscopic ulcers in patients requiring long-term NSAID therapy.[40] PPIs are more effective than H2-blockers at standard dosages in reducing the risk of gastric and duodenal ulcer, and are superior to misoprostol in preventing duodenal but not gastric lesions.[41]

**Table 3**
**Common medications used for peptic ulcer disease**

| Class | Medication | Typical Dose | Precautions |
|---|---|---|---|
| Histamine -2 Receptor blocker | Cimetidine | 400 mg BID | High incidence of side effects and potential for drug interactions due to inhibition of CYP450 |
| | Ranitidine | 150 mg BID | — |
| | Nizatidine | 150 mg BID | — |
| | Famotidine | 20 mg BID | — |
| Proton pump inhibitors | Omeprazole | 20–40 mg daily | Altered metabolism of medications through CYP450 |
| | Lansoprazole | 15–30 mg daily | |
| | Pantoprazole | 40 mg BID | |
| | Rabeprazole | 20–60 mg daily | Inhibits absorption of vitamin B12 |
| | Esomeprazole | 20–40 mg daily | |
| Prostaglandins | Misoprostol | 200 μg QID | Dose-dependent diarrhea and abdominal pain. Avoid in fertile women and during pregnancy |
| Other medications | Sucralfate | 1 g QID | Contains aluminum, should be avoided in patients with renal failure. Can prevent absorption of other medications |

Aspirin is commonly recommended to reduce the risk of cardiovascular events. Several factors have been identified to increase the risk of patients to develop aspirin-associated GI bleeding. These include a history of previous GI ulcer, ulcer complications, dyspepsia, H pylori infection, and simultaneous use of aspirin with NSAIDs or clopidogrel.[42] The use of enteric-coated or buffered aspirin does not signif- icantly decrease the risk of ulcer complications due to its systemic effect. Combining a PPI with aspirin significantly reduces the risk recurrent ulcer bleeding.

Weight loss, anemia, recurrent vomiting, dysphasia, jaundice, blood in the stool, or melena indicate serious complications, and a repeat EGD should be performed.[18]

When H pylori is present in patients with PUD, treatment should focus on eradi- cating H pylori. The US Food and Drug Administration (FDA) approved treatment regi- mens recommend initial treatment of H pylori for 10 to 14 days with one of the following regimens[43]:

Omeprazole 40 mg daily plus clarithromycin 500 mg 3 times daily for 2 weeks, then omeprazole 20 mg daily for 2 weeks

Ranitidine bismuth citrate 400 mg twice daily plus clarithromycin 500 mg three times daily for 2 weeks, then ranitidine bismuth citrate 400 mg twice daily for 2 weeks;

Bismuth subsalicylate 525 mg 4 times daily plus metronidazole 250 mg 4 times daily plus tetracycline 500 mg 4 times daily for 2 weeks plus H2 receptor antag- onist therapy as directed for 4 weeks;

Lansoprazole 30 mg twice daily plus amoxicillin 1 g twice daily plus clarithromycin 500 mg 3 times daily for 10 days

Lansoprazole 30 mg 3 times daily plus amoxicillin 1 g 3 times daily for 2 weeks

Rantidine bismuth citrate 400 mg twice daily plus clarithromycin 500 mg twice daily for 2 weeks, then ranitidine bismuth citrate 400 twice daily for 2 weeks

Omeprazole 20 mg twice daily plus clarithromycin 500 mg twice daily plus amox- icillin 1 g twice daily for 10 days

Lansoprazole 30 mg twice daily plus clarithromycin 500 mg twice daily, amoxicillin 1 g twice daily or metronidazole (400 or 500 mg) twice daily, 14-day treatment; A 7-day treatment may be acceptable where local studies show that it is effective.

Overall triple therapy for 14 days has been shown to be more effective at eradication of H pylori than dual therapy.[44] A recent meta-analysis did not find a difference in H pylori eradication rate between quadruple (PPI + bismuth + metronidazole + tetra- cycline for 10–14 days) and triple therapy (PPI + clarithromycin + azithromycin for 7–14 days).[45] Sequential therapy for H pylori (refers to adding more antibiotics to the treat- ment regimen but giving them in sequence rather than giving all 4 drugs together) has been found to be more effective than standard therapy in eradicating the bacteria and preventing recurrence.[46] The same first choice H pylori treatments are recommended worldwide, although different doses may be appropriate. H pylori eradication is of value in chronic NSAID users but is insufficient to prevent NSAID related ulcer disease completely.

A thorough review of natural supplements and therapies for gastrointestinal disor- ders has been detailed in a previous issue (Michelfelder 2010).[47] Using probiotics increases the efficacy of H pylori eradication regimens. Probiotics are live microorgan- isms that confer a health benefit on the host when administered in adequate amounts. Saccharomyces boulardii is a nonpathogenic yeast, which, when added to the standard H pylori eradication regimen in children, enhanced its effects and reduced significantly the incidence of side effects.[48] Using bovine lactoferrin or fermented milk-based probiotics with standard triple therapy could also improve the standard eradication therapy for *H pylori* infection.[49–51] Bovine lactoferrin is a multifunctional iron-binding glycoprotein that is found in the milk and mucosal secretions, and it appears to be an important factor in the host's defense against a wide range of bacteria by preventing of iron use as well as attachment of bacteria to epithelial cells.

## TAKE HOME

PUD is due mostly to the widespread use of low-dose aspirin, and NSAIDs. It occurs mostly in older patients and those with comorbidities.

Causes of non-*H pylori* non-NSAID ulcers are the use of antiplatelet agents, stress, *H heilmanii*, cytomegalovirus infections, Behcet disease, Zollinger Ellison syndrome, Crohn disease, and cirrhosis with portal hypertension.

Pain awakening the patient from sleep between 12 and 3 a.m. affects two-thirds of DU patients and one-third of gastric ulcer patients.

Older adults(>80 years old) with PUD often do not present with abdominal pain; instead, epigastric pain, nausea and vomiting are among their most common presenting symptoms.

Approximately 80% to 85% of upper GI bleeding stops spontaneously with supportive therapy.

Perforated duodenal ulcer is a medical and surgical emergency.

Risk factors that increase mortality following perforation are severe comorbidity, shock on admission, and delayed presentation for more than 24 hours.

Subjects with symptoms of gastric outlet obstruction should be investigated for malignancy (66%).

## ACKNOWLEDGMENTS

The author wishes to thank Dr Hamideh Sadighzadeh for her diligent assistance in literature review and analysis.

## REFERENCES

1. Aro P, Storskrubb T, Ronkainen J, et al. Peptic ulcer disease in a general adult population: the Kalixanda study: a random population-based study. Am J Epidemiol 2006;163(11):1025–34.
2. Garrow D, Delegge MH. Risk factors for gastrointestinal ulcer disease in the US population. Dig Dis Sci 2010;55(1):66–72.
3. Sung JJY, Kuiperse J, El-Serag HB. Systematic review: the global incidence and prevalence of peptic ulcer disease. Aliment Pharmacol Ther 2009;29:938–46.
4. Kusters JG, van Vliet AH, Kuipers EJ. Pathogenesis of Helicobacter pylori Infection. Clinical Microbilology Reviews 2006;19(3):449–90.
5. Sonnenberg A. Time trends of ulcer mortality in Europe. Gastroenterology 2007; 132(7):2320–7.
6. Kitchens DH, Binkley CJ, Wallace DL, et al. *Heficobacter pyfori* infection in people who are intellectually and developmentally disabled: a review. Spec Care Dentist 2007;27(4):127–33.
7. Manuel D, Cutler A, Goldstein J, et al. Decreasing prevalence combined with increasing eradication of Helicobacter pylori infection in the United States has not resulted in fewer hospital admissions for peptic ulcer disease-related complications. Aliment Pharmacol Ther 2007;25(12):1423–7.

8. Post PN, Kuipers EJ, Meijer GA. Declining incidence of peptic ulcer but not of its complications: a nationwide study in The Netherlands. Aliment Pharmacol Ther 2006;23(11):1587–93.

9. Kang JY, Elders A, Majeed A, et al. Recent trends in hospital admissions and mortality rates for peptic ulcer in Scotland 1982–2002. Aliment Pharmacol Ther 2006;24(1):65–79.

10. Makola D, Peura DA, Crowe SE. *Helicobacter pylori* infection and related gastrointestinal diseases. J Clin Gastroenterol 2007;41(6):548–58.

11. Hobsley M, Tovey FI, Holton J. Precise role of *H pylori* in duodenal ulceration. World J Gastroenterol 2006;12(40):6413–9.

12. Bardou M, Barkun AN. Preventing the gastrointestinal adverse effects of nonsteroidal anti-inflammatory drugs: from risk factor identification to risk factor intervention. Joint Bone Spine 2010;77(1):6–12.

13. Boers M, Tangelder MJ, van Ingen H, et al. The rate of NSAID-induced endoscopic ulcers increases linearly but not exponentially with age: a pooled analysis of 12 randomised trials. Ann Rheum Dis 2007;66(3):417–8.

14. Layton D, Souverein PC, Heerdink ER, et al. Evaluation of risk profiles for gastrointestinal and cardiovascular adverse effects in nonselective NSAID and COX-2 inhibitor users: a cohort study using pharmacy dispensing data in The Netherlands. Drug Saf 2008;31(2):143–58.

15. Hooper L, Brown TJ, Elliott R, et al. The effectiveness of five strategies for the prevention of gastrointestinal toxicity induced by non-steroidal anti-inflammatory drugs: systematic review. BMJ 2004;329(7472):948.

16. Laine L, Curtis CS, Cryer B, et al, for the MEDAL Steering Committee. Assessment of upper gastrointestinal safety of etoricoxib and diclofenac in patients with osteoarthritis and rheumatoid arthritis in the Multinational Etoricoxib and Diclofenac Arthritis Long-term (MEDAL) programm: a randomised comparison. Lancet 2007;369(9560):465–73.

17. Goldstein JL, Lowry SC, Lanza FL, et al. The impact of low-dose aspirin on endoscopic gastric and duodenal ulcer rates in users of a non-selective nonsteroidal anti-inflammatory drug or a cyclo-oxygenase-2-selective inhibitor. Aliment Pharmacol Ther 2006;23(10):1489–98.

18. Ramakrishnan K, Salinas RC. Peptic ulcer disease. Am Fam Physician 2007; 76(7):1005–12.

19. Barkun A, Leontiadis G. Systematic review of the symptom burden, quality-of-life impairment, and costs associated with peptic ulcer disease. Am J Med 2010; 123(4):358–66.

20. Hilton D, Iman N, Burke GJ, et al. Absence of abdominal pain in older persons with endoscopic ulcers: a prospective study. Am J Gastroenterol 2001;96(2): 380–4.

21. Lu CL, Chang SS, Wang SS, et al. Silent peptic ulcer disease: frequency, factors leading to silence, and implications regarding the pathogenesis of visceral symptoms. Gastrointest Endosc 2004;60(1):34–8.

22. Yuan Y, Padol IT, Hunt RH. Peptic ulcer disease today. Nat Clin Pract Gastroenterol Hepatol 2006;3(2):80–9.

23. Franceschi M, Di Mario F, Leandro G, et al. Acid-related disorders in the elderly. Best Pract Res Clin Gastroenterol 2009;23(6):839–48.

24. Nahon S, Pariente A, Faroux R, et al, Association Nationale des Gastroentérologues des Hôpitaux Généraux. Prognosis of upper gastrointestinal bleeding in the oldest-old patients: a post hoc analysis of a prospective study. J Am Geriatr Soc 2010;58(5):989–90.

25. Sung JJ, Tsoi KK, Ma TK, et al. Causes of mortality in patients with peptic ulcer bleeding: a prospective cohort study of 10,428 cases. Am J Gastroenterol 2010;105(1):84–9.
26. Nahon S, Pariente A, Nalet B, et al, group of investigators of the ANGH (Association Nationale des Gastroentérologues des Hôpitaux Généraux). Causes of mortality related to peptic ulcer bleeding in a prospective cohort of 965 French patients: a plea for primary prevention. Am J Gastroenterol 2010;105(8):1902–3.
27. Laine L, McQuaid KR. Endoscopic therapy for bleeding ulcers: an evidence-based approach based on meta-analyses of randomized controlled trials. Clin Gastroenterol Hepatol 2009;7(1):33–47.
28. Sung JY. Current management of peptic ulcer bleeding. Nat Clin Pract Gastroenterol Hepatol 2006;3(1):24–32.
29. Cheung FK, Lau JY. Management of massive peptic ulcer bleeding. Gastroenterol Clin North Am 2009;38(2):231–43.
30. Lau JY, Sung JJ, Lam YH, et al. Endoscopic retreatment compared with surgery in patients with recurrent bleeding after initial endoscopic control of bleeding ulcers. N Engl J Med 1999;340(10):751–6.
31. Svanes C. Trends in perforated peptic ulcer: incidence, etiology, treatment, and prognosis. World J Surg 2000;24(3):277–83.
32. Ng EK, Lam YH, Sung JJ, et al. Eradication of *Helicobacter pylori* prevents recurrence of ulcer after simple closure of duodenal ulcer perforation: randomized controlled trial. Ann Surg 2000;231(2):153–8.
33. Bhogal RH, Athwal R, Durkin D, et al. Comparison between open and laparoscopic repair of perforated peptic ulcer disease. World J Surg 2008;32(11):2371–4.
34. Boey J, Choi SK, Poon A, et al. Risk stratification in perforated duodenal ulcers. A prospective validation of predictive factors. Ann Surg 1987;205(1):22–6.
35. Donovan AJ, Berne TV, Donovan JA. Perforated duodenal ulcer: an alternative therapeutic plan. Arch Surg 1998;133(11):1166–71.
36. Shone DN, Nikoomanesh P, Smith-Meek MM, et al. Malignancy is the most common cause of gastric outlet obstruction in the era of H2 blockers. Am J Gastroenterol 1995;90(10):1769–70.
37. Jaffin BW, Kaye MD. The prognosis of gastric outlet obstruction. Ann Surg 1985; 201(2):176–9.
38. Kozarek RA, Botoman VA, Patterson DJ. Long-term follow-up in patients who have undergone balloon dilation for gastric outlet obstruction. Gastrointest Endosc 1990;36(6):558–61.
39. Yusuf TE, Brugge WR. Endoscopic therapy of benign pyloric stenosis and gastric outlet obstruction. Curr Opin Gastroenterol 2006;22(5):570–3.
40. Brown TJ, Hooper L, Elliott RA, et al. A comparison of the cost-effectiveness of five strategies for the prevention of nonsteroidal anti-inflammatory drug-induced gastrointestinal toxicity: a systematic review with economic modelling. Health Technol Assess 2006;10(38):1–183.
41. Lazzaroni M, Porro GB. Management of NSAID-induced gastrointestinal toxicity: focus on proton pump inhibitors. Drugs 2009;69(1):51–69.
42. Lanas A, Scheiman J. Low-dose aspirin and upper gastrointestinal damage: epidemiology, prevention and treatment. Curr Med Res Opin 2007;23(1):163–73.
43. Helicobacter pylori and peptic ulcer disease. The key to cure. Available at: http://www.cdc.gov/ulcer/keytocure.htm#treatment. Accessed June 20, 2011.
44. Malfertheiner P, Megraud F, O'Morain C, et al. Current concepts in the management of *Helicobacter pylori* infection: the Maastricht III consensus report. Gut 2007;56(6):772–81.

45. Luther J, Higgins PD, Schoenfeld PS, et al. Empiric quadruple vs. triple therapy for primary treatment of *Helicobacter pylori* infection: systematic review and meta-analysis of efficacy and tolerability. Am J Gastroenterol 2010;105(1):65–73.
46. Jafri NS, Hornung CA, Howden CW. Meta-analysis: sequential therapy appears superior to standard therapy for *Helicobacter pylori* infection in patients naive to treatment. Ann Intern Med 2008;148(12):923–31.
47. Michelfelder AJ, Lee KC, Bading EM, et al. Integrative medicine and gastrointestinal disease. Clinics in Office Practice. Prim Care 2010;37(2):255–67.
48. Hurduc V, Plesca D, Dragomir D, et al. A randomized open trial evaluating the effect of *Saccharomyces boulardii* on the eradication rate of *Helicobacter pylori* infection in children. Acta Paediatr 2009;98(1):127–31.
49. Sachdeva A, Nagpal J. Meta-analysis: efficacy of bovine lactoferrin in *Helicobacter pylori* eradication. Aliment Pharmacol Ther 2009;29(7):720–30.
50. de Bortoli N, Leonardi G, Ciancia E, et al. *Helicobacter pylori* eradication: a randomized prospective study of triple therapy plus lactoferrin and probiotics. Am J Gastroenterol 2007;102(5):951–6.
51. Sachdeva A, Nagpal J. Effect of fermented milk-based probiotic preparations on *Helicobacter pylori* eradication: a systematic review and meta-analysis of randomized–controlled trials. Eur J Gastroenterol Hepatol 2009;21(1):45–53.

# Selected Disorders of Malabsorption

Zafreen Siddiqui, MD*, Amimi S. Osayande, MD

**KEYWORDS**

- Celiac • Pernicious anemia • Lactose intolerance
- Lactase deficiency • Vitamin $B_{12}$ • Sprue

Malabsorption syndrome encompasses numerous clinical entities that result in chronic diarrhea, abdominal distention, and failure to thrive. Some of these disorders may be congenital or acquired. Some of the congenital disorders include cystic fibrosis and Shwachman-Diamond syndrome, which may cause amylase deficiency; the rare congenital lactase deficiency; glucose-galactose malabsorption; sucrase-isomaltase deficiency; and adult-type hypolactasia or acquired: the most common being lactose intolerance, typically secondary to a damage of the mucosa, such as from a viral enteritis, pernicious anemia, and conditions that cause mucosal atrophy, such as celiac disease. Malabsorption disorders arise from defects anywhere in the process of transportation of nutrients from the intestine to the bloodstream. The pathology may be due to impairment in absorption or digestion of food nutrients resulting in nutritional deficiency, gastrointestinal symptoms, and in some patients extragastrointestinal symptoms. Treatment is aimed at correcting the deficiencies and symptoms to improve the quality of life.

Some of the most common disorders of malabsorption—celiac disease, pernicious anemia, and lactase deficiency—are discussed in this article.

## CELIAC DISEASE

Celiac disease is a disorder of absorption related to an immunologic reaction to gluten[1] or other related proteins in the diet. These proteins are found mostly in wheat products. This condition is also known as celiac sprue, nontropical sprue, gluten-sensitive enteropathy, and Gee-Thaysen disease,[2] named after the physician who first described it in 1888. It is primarily a disease of the proximal small intestinal epithelium[1]; however, other organs that may be affected include central nervous system and skin, even in the absence of gastrointestinal involvement.[3] Causes of celiac disease include genetic predisposition,[1] toxic effects of gluten/gliaden (a glycoprotein component of gluten),[1] immune reaction to gluten,[1] and exposure to adenovirus type 12.[4]

Department of Family and Community Medicine, University of Texas Southwestern Medical Center, 5909 Harry Hines Boulevard, Suite 100, Dallas, TX 75390-9067, USA
* Corresponding author.
*E-mail address:* Zafreen.Siddiqui@UTSouthwestern.edu

Prim Care Clin Office Pract 38 (2011) 395–414
doi:10.1016/j.pop.2011.05.002
0095-4543/11/$ – see front matter © 2011 Published by Elsevier Inc.

Likely risk factors include a positive family history, irritable bowel syndrome,[5] type 1 diabetes mellitus,[6] and persistent elevations in liver transaminases.[7] Some studies suggest that the introduction of gluten-containing foods (wheat, barley, and rye) during the first 3 months of life (or possibly after 7 months of age) may also be associated with increased risk of developing celiac disease.[8]

### Epidemiology

Approximately 1% of the general Western population is estimated to have celiac disease. The age of presentation varies, based on if defects are congenital, with onset of symptoms shortly after birth, or if they are acquired, with onset of symptoms at any age. The classic presentation is in infancy, ages 4 to 24 months, when cereals are added to the diet. Failure to thrive is the presenting symptom. Peak incidence occurs in adults aged 40 to 50 years,[9] with some diagnoses made after age 60 years.[10] Women seem more commonly affected than men, at a rate of 3.33:1.[11] Prevalence is increased up to 20% in first-degree relatives and patients diagnosed with certain medical conditions: 3% to 6% in patients with type 1 diabetes mellitus, 1% to 3% of patients with osteoporosis, and 10% to 15% of patients with symptomatic anemia.[12] Introduction of immunoglobulin A endomysial antibody testing for celiac disease has resulted in early age of detection with increasing incidence in children.[13] Within the United States, the prevalence is 0.75% among persons not at risk for celiac disease, 4.5% among first-degree relatives of celiac disease patients, 2.6% among second-degree relatives of celiac disease patients, and 1.8% among patients with gastrointestinal symptoms or disorders associated with celiac disease.[14]

### Physiology of the Normal Colon

When viewed through a light microscope, the luminal surface of the proximal small intestine has abundant well-developed villi with height relative to crypt depth of 4:1. Histologically, the villi are covered with tall columnar epithelial cells and basal nuclei with occasional goblet cells and scattered lymphocytes between them. The lamina propria normally contains a scattering of plasma cells, lymphocytes, macrophages, and occasional eosinophils and mast cells.

### Pathophysiology of Celiac Disease

In contrast to the normal epithelium, the luminal surface of small intestinal biopsy shows loss of villi with flat mucosal surface accentuated by ridges of crypt openings. In severe disease, the ratio of villi height to crypt depth may be reduced to 1:1. The complete loss of villi is accompanied by the presence of markedly abnormal squamoid surface epithelial cells. There is an increase in the number of intraepithelial lymphocytes and plasma cells in the lamina propria and striking crypt hypertrophy with increase in the crypt mitosis. Pathologic changes in less severe celiac disease are not as marked and can be characterized by increased numbers of intraepithelial lymphocytes and less extensive villous atrophy and crypt hypertrophy, termed *subtotal villous atrophy*.

### Disease Pathogenesis

Disease pathogenesis involves interactions among environmental, genetic, and immunologic factors.

### Environmental factors

Celiac disease is activated and triggered by proteins in the dietary cereal grains; gliadin from wheat, hordeins from barley, and secalins from rye. These peptides have high glutamine and proline content, are very immunogenic, and are resistant to intestinal chymotrypsin, pepsin, and brush border enzymes, resulting in the accumulation of relatively large peptide fragments (as many as 50 amino acids in length). Failure to digest these and other proteins might be exaggerated in the small intestine of individuals with active disease who manifest epithelial cell brush border injury and accompanying pancreatic dysfunction. It is possible that susceptible patients have a genetically weak intestinal mucosal barrier.

Exposure to adenovirus type 12 is also linked with celiac disease because it shares a sequence of 8 to 12 amino acids with the toxic gliadin fraction.

### Genetic factors
Genetic studies show strong association with specific HLA class 11 genotype.[15] HLA contribution to development of celiac disease among siblings is 36%. Homozygosity for HLA-DQ2 is associated with an increased risk for refractory celiac disease and enteropathy-associated T-cell lymphoma, disease processes linked with HLA-DQ2 and/or HLA-DQ8 gene locus. In addition, type 1 diabetes mellitus and celiac disease have common genetic risk regions. A particular association was found with chromosome 15q26, which contains a type 1 diabetes mellitus susceptibility locus.[16]

### Immunologic factors
**Humoral immunity**  Serologic studies show positive ELISA for IgA antibodies to gliadin and endomysium, which is a component of the smooth muscle connective tissue, the presence of which is virtually path gnomonic for celiac disease.[17] The target autoantigen contained within the endomysium was identified as tissue transglutaminase (tTG), an intracellular enzyme, which is released by inflammatory and endothelial cells and fibroblasts in response to mechanical irritation or inflammation. tTG supports the bioactivation of transforming growth factor $\beta1$, which is required for epithelial differentiation, a process that is impaired in celiac disease.[18]

### Cellular immunity
After tTG is secreted, it crosslinks glutamine-rich proteins, such as gluten proteins from wheat. It may also deamidate glutamine residues in gluten to glutamic acid. The deamidation produces a negative charge in gluten peptides, which increases their binding to HLA-DQ2 and HLA-DQ8, thereby potentiating their capacity to stimulate T-cells.[19]

Initial studies suggested that in adult patients, the dominant epitope responsible for the T-cell response seemed to be a deamidated glutamine residue of $\alpha$-gliadin. In comparison with adults, in younger patients there may be broad group of different glutenin peptides that activate the disease; hence, they have less restricted T-cell response with reactivity to a more diverse glutamine set of gliadin and glutenin.[20] One of the common features is the recognition of epitopes in gliadin located in regions rich in proline residues that is particularly resistant to gastrointestinal peptidases.[21] Enterocytes from patients with celiac disease also showed only limited digestion of peptide 31–49 of A-gliadin, a peptide that is not recognized by HLA-DQ2/DQ8. The high stability against proteolysis or the incomplete degradation of these gliadin peptides favors them as important initiators of the inflammatory response and toxic effects.[22]

### Innate immunity
In addition to the activation of T cells, innate response to gliadin is also involved in triggering the immune response in genetically predisposed individuals.[23] This results in initiation of the innate immune response in monocytes, macrophages, intestinal epithelial cells, and dendritic cells via unknown receptors and mechanisms. The innate

immune system uses the pattern recognition to provide an early response to the stimuli, such as RNA, DNA, lipopolysaccharide, and viral proteins, in contrast to the adaptive immune system, which depends on the HLA presentation cell recognition and expansion.[17]

### History and Physical Examination Findings in Celiac Disease

Presenting complaints of patients identified with celiac disease include chronic diarrhea; weight loss; weakness and fatigue; stool abnormalities, including pale, bulky, frothy, floating, or fouls-smelling stools; abdominal bloating; failure to thrive in children; and vomiting.[1] Three percent of patients with celiac disease come with presenting complaint of abdominal pain.[24]

The physical examination findings depend on the age at presentation and the severity of the disease.[25] In general, children or infants may present with signs of malabsorption as evidenced by poor weight gain or growth retardation and failure to thrive as well as irritability.[1] Some adults may appear normal, whereas in some, short stature, muscle wasting, or pallor may be obvious. Patients with celiac disease are usually thin although a few cases of obese patients have been reported.[26]

#### Mucous membranes
Relevant findings of celiac disease are usually in the mucosal membranes—mucosal pallor, geographic or fissured tongue, aphthous stomatitis, atrophic glossitis, and cheilitis.[27] Dental enamel defects affecting the secondary dentition are also seen in both adults and children.[28]

#### Abdomen
Examination of the abdomen may reveal abdominal distention and hyperactive bowel sounds.[25]

#### Skin
Dermatologic findings in celiac disease may include xerosis, vitiligo, keratosis pilaris, and a psoriasiform rash.[27] Dermatitis herpetiformis, seen in less than in 10% of patients,[25] is characterized by large symmetric groups of blisters, urticarial plaques, vesicles, and excoriated erythematous base. It usually affects the extensor surface of the extremities, scalp, and trunk and is regarded as a cutaneous variant of celiac disease.[25]

#### Neurologic
Patients may display hypotonia, cerebellar ataxia, peripheral neuropathy, seizures, and possibly cognitive impairment.[29,30]

#### Psychiatric
Psychiatric manifestations of celiac disease include developmental delay and learning disorders.[31]

### Diagnosis of Celiac Disease

Definitive diagnosis of celiac disease is made by small intestinal biopsy; however, a high index of suspicion usually precedes this, based on history and physical examination in conjunction with blood testing (discussed later).

### Who Should be Tested?

Testing for celiac disease should be considered in high-risk patients, including adult patients with chronic gastrointestinal symptoms and/or autoimmune disorders as well as symptomatic first-degree relatives of patients with celiac disease.[32]

The diagnosis should also be considered in infants and children with failure to thrive, persisting gastrointestinal symptoms, and asymptomatic conditions associated with celiac disease (type 1 diabetes mellitus, autoimmune thyroiditis, Down syndrome, Turner syndrome, Williams syndrome, selective IgA deficiency, and first-degree relatives of celiac patients). Testing is recommended for asymptomatic children who belong to groups at risk, beginning at approximately 3 years of age and provided they have had an adequate gluten-containing diet for at least 1 year before testing.[33] Serologic tests are

1. IgA tTG antibody—sensitivity 92.8% and specificity 98.1%[34]
2. IgA endomysial antibody—sensitivity 93% and specificity 99.7%[34]; false-negative results for antiendomysium (EMA) may occur before 2 years of age.[35]
3. IgA and IgG antigliadin antibodies have been used; however, studies have shown them less sensitive or specific compared with IgA EMA and IgA gluten-sensitive enteropathy tTG.[36] Patients with and without gastrointestinal inflammation from other causes may test positive for antigliadin antibodies.[37] IgA antigliadin antibody, however, is the most useful serologic marker in symptomatic children younger than 2 years of age. IgG antigliadin antibody is useful in the small percentage of patients with celiac sprue who have coexisting IgA deficiency.[38] Otherwise, measurement of IgA antibody to human tTG is recommended for initial testing for CD, based on practical considerations, including accuracy, reliability, and cost.[33]

These serologic tests can be performed with high diagnostic accuracy using rapid commercial assays. Serum-based rapid assay for IgA or IgG anti–human-transglutaminase antibodies have 100% sensitivity and 95% specificity, and blood drop–based rapid assay for IgA anti–human-transglutaminase antibodies have 90% sensitivity and 100% specificity.[39]

Combinations of antibodies may reduce the need for small-bowel biopsy.[40] In one study, a combination of antigliadin and EMA antibody tests had 100% sensitivity and 100% negative predictive value,[41] whereas false-positive results tended.

False-negative results are seen in patients with mild enteropathy, children under 2 years of age, and patients with IgA deficiency. Approximately 1% to 2% of patients with celiac disease have selective IgA deficiency.[42] The IgA EMA and IgA tTG (antitransglutaminase antibodies) serology tests yield false-negative results in untreated celiac disease in this group of patients. Total serum IgA should be measured in addition to IgA EMA or IgA tTG, especially when there is heightened clinical suspicion for celiac disease and IgA markers are negative.

### Hematologic and Biochemical Tests

Findings consistent with celiac disease include iron deficiency anemia and mineral and vitamin deficiencies, including decreased levels of calcium, albumin, cholesterol, iron, magnesium, zinc, carotenes, and vitamin A.[43]

The 72-hour fecal fat and d-xylose absorption test[1] are tests of intestinal absorption that have been used in the past but have not been shown to provide a specific diagnosis. These tests are normal in many patients with mild-to-moderate enteropathy.[44] Consequently, they are no longer important tools in cases of suspected celiac disease.[45]

### Imaging

Small intestinal radiographs may show malabsorption features, such as dilatation of the small intestines. Bone radiographs may show demineralization. CT and MRI may be ordered when complications, such as lymphoma or carcinoma, are suspected. In these cases, thickening of the small bowel is observed.[46] Imaging should be considered to evaluate patients with symptoms, such as marked weight loss, diarrhea, or abdominal pain.

## Pathology

Characteristic jejunal or distal duodenal biopsy findings in celiac disease[1]:

1. Loss of villi, due to lymphocytic infiltration—84% sensitivity and 88% specificity for early-stage celiac disease[47]
2. Flattening of mucosa
3. Lymphocytes and plasma cells in lamina propria
4. Increased mitoses in crypts.

Definitive diagnosis of celiac disease is made with 3 sequential small intestinal biopsies taken at different times during evaluation[1] with findings of

5. Flattened mucosa at presentation
6. Recovery of villi after gluten-free diet for 12 months
7. Flattening on gluten rechallenge.

In spite of these guidelines, the accuracy of available serologic tests has reduced the need for multiple biopsies. Small intestinal biopsy is reserved for selected patients who have an unsatisfactory or indeterminate clinical response to a strict gluten-free diet. Gluten challenge should be initiated in consultation with a specialist and with caution, because patients are sometimes extremely sensitive to gluten. A gluten challenge may also be considered in patients whose diagnoses were made based on small intestinal biopsy in childhood without the benefit of IgA EMA testing. This is of great importance because some transient childhood enteropathies have been seen to mimic celiac disease histologically.[48]

## Management

### Treatment plan

Celiac disease is treated by eliminating gluten-containing foods from the diet. Gluten-containing foods include wheat, rye, oats, and barley. An intake of 10 mg to 36 mg of gluten per day may result in mucosal abnormalities.[49] All initial serology testing and biopsies should be performed before starting gluten restriction. After placing a patient on a gluten-free diet, tTG antibody levels should be measured because lowering in the titer is associated with adherence to a gluten-free diet.[50]

The most common reasons for a lack of response to therapy are poor compliance and inadvertent gluten ingestion. A meticulous dietary history should be obtained and dietary counseling done with an experienced dietitian in patients who continue to have symptoms or persistent histologic abnormalities. It should also be done in those in whom serum antibody titers have not declined. Trace amounts of gluten may be contained in products that are labeled as gluten-free; however, the small amount of gluten contained in these products should not result in refractory disease.

The toxicity of oats is less clear because some studies suggest that pure oat flour can be tolerated without disease recurrence.[51] Moderate intake of oats seems safe in most children with celiac disease[52] and wheat-based starches may not be harmful.[53] A reasonable approach is to limit oat consumption to 50 to 60 g/day (approximately 2 oz) in patients with mild disease on presentation or in patients whose disease is in remission after a stringent gluten-free diet. Patients should be followed carefully for clinical or serologic evidence of disease recurrence after reintroducing oats. Patients with severe disease should completely avoid oats because oat products obtained in the store are frequently contaminated with small amounts of other cereals.[54]

Asymptomatic patients may also have micronutrient deficiencies that present clinically, such as bone loss due to vitamin D deficiency.[55] A patient's nutritional status should be considered so that nutritional and caloric deficiencies can be adequately supplemented. Specific dietary deficiencies, such as iron, folic acid, calcium, vitamin D, and vitamin $B_{12}$ deficiency, should be corrected. A gluten-free diet may lead to constipation due to decreased fiber in the diet. This usually responds to fiber supplementation with psyllium seed husks.

Osteopenia or osteoporosis is common in celiac disease and can occur in patients without gastrointestinal symptoms.[56] Patients diagnosed with celiac disease should be evaluated for bone loss using a dual-energy x-ray absorptiometry (DXA) scan. Monitoring by repeat DXA scan after 1 year is useful in patients with osteopenia because it permits estimation of the rate of change of bone mineral density.[57] Vitamin D deficiency may also cause secondary hyperparathyroidism resulting in bone loss. This may be partially reversed with a gluten-free diet because loss of bone density in the peripheral skeleton may persist despite apparent normalization at axial skeletal sites. Patients with advanced disease may have bone pain, pseudofractures, or deformity, but the majority of patients are asymptomatic or have only raised serum levels of alkaline phosphatase or hypocalcaemia.[57]

Celiac disease is associated with hyposplenism. Prophylactic administration of pneumococcal vaccine is recommended.

### Follow-up

There is a variable response to a gluten-free diet. Approximately 70% of patients have noticeable clinical improvement within 2 weeks.[58] Symptoms improve faster than histology, especially when biopsies are obtained in the proximal intestine. A possible explanation is that the less severely damaged distal small intestine recovers faster than the proximal intestine, which is usually more severely affected due to relatively increased exposure to gluten.[59]

Patients with positive IgA endomysial antibody and gluten sensitivity, but who have a normal small bowel biopsy, are considered to have latent celiac disease. Such patients are currently not advised to have a gluten-free diet but should continue to be monitored and rebiopsied if symptoms develop. Histologically evident celiac disease should be adequately evaluated in such patients with multiple intestinal biopsies, however, because the histologic abnormalities can be patchy.[60]

Patients with refractory sprue fall into 2 clinical categories[61]: patients who have no initial response to a gluten-free diet and patients who experience initial clinical improvement on a gluten-free diet but after a period of remission develop disease refractory to gluten abstinence.

Refractory sprue has also been subdivided into 2 immunologic categories[62]:

Type 1, in which there is a normal population of intraepithelial lymphocytes: these patients have a less severe presentation and a much better prognosis than patients with type 2 disease.

Type 2, in which there is an aberrant or premalignant population of intraepithelial lymphocytes. This can progress to enteropathy-associated T-cell lymphoma, which may present clinically as ulcerative jejunitis.[63]

Diagnosis can be established on biopsy; CT and fludeoxyglucose F 18–positron emission tomography scanning also help identify suspicious areas.[64]

Refractory sprue (in particular, type 2) can be severe and associated with progressive malabsorption and death. Some patients develop subepithelial collagen deposition, a condition referred to as collagenous sprue.[65]

The cause of refractory sprue is unknown. It is possible that some patients with this condition develop sensitivity to a dietary constituent other than gluten. Treatment is focused on immunosuppression, with use of corticosteroids.

In severely ill patients, higher-dose hydrocortisone (100 mg intravenously every 6 hours) is used. Oral dosing (such as 40 to 60 mg of prednisone daily) can be used in patients who are tolerating an oral diet. After a few weeks, the dose can be reduced by 5 to 10 mg per day in responding patients and subsequently tapered to the lowest dose that keeps the patient in remission.[66] Other medications that have been tried are azathioprine,[67] oral budesonide,[68] and intravenous cyclosporine.[69]

Other autoimmune disorders associated with celiac disease include type 1 diabetes mellitus, connective tissue diseases, Hashimoto thyroiditis, and Graves disease. These seem related to the duration of exposure to gluten.[70]

Mothers with untreated celiac disease are at increased risk for having low-birth-weight newborns and preterm births and as such should be closely monitored.[71]

---

**Key Points for Primary Care**

- Test for celiac disease in symptomatic patients who are at high risk.[32] These patients include patients with chronic gastrointestinal symptoms and/or autoimmune disorders and first-degree relatives. Test infants/children with failure to thrive, persisting gastrointestinal symptoms, and asymptomatic conditions associated with celiac disease[33,72] (grade A recommendation).

- Use serologic screening for IgA tTG antibody for the initial detection of celiac disease[32] (grade A recommendation).

- Avoid recommending a gluten-free diet unless the diagnosis of celiac sprue is firmly established.[1] It is expensive and may limit patients socially. On confirmation of celiac disease, strict lifelong adherence to the diet is recommended.[32] Consider involving an experienced dietician and support group in patient care[33,72] (grade A recommendation).

- Treat nutritional deficiencies with special attention to iron, folate, and vitamin $B_{12}$[32] (grade A recommendation).

- Consider screening for other conditions associated with celiac disease. If found, treat conditions and provide prophylaxis against predisposing infections[32] (grade A recommendation).

---

## PERNICIOUS ANEMIA

Pernicious anemia is form of megaloblastic anemia also known as Biermer anemia, Addison anemia, or Addison-Biermer anemia. It results from decreased absorption of vitamin $B_{12}$ due to lack of gastric intrinsic factor (IF), which may be as a result of atrophic gastritis or autoimmune parietal cell loss. It is common and often undiagnosed in the elderly.[73]

The most common source of vitamin $B_{12}$ or cyanocobalamine for humans is animal products (meat and dairy products); therefore, adequate absorption of cobalamin depends on sufficient dietary intake. The usual Western diet contains 5 μg to 7 μg of cobalamin per day; 6 μg to 9 μg per day is the minimum daily requirement.[74] The total body stores of cobalamin are 2 mg to 5 mg, approximately one-half of which is in the liver. Due to high stores of this vitamin, it takes years to develop vitamin $B_{12}$ deficiency after cessation of dietary absorption.[74]

## Epidemiology

Approximately 1.9% of people over age 60 have undiagnosed and untreated pernicious anemia.[73] It is most common in whites of Northern European ancestry. The average age of diagnosis is approximately 60 years. Under age 30, it is usually associated with other autoimmune diseases.[75]

## Pathophysiology

IF antibodies is produced from the parietal cells of the stomach. Antibodies to IF seem to inhibit acid production of parietal cells but do not seem to interact with gastrin receptors. Autoantibodies to the IF are a major cause of vitamin $B_{12}$ deficiency and are present in 70% of patients with pernicious anemia.[76] They are divided in 2 types: type I, which blocks attachment of vitamin $B_{12}$ to IF, and type II, which blocks $B_{12}$ IF complex to the ileal receptor.

Autoantibody to gastric parietal cells is found in 90% of patients with pernicious anemia; it is directed against the hydrogen-potassium-adenosine triphosphatase on the cell membrane, leading to decline in number of parietal cells and IF production. It leads to chronic atrophic gastritis and gastric atrophy. Autoimmune atrophic gastritis also promotes vitamin $B_{12}$ deficiency by causing decreased production of pepsin and decreased IF release from available parietal cells.[73]

Other causes of gastritides causing pernicious anemia include: nonautoimmune gastric atrophy, for example, from achlorhydria or *Helicobacter pylori* infection; gastritis secondary to long-term ingestion of biguanides, antacids, $H_2$ receptor antagonists, and proton pump inhibitors; chronic alcoholism; and pancreatic exocrine deficiency.

Differential diagnoses of pernicious anemia include other causes of vitamin $B_{12}$ deficiency, such as impaired vitamin $B_{12}$ absorption after gastrectomy or gastric bypass surgery and intestinal bacterial overgrowth secondary to antibiotic treatment. Rare cases of exacerbation of vitamin $B_{12}$ deficiency have been reported at high doses of folic acid supplementation.[77]

## History and Physical Examination Finding in Pernicious Anemia

Anemia may present with complaints of fatigue, low-grade fever, weight loss due to anorexia, lightheadedness, personality changes, unsteady gait, pallor, and palpitations. Neurologic complaints include paresthesias, loss of position and vibration senses, memory impairment, depression, dementia, psychosis, pain, and impaired micturition due to involvement of spinal cord.[78]

The physical examination findings are as follows:

Dermatologic findings include pallor and occasionally depigmentation due to coexisting autoimmune antibodies. Patients are rarely jaundiced due to impaired erythropoesis.

On examination of the head, the tongue may be swollen and red, a condition known as atrophic glossitis. Abdominal examination may show tenderness secondary to atrophic gastritis.

Neurologic findings include impaired sensation in the fingers or toes, decreased vibrations in toes distal sensory loss (posterior column), absent ankle reflex, increased knee reflex response, and extensor plantar response as a result of subacute combined degeneration of cord, a complication of severe chronic pernicious anemia. Psychiatric manifestations of pernicious anemia include personality change or memory loss.

Cardiac examination may show low blood pressure and rapid heart rate.[79]

### Diagnosis of Pernicious Anemia

Diagnosis is made by measuring anti-IF antibody and serum gastrin levels. This has a specificity of 90% to 95% but does not diagnose bacterial overgrowth of gut.[80] Gastrin levels are usually increased. Other causes of anemia should be ruled out using biochemical tests, including complete blood count, basic metabolic panel, thyroid function tests, and liver function tests.

Hematologic findings in pernicious anemia include macrocytosis, which is mean corpuscular volume (MCV) greater than 97 μm. Ideally this should be compared with the patient's baseline MCV. Other findings include low reticulocyte count, decreased vitamin $B_{12}$ (falsely low in severe folate deficiency; falsely increased or normal in severe liver disease), leukopenia, mild thrombocytopenia, and pancytopenia.

Blood chemistry findings are those of increased lactate dehydrogenase (LDH), increased bilirubin levels (as a result of hemolysis secondary to abnormal DNA synthesis), and increased methylmalonic acid and total homocysteine levels.

Blood film findings on peripheral smear include megaloblasts, teardrop cells, Cabot ring (spindle remnant), and hypersegmented polymorphonucleocytes (>6 lobes), which may be falsely elevated in renal insufficiency.

Bone marrow findings show intense erythroid hyperplasia with abnormal morphology; macroovalocytes and occasional megaloblasts can be seen as well as hypersegmented polymorphonucleocytes (>5% with 5 or more lobes or >1% with 6 or more lobes).

Urine chemistry shows methylmalonic acid in urine.

The Schilling test is not commonly used because it has unacceptable rates of false-positive and false-negative results.[81] It is only recommended when antiintrinsic antibodies are normal and differentiates vitamin $B_{12}$ deficiency due to pernicious anemia from those who have an intestinal lesion causing malabsorption. It is done in 2 stages:

In stage I, 1 μg of radiolabeled vitamin $B_{12}$ is given orally; 1 hour after the test dose, a 1000-μg flushing dose of nonradioactive vitamin $B_{12}$ is given to saturate vitamin $B_{12}$ binders (transcobalamines). A 24-hour urine is collected to determine how much radiolabeled vitamin $B_{12}$ is excreted. Normal is 8% to 35%. Reduced urinary excretion (<5%) in the presence of normal kidney function supports the diagnosis of decreased absorption of vitamin $B_{12}$.

Stage II is done only if stage I is abnormal. Stage I is repeated, except with the addition of added oral IF, which should normalize vitamin $B_{12}$ absorption in pernicious anemia but not intestinal malabsorption[81] and the process is repeated.

### Treatment

Synthetic vitamin $B_{12}$ (cyanocobalamin) is given by injection, 1000 μg intramuscularly. This is done every week for 6 weeks, then 500 to 1000 μg/month indefinitely. There is no risk of overtreatment, because cyanocobalamin is inexpensive and nontoxic and excess is excreted in urine.[82]

Intranasal vitamin $B_{12}$ gel (cyanocobalamin gel) is available for use after hematologic parameters have been normalized by intramuscular vitamin $B_{12}$ use. The dose is 1 spray every week. Patients should be advised regarding side effects of headache, nausea, and rhinitis.[83]

Oral vitamin $B_{12}$ replacement is given in large oral doses (1000 μg/d) and may correct vitamin $B_{12}$ deficiency even in patients with IF deficiency.[82]

Oral vitamin $B_{12}$, 1000 μg twice daily versus intramuscular vitamin $B_{12}$ on 7 days over 3 months showed comparable hematologic and neurologic responses in comparison trial; serum concentrations were 3 times higher with oral than intramuscular regimen.[84]

Sublingual vitamin $B_{12}$ replacement may be shown effective in preliminary studies.[85]

Response to treatment should be assessed. Parameters that indicate adequate response include reticulocytosis, which should occur in 3 to 4 days; rise in hemoglobin concentration should occur within 10 days; and normalization in 8 weeks as well as correction of MCV. Fall of serum LDH levels should occur within 2 days and hypersegmented polymorphonucleocytes expected to disappear in 10 to 14 days. Serum potassium should be monitored for severe hypokalemia during early response due to marked increased use in hematopoiesis.

Other conditions associated with pernicious anemia include autoimmune thyroiditis and adrenalitis; 5% to 10% of patients have hypothyroidism, and fewer than 5% of patients with hyperthyroidism have associated atrophic body gastritis.[75]

## Complications

Intestinal metaplasia may lead to 3 times risk of gastric carcinoma,[76,86] gastric carcinoid (more common than gastric cancer), cardiac failure due to hypoxia, iron overload, leukopenia, thrombocytopenia, and subacute combined degeneration of spinal cord (early complications— insidious paraparesis, ataxia, numbness, tingling of legs, and spasticity of the arms, and late complications—complete paraplegia with anesthesia) are possible complications. Recovery generally occurs in early stage of subacute combined degeneration of the spinal cord.

## Referral Criteria

Referral to a gastroenterologist should be done for patients with atrophic gastritis (pernicious anemia) who develop unexplained worsening of their dyspepsia as well as for any patient with pernicious anemia who has gastric symptoms and/or coexistent iron deficiency. There may be an increased risk of gastric cancer as well as gastric carcinoid tumors in patients with pernicious anemia. The risk seems highest within the first year of diagnosis.[86,87]

---

**Key Points for Primary Care**

- MCV should return to normal or else other causes of anemia should be considered.
- A single endoscopy should be considered to identify prevalent lesions (gastric cancer and carcinoid tumors) in patients with pernicious anemia, but there are insufficient data to support routine subsequent endoscopic surveillance for these patients.[88]
- Consider thyroid function screening annually.

---

## LACTASE DEFICIENCY

Lactase deficiency is a common condition associated with deficiency of intestinal lactase and malabsorption of dietary lactose. It manifests as lactose intolerance, which is the inability or insufficient ability to digest lactose, a sugar found in milk and milk products[89] and the primary carbohydrate in mammal milk. This inability results in the presence of one or more gastrointestinal symptoms after the ingestion of lactose. These symptoms include bloating, flatulence, nausea, abdominal pain, and/or diarrhea.

Lactase phlorizin hydrolase (lactase) is the intestinal brush border enzyme responsible for breaking lactose down into its component parts of glucose and galactose. It is found in the villi of the small intestine.

Lactose intolerance can also occur as a result of an imbalance between the amount of lactose ingested and the hydrolytic capacity of the lactase resulting in gastrointestinal symptoms. Such patients may be described as having lactose malabsorption.

Lactase deficiency is classified as follows.

### Primary Lactase Deficiency

Primary lactase deviciency is the most common form of lactose malabsorption, characterized by the relative or absolute absence of lactase. It develops over time, usually after age 2 when the body begins to produce less lactase,[89] and continues into childhood with age of symptoms presenting later in life although this varies in different racial groups.

### Secondary Lactase Deficiency

Secondary lactase deficiency results from injury to small bowel mucosa. The etiology of secondary lactose intolerance includes any gastrointestinal illness that causes significant damage to the brush borders of the small intestines[90] or significantly increases bowel transit time.

Causes of secondary lactose intolerance are:

1. Celiac disease
2. Whipple disease
3. Carcinoid syndrome
4. Cystic fibrosis
5. Diabetic gastropathy
6. HIV enteropathy
7. Regional enteritis
8. Kwashiorkor
9. Zollinger-Ellison syndrome
10. Radiation gastritis
11. Drugs (eg, colchicines).

### Congenital Lactase Deficiency

Congenital lactase deficiency is described as a congenital absence of lactase and is extremely rare. It manifests as intractable diarrhea as soon as human milk or lactose-containing formula is introduced. Intestinal biopsy reveals normal histologic characteristics but low or completely absent lactase concentrations.[91,92] Unless it is recognized and treated quickly, this condition is life threatening because of dehydration and electrolyte losses. Treatment is simply removal and substitution of lactose from the diet with a commercial lactose-free formula.[89]

### Epidemiology

Primary lactase deficiency typically presents in late adolescence and adulthood. Ethnic groups with greater than 50% prevalence of this condition include 95% to 100% of Asian populations, 80% to 100% of Native American populations, 60% to 80% of Ashkenazi Jews and African American populations, 50% to 80% of Hispanic populations, and 60% to 70% of Southern Indian subcontinent populations. Only 6% to 22% of the American white population suffers from primary lactase deficiency.[93]

### Physiology and Pathophysiology

The lactase enzyme is located in the brush border of the small intestinal cells. It is responsible for the breakdown of dietary lactose into its constituent parts of glucose and galactose, which are then transported across the cell membranes.[90] There is a normal developmental decline in lactase levels that occur after weaning with humans and a continuous decrease through adulthood. As much as 90% to 95% of birth quantities of lactase with different racial variations may be lost by early childhood.[90] In the absence or deficiency of lactase, the unabsorbed sugars generate an osmotic load, which draws fluid into the intestinal lumen causing loose stools.[94]

Bacteria that are located in the colon metabolize lactose, causing the production of volatile fatty acids and gases, such as methane, hydrogen, and carbon dioxide, all of which result in flatulence and bloating.

Approximately 12 g to 18 g (8–12 oz) of milk are sufficient to result in symptoms in patients with primary adult lactose deficiency. Smaller quantities may produce symptoms without diarrhea while larger quantities produce more symptoms.

Lactose content of some common dairy products[89]:

1. Whole milk (8 ounces): 12.8 g
2. Reduced-fat milk (8 ounces): 12.2 g
3. Plain low-fat yogurt (8 ounces): 8.4 g
4. Vanilla ice cream (4 ounces): 4.9 g
5. Small curd cottage cheese (8 ounces): 1.4 g
6. Cheddar cheese (1 ounce): 0.07 g
7. Swiss cheese (1 ounce): 0.02 g.

Other factors contributing to worsened symptoms include faster transit and gastric emptying time and suitable microflora in the colon.

### Clinical Manifestations

Individual symptoms vary and depend on the amount of lactose consumed. They usually occur approximately 2 hours after ingestion of lactose[90] and are not necessarily correlated with the degree of intestinal lactase deficiency.[94] They may include abdominal pain, bloating, cramping, diarrhea, and flatulence. Several factors affect the severity of the symptoms and include the ethnicity and age, with older patients being more susceptible.

There are no physical findings definitive for lactose intolerance; however, hyperactive bowel sounds and abdominal distension may be present.

### Diagnosis

Diagnosis is made by clinical history and dietary manipulation involving trial of lactose avoidance. During a diagnostic lactose-free diet, it is important that all sources of lactose be eliminated. This involves the reading of food labels to identify hidden sources of lactose.[94]

Foods with significant amounts of lactose[89]:

1. Bread and other baked goods
2. Waffles, pancakes, biscuits, and cookies and mixes to make them
3. Processed breakfast foods, such as doughnuts, frozen waffles and pancakes, toaster pastries, and sweet rolls
4. Processed breakfast cereals and nonfat dry milk powder
5. Instant potatoes, soups, and breakfast drinks, milk, curds, whey, milk by-products, and dry milk solids
6. Potato chips, corn chips, and other processed snacks
7. Processed meats, such as bacon, sausage, hot dogs, and lunchmeats
8. Margarine

9. Salad dressings
10. Liquid and powdered milk–based meal replacements
11. Protein powders and bars
12. Candies
13. Nondairy liquid and powdered coffee creamers
14. Nondairy whipped toppings.

Checking the ingredients on food labels is helpful in finding possible sources of lactose in food products. If any of the food labels includes words like whey, curds, milk by- products the product contains lactose. Bread, baked goods, waffles, biscuits, processed cereals, instant potatoes, breakfast or protein drinks or bars, corn chips, potato chips, margarine, hot dogs, salads, and candies contain lactose.[89]

The lactose breath hydrogen test may be used in diagnosis. It is based on the principle that carbohydrate in the colon is detectable in pulmonary excretion of hydrogen and other gases.[93] This test involves ingestion of oral lactose (2 g/kg; maximum 25 g, equivalent to 16 oz milk) after an overnight fast. The amount of hydrogen in expired air is measured for 2 to 3 hours after the ingestion of lactose. An increase (>20 ppm) in expired hydrogen after 60 minutes is diagnostic of lactose intolerance.

The lactose breath hydrogen test is positive in 90% of patients with lactose malabsorption. False-negative results occur in cases of absence of bacterial flora, recent use of oral antibiotics, or recent high colonic enema. False-positive results characterized by increased breath hydrogen secretion unrelated to lactose may be obtained during sleep or exercise or with previous use of aspirin and with smoking. The lactose tolerance test has been used for diagnoses in the past but is no longer recommended due to unacceptable rates of false-positive and false-negative results.

Differential diagnosis of lactose malabsorption includes any of the malabsorption syndromes and may include irritable bowel syndrome, inflammatory bowel disease, infectious diarrhea, celiac disease, diverticulitis, and parasitic infections. These may be ruled out by stool testing for parasites or pH, blood testing for celiac disease or IgA deficiency, or biopsy as necessary.[94]

### Management of Primary Lactase Deficiency

Treatment should only be initiated in the presence of symptoms of intolerance. The intensity of symptoms varies in different people and as such it is recommended that individuals tailor their intake to the threshold at which symptoms occur. Milk intake for most patients is limited to less than 8 to 12 oz/day, and lactose hydrolyzed milk may reduce symptoms[95] (grade B). Complete exclusion of milk and dietary products from the diet has had no benefit, instead resulting in serious nutritional consequences. As a result, patients are advised to maintain a calcium intake of 1200 to 1500 mg/day[90] (grade A).

Other modifications that help with reduction of symptoms include consuming lactose-containing beverages with food[96] (grade B); use of lactase enzyme tablets and consumption of yogurt, which is thought as effective as lactase hydrolyzed milk (grade B); or consumption of milk products treated with lactobacillus or yogurt cultures[97] (grade B). Some medications that have been considered in reduction of symptoms include loperamide[98] (grade B) but this is not recommended due to symptoms of constipation. Propantheline has also been suggested[99] (grade B); however, both recommendations are based on small clinical trials.

### Counseling

Patients need to be counseled and reassured that ingestion of lactose does not cause permanent damage and they do not need to be on a totally lactose-free or severely restricted diet.[90] Dairy products should not be totally eliminated because they provide key nutrients, such as calcium, vitamins A and D, riboflavin, and phosphorus; in addition, other milk forms that are plant based—soy and rice—may be substituted. Adequate calcium intake may also be provided in the form of calcium supplementation.[90] Other necessary counseling should include the need to avoid foods that contain lactose as fillers and to distinguish certain foods that are hidden sources of lactose.

### Referral Criteria

Persistent symptoms after a 2-week trial of dietary modifications should raise consideration of secondary lactose deficiency or other gastrointestinal pathology as a cause for symptoms, at which time a gastroenterologist should be consulted.

Tests, such as the hydrogen breath tests and blood and stool tests, may be done in conjunction with a gastroenterologist to ensure accurate interpretation of results.[94]

---

**Key Points for Primary Care**

- Diagnosis of lactose intolerance can be achieved easily with dietary elimination and challenge (grade A).

- Treatment of lactose intolerance by elimination of milk and other dairy products is not usually necessary given newer approaches to lactose intolerance, including the use of partially digested products[100,101] (grade B).

- If lactose-free diets are used for treatment of lactose intolerance, diets should include a good source of calcium and/or calcium supplementation to meet daily recommended intake levels (grade A).

- Patients with secondary lactose intolerance require further investigation to identify the primary problem. Effective treatment of the underlying condition may not only ameliorate symptoms but also improve lactose intolerance (grade A).

- A gradual re-introduction of dairy products considering the individual threshold dose to assure an adequate intake of essential nutritional substances may be undertaken[102] (grade B).

---

### ACKNOWLEDGMENTS

The author would like to thank Jay Morro, DVM, MPH; Emeka Ohagi, MS, MPH; M. Raza Khan, MD; and Laura Snell, MPH, for their contributions to this work.

### REFERENCES

1. Farrell RJ, Kelly CP. Celiac sprue. N Engl J Med 2002;346(3):180–8.
2. Venes D, Taber CW, editors. Taber's cyclopedic medical dictionary. 21st edition. Illustrated in full color. Philadelphia: F. A. Davis Co; 2009.
3. Hadjivassiliou M, Grunewald RA, Davies-Jones GA. Idiopathic cerebellar ataxia associated with celiac disease: lack of distinctive neurological features. J Neurol Neurosurg Psychiatry 1999;67(2):257.
4. Kagnoff MF, Austin RK, Hubert JJ, et al. Possible role for a human adenovirus in the pathogenesis of celiac disease. J Exp Med 1984;160(5):1544–57.
5. Sanders DS, Carter MJ, Hurlstone DP, et al. Association of adult coeliac disease with irritable bowel syndrome: a case-control study in patients fulfilling ROME II criteria referred to secondary care. Lancet 2001;358(9292): 1504–8.

6. Barera G, Bonfanti R, Viscardi M, et al. Occurrence of celiac disease after onset of type 1 diabetes: a 6-year prospective longitudinal study. Pediatrics 2002;109(5): 833–8.

7. Lo Iacono O, Petta S, Venezia G, et al. Anti-tissue transglutaminase antibodies in patients with abnormal liver tests: is it always coeliac disease? Am J Gastroenterol 2005;100(11):2472–7.

8. Norris JM, Barriga K, Hoffenberg EJ, et al. Risk of celiac disease autoimmunity and timing of gluten introduction in the diet of infants at increased risk of disease. JAMA 2005;293(19):2343–51.

9. Feighery C. Fortnightly review: coeliac disease. BMJ 1999;319(7204):236–9.

10. Hankey GL, Holmes GK. Coeliac disease in the elderly. Gut 1994;35(1):65–7.

11. Ciacci C, Cirillo M, Sollazzo R, et al. Gender and clinical presentation in adult celiac disease. Scand J Gastroenterol 1995;30(11):1077–81.

12. Dube C, Rostom A, Sy R, et al. The prevalence of celiac disease in average-risk and at-risk Western European populations: a systematic review. Gastroenterolog 2005;128(4 Suppl 1):S57–67.

13. McGowan KE, Castiglione DA, Butzner JD. The changing face of childhood celiac disease in north america: impact of serological testing. Pediatrics 2009; 124(6):1572–8.

14. Fasano A, Berti I, Gerarduzzi T, et al. Prevalence of celiac disease in at-risk and not-at-risk groups in the United States: a large multicenter study. Arch Intern Med 2003;163(3):286–92.

15. Pietzak MM, Schofield TC, McGinniss MJ, et al. Stratifying risk for celiac disease in a large at-risk United States population by using HLA alleles. Clin Gastroenterol Hepatol 2009;7(9):966–71.

16. Petronzelli F, Bonamico M, Ferrante P, et al. Genetic contribution of the HLA region to the familial clustering of coeliac disease. Ann Hum Genet 1997;61(Pt 4):307–17.

17. Pittschieler K, Ladinser B. Coeliac disease: screened by a new strategy. Acta Paediatr Suppl 1996;412:42–5.

18. Vader W, Kooy Y, Van Veelen P, et al. The gluten response in children with celiac disease is directed toward multiple gliadin and glutenin peptides. Gastroenterology 2002;122(7):1729–37.

19. Esposito C, Paparo F, Caputo I, et al. Anti-tissue transglutaminase antibodies from coeliac patients inhibit transglutaminase activity both in vitro and in situ. Gut 2002;51(2):177–81.

20. Maki M, Mustalahti K, Kokkonen J, et al. Prevalence of Celiac disease among children in Finland. N Engl J Med 2003;348(25):2517–24.

21. Matysiak-Budnik T, Candalh C, Dugave C, et al. Alterations of the intestinal transport and processing of gliadin peptides in celiac disease. Gastroenterology 2003;125(3):696–707.

22. Lammers KM, Lu R, Brownley J, et al. Gliadin induces an increase in intestinal permeability and zonulin release by binding to the chemokine receptor CXCR3. Gastroenterology 2008;135(1):194–204, e193.

23. Maiuri L, Ciacci C, Ricciardelli I, et al. Association between innate response to gliadin and activation of pathogenic T cells in coeliac disease. Lancet 2003; 362(9377):30–7.

24. Sanders DS, Hopper AD, Azmy IA, et al. Association of adult celiac disease with surgical abdominal pain: a case-control study in patients referred to secondary care. Ann Surg 2005;242(2):201–7.

25. McPhee SJ, Papadakis MA. Current medical diagnosis & treatment 2010. London. 49th edition. New York: McGraw-Hill Medical; 2010.

26. Furse RM, Mee AS. Atypical presentation of coeliac disease. BMJ 2005; 330(7494):773–4.
27. Seyhan M, Erdem T, Ertekin V, et al. The mucocutaneous manifestations associated with celiac disease in childhood and adolescence. Pediatr Dermatol 2007; 24(1):28–33.
28. Aine L, Maki M, Collin P, et al. Dental enamel defects in celiac disease. J Oral Pathol Med 1990;19(6):241–5.
29. Hu WT, Murray JA, Greenaway MC, et al. Cognitive impairment and celiac disease. Arch Neurol 2006;63(10):1440–6.
30. Lionetti E, Francavilla R, Maiuri L, et al. Headache in pediatric patients with celiac disease and its prevalence as a diagnostic clue. J Pediatr Gastroenterol Nutr 2009;49(2):202–7.
31. Zelnik N, Pacht A, Obeid R, et al. Range of neurologic disorders in patients with celiac disease. Pediatrics 2004;113(6):1672–6.
32. AGA Institute. AGA Institute Medical Position Statement on the Diagnosis and Management of Celiac Disease. Gastroenterology 2006;131(6):1977–80.
33. Hill ID, Dirks MH, Liptak GS, et al. Guideline for the diagnosis and treatment of celiac disease in children: recommendations of the North American Society for Pediatric Gastroenterology, Hepatology and Nutrition. J Pediatr Gastroenterol Nutr 2005;40(1):1–19.
34. Lewis NR, Scott BB. Systematic review: the use of serology to exclude or diagnose coeliac disease (a comparison of the endomysial and tissue transglutaminase antibody tests). Aliment Pharmacol Ther 2006;24(1):47–54.
35. Kwiecien J, Karczewska K, Lukasik M, et al. Negative results of antiendomysial antibodies: long term follow up. Arch Dis Child 2005;90(1):41–2.
36. Kelly CP, Feighery CF, Gallagher RB, et al. Mucosal and systemic IgA anti-gliadin antibody in celiac disease. Contrasting patterns of response in serum, saliva, and intestinal secretions. Dig Dis Sci 1991;36(6):743–51.
37. Uibo O, Uibo R, Kleimola V, et al. Serum IgA anti-gliadin antibodies in an adult population sample. High prevalence without celiac disease. Dig Dis Sci 1993; 38(11):2034–7.
38. Fotoulaki M, Nousia-Arvanitakis S, Augoustidou-Savvopoulou P, et al. Clinical application of immunological markers as monitoring tests in celiac disease. Dig Dis Sci 1999;44(10):2133–8.
39. Nemec G, Ventura A, Stefano M, et al. Looking for celiac disease: diagnostic accuracy of two rapid commercial assays. Am J Gastroenterol 2006;101(7):1597–600.
40. Hadithi M, von Blomberg BM, Crusius JB, et al. Accuracy of serologic tests and HLA-DQ typing for diagnosing celiac disease. Ann Intern Med 2007;147(5): 294–302.
41. Russo PA, Chartrand LJ, Seidman E. Comparative analysis of serologic screening tests for the initial diagnosis of celiac disease. Pediatrics 1999;104(1 Pt 1):75–8.
42. Cataldo F, Marino V, Bottaro G, et al. Celiac disease and selective immunoglobulin A deficiency. J Pediatr 1997;131(2):306–8.
43. Ackerman Z, Eliakim R, Stalnikowicz R, et al. Role of small bowel biopsy in the endoscopic evaluation of adults with iron deficiency anemia. Am J Gastroenterol 1996;91(10):2099–102.
44. Uil JJ, van Elburg RM, Mulder CJ, et al. The value of the D-xylose test compared with the differential sugar absorption test in recognizing coeliac disease. Neth J Med 1996;49(2):68–72.
45. Kelly CP, Feighery CF, Gallagher RB, et al. Diagnosis and treatment of gluten-sensitive enteropathy. Adv Intern Med 1990;35:341–63.

46. Rubesin SE, Herlinger H, Saul SH, et al. Adult celiac disease and its complications. Radiographics 1989;9(6):1045–66.
47. Jarvinen TT, Collin P, Rasmussen M, et al. Villous tip intraepithelial lymphocytes as markers of early-stage coeliac disease. Scand J Gastroenterol 2004;39(5):428–33.
48. Trier JS. Diagnosis of celiac sprue. Gastroenterology 1998;115(1):211–6.
49. Akobeng AK, Thomas AG. Systematic review: tolerable amount of gluten for people with coeliac disease. Aliment Pharmacol Ther 2008;27(11):1044–52.
50. Fabiani E, Catassi C. The serum IgA class anti-tissue transglutaminase antibodies in the diagnosis and follow up of coeliac disease. Results of an international multi-centre study. International Working Group on Eu-tTG. Eur J Gastroenterol Hepatol 2001;13(6):659–65.
51. Janatuinen EK, Pikkarainen PH, Kemppainen TA, et al. A comparison of diets with and without oats in adults with celiac disease. N Engl J Med 1995; 333(16):1033–7.
52. Hogberg L, Laurin P, Falth-Magnusson K, et al. Oats to children with newly diagnosed coeliac disease: a randomised double blind study. Gut 2004;53(5):649–54.
53. Kaukinen K, Salmi T, Collin P, et al. Clinical trial: gluten microchallenge with wheat-based starch hydrolysates in coeliac disease patients - a randomized, double-blind, placebo-controlled study to evaluate safety. Aliment Pharmacol Ther 2008;28(10):1240–8.
54. Lundin KE, Nilsen EM, Scott HG, et al. Oats induced villous atrophy in coeliac disease. Gut 2003;52(11):1649–52.
55. Shaker JL, Brickner RC, Findling JW, et al. Hypocalcemia and skeletal disease as presenting features of celiac disease. Arch Intern Med 1997;157(9):1013–6.
56. Meyer D, Stavropolous S, Diamond B, et al. Osteoporosis in a north american adult population with celiac disease. Am J Gastroenterol 2001;96(1):112–9.
57. Scott EM, Gaywood I, Scott BB. Guidelines for osteoporosis in coeliac disease and inflammatory bowel disease. British Society of Gastroenterology. Gut 2000; 46(Suppl 1):i1–8.
58. Pink IJ, Creamer B. Response to a gluten-free diet of patients with the coeliac syndrome. Lancet 1967;1(7485):300–4.
59. Macdonald WC, Brandborg LL, Flick AL, et al. Studies of Celiac Sprue. Iv. The Response of the Whole Length of the Small Bowel to a Gluten-Free Diet. Gastroenterology 1964;47:573–89.
60. Selby PL, Davies M, Adams JE, et al. Bone loss in celiac disease is related to secondary hyperparathyroidism. J Bone Miner Res 1999;14(4):652–7.
61. Carroccio A, Iacono G, Lerro P, et al. Role of pancreatic impairment in growth recovery during gluten-free diet in childhood celiac disease. Gastroenterology 1997;112(6):1839–44.
62. Trier JS, Falchuk ZM, Carey MC, et al. Celiac sprue and refractory sprue. Gastroenterology 1978;75(2):307–16.
63. Ryan BM, Kelleher D. Refractory celiac disease. Gastroenterology 2000;119(1): 243–51.
64. Bagdi E, Diss TC, Munson P, et al. Mucosal intra-epithelial lymphocytes in enteropathy-associated T-cell lymphoma, ulcerative jejunitis, and refractory celiac disease constitute a neoplastic population. Blood 1999;94(1):260–4.
65. Gao Y, Kristinsson SY, Goldin LR, et al. Increased risk for non-Hodgkin lymphoma in individuals with celiac disease and a potential familial association. Gastroenterology 2009;136(1):91–8.
66. Baker AL, Rosenberg IH. Refractory sprue: recovery after removal of nongluten dietary proteins. Ann Intern Med 1978;89(4):505–8.

67. Maurino E, Niveloni S, Chernavsky A, et al. Azathioprine in refractory sprue: results from a prospective, open-label study. Am J Gastroenterol 2002;97(10):2595–602.
68. Daum S, Ipczynski R, Heine B, et al. Therapy with budesonide in patients with refractory sprue. Digestion 2006;73(1):60–8.
69. Wahab PJ, Crusius JB, Meijer JW, et al. Cyclosporin in the treatment of adults with refractory coeliac disease–an open pilot study. Aliment Pharmacol Ther 2000;14(6):767–74.
70. Ventura A, Magazzu G, Greco L. Duration of exposure to gluten and risk for autoimmune disorders in patients with celiac disease. SIGEP Study Group for Autoimmune Disorders in Celiac Disease. Gastroenterology 1999;117(2):297–303.
71. Norgard B, Fonager K, Sorensen HT, et al. Birth outcomes of women with celiac disease: a nationwide historical cohort study. Am J Gastroenterol 1999;94(9): 2435–40.
72. Coeliac disease: recognition and assessment of coeliac disease. 2009. Available at: http://www.nice.org.uk/nicemedia/pdf/CG86FullGuideline.pdf. Accessed August 16, 2010.
73. Carmel R. Prevalence of undiagnosed pernicious anemia in the elderly. Arch Intern Med 1996;156(10):1097–100.
74. Green R, Kinsella LJ. Current concepts in the diagnosis of cobalamin deficiency. Neurology 1995;45(8):1435–40.
75. Centanni M, Marignani M, Gargano L, et al. Atrophic body gastritis in patients with autoimmune thyroid disease: an underdiagnosed association. Arch Intern Med 1999;159(15):1726–30.
76. Pruthi RK, Tefferi A. Pernicious anemia revisited. Mayo Clin Proc 1994;69(2): 144–50.
77. Campbell NR. How safe are folic acid supplements? Arch Intern Med 1996; 156(15):1638–44.
78. Toh BH, van Driel IR, Gleeson PA. Pernicious anemia. N Engl J Med 1997; 337(20):1441–8.
79. Dang CV. Runner's anemia. JAMA 2001;286(6):714–6.
80. Lahner E, Norman GL, Severi C, et al. Reassessment of intrinsic factor and parietal cell autoantibodies in atrophic gastritis with respect to cobalamin deficiency. Am J Gastroenterol 2009;104(8):2071–9.
81. Lindgren A, Bagge E, Cederblad A, et al. Schilling and protein-bound cobalamin absorption tests are poor instruments for diagnosing cobalamin malabsorption. J Intern Med 1997;241(6):477–84.
82. Berlin H, Berlin R, Brante G. Oral treatment of pernicious anemia with high doses of vitamin B12 without intrinsic factor. Acta Med Scand 1968;184(4): 247–58.
83. Slot WB, Merkus FW, Van Deventer SJ, et al. Normalization of plasma vitamin B12 concentration by intranasal hydroxocobalamin in vitamin B12-deficient patients. Gastroenterology 1997;113(2):430–3.
84. Elia M. Oral or parenteral therapy for B12 deficiency. Lancet 1998;352(9142): 1721–2.
85. Delpre G, Stark P, Niv Y. Sublingual therapy for cobalamin deficiency as an alternative to oral and parenteral cobalamin supplementation. Lancet 1999; 354(9180):740–1.
86. Hsing AW, Hansson LE, McLaughlin JK, et al. Pernicious anemia and subsequent cancer. A population-based cohort study. Cancer 1993;71(3):745–50.
87. Brinton LA, Gridley G, Hrubec Z, et al. Cancer risk following pernicious anaemia. Br J Cancer 1989;59(5):810–3.

88. Hirota WK, Zuckerman MJ, Adler DG, et al. ASGE guideline: the role of endoscopy in the surveillance of premalignant conditions of the upper GI tract. Gastrointest Endosc 2006;63(4):570–80.

89. Sibley E, Fisher R, Pennington J. Lactose intolerance. 2009. Available at: http://digestive.niddk.nih.gov/ddiseases/pubs/lactoseintolerance/. Accessed May 5, 2010.

90. Swagerty DL Jr, Walling AD, Klein RM. Lactose intolerance. Am Fam Physician 2002;65(9):1845–50.

91. Asp NG, Dahlqvist A, Kuitunen P, et al. Complete deficiency of brush-border lactase in congenital lactose malabsorption. Lancet 1973;2(7824):329–30.

92. Freiburghaus AU, Schmitz J, Schindler M, et al. Protein patterns of brush-border fragments in congenital lactose malabsorption and in specific hypolactasia of the adult. N Engl J Med 1976;294(19):1030–2.

93. Arola H. Diagnosis of hypolactasia and lactose malabsorption. Scand J Gastroenterol Suppl 1994;202:26–35.

94. Heyman MB. Lactose intolerance in infants, children, and adolescents. Pediatrics 2006;118(3):1279–86.

95. Reasoner J, Maculan TP, Rand AG, et al. Clinical studies with low-lactose milk. Am J Clin Nutr 1981;34(1):54–60.

96. Martini MC, Savaiano DA. Reduced intolerance symptoms from lactose consumed during a meal. Am J Clin Nutr 1988;47(1):57–60.

97. Lin MY, Yen CL, Chen SH. Management of lactose maldigestion by consuming milk containing lactobacilli. Dig Dis Sci 1998;43(1):133–7.

98. Szilagyi A, Torchinsky A, Calacone A. Possible therapeutic use of loperamide for symptoms of lactose intolerance. Can J Gastroenterol 2000;14(7):581–7.

99. Peuhkuri K, Vapaatalo H, Nevala R, et al. Influence of the pharmacological modification of gastric emptying on lactose digestion and gastrointestinal symptoms. Aliment Pharmacol Ther 1999;13(1):81–6.

100. Medow MS, Thek KD, Newman LJ, et al. Beta-galactosidase tablets in the treatment of lactose intolerance in pediatrics. Am J Dis Child 1990;144(11):1261–4.

101. Sanders ME, Klaenhammer TR. Invited review: the scientific basis of Lactobacillus acidophilus NCFM functionality as a probiotic. J Dairy Sci 2001;84(2):319–31.

102. Hertzler SR, Savaiano DA. Colonic adaptation to daily lactose feeding in lactose maldigesters reduces lactose intolerance. Am J Clin Nutr 1996;64(2):232–6.

# Inflammatory Bowel Disease

Anne Walsh, MMSc, PA-C[a,b,c,]*, John Mabee, PhD, PA-C[a,b],
Kashyap Trivedi, MD[c]

**KEYWORDS**

- Inflammatory bowel disease • Crohn disease • Ulcerative colitis

Crohn disease (CD) and ulcerative colitis (UC) are the most common forms of inflammatory bowel disease (IBD) likely to be encountered in primary care. Because IBD is a chronic, systemic inflammatory illness with a characteristically waxing and waning course, patients may manifest unpredictable intestinal symptom flares as well as various nongastrointestinal symptoms and complications. As a disease whose overall incidence is increasing and whose diagnosis is often delayed, with sufferers being primarily young adults, the burden placed on health care utilization by IBD is substantial. Patient-centered care is essential for positive outcomes, and should include long-term continuity with an empathetic primary care provider who can provide skillful coordination of the requisite multidisciplinary approach. Early primary care suspicion of the diagnosis and referral to expert gastroenterologists for confirmation and medical management is essential. Coordinating interdisciplinary consultations involving colorectal surgeons, radiologists, stoma therapists, psychologists, and rheumatologists, in combination with comprehensive patient education, is key to decreasing overall morbidity, mortality, and health care costs associated with this lifelong condition.

## EPIDEMIOLOGY

In North America, the incidence rates for CD range from 3.1 to 14.6 per 100,000 person-years, and for UC from 2.2 to 14.3 per 100,000 person-years. Prevalence of CD ranges from 26 to 199 per 100,000 persons, and for UC from 37 to 246 per 100,000 persons.[1] Estimating a combined population of 343 million persons in the United States[2] and Canada[3] in 2010, between 10,600 and 50,100 persons will be

[a] Department of Family Medicine, University of Southern California, 1975 Zonal Avenue, KAM-B33, Los Angeles, CA 90033, USA
[b] KSOM-USC Primary Care Physician Assistant Program, 1000 South Fremont, Unit 7, Building A11, Room 150, Alhambra, CA 91803, USA
[c] Hertz and Associates in Gastroenterology, 4132 Katella Avenue, Suite 200, Los Alamitos, CA 90720, USA
* Corresponding author. Department of Family Medicine, 1975 Zonal Avenue, KAM-B33, Los Angeles, CA 90033.
E-mail address: annewals@usc.edu

Prim Care Clin Office Pract 38 (2011) 415–432
doi:10.1016/j.pop.2011.06.001
0095-4543/11/$ – see front matter © 2011 Elsevier Inc. All rights reserved.

primarycare.theclinics.com

newly diagnosed with CD each year, and as many as 682,600 persons may have this disease. Similarly, between 7550 and 49,050 persons will be newly diagnosed with UC each year, and as many as 843,800 persons may have this disease.

The considerable variation in reported IBD incidence is likely due to its complex nature and range of factors thought to play a role in disease genesis. While many studies have focused on Caucasian populations, the incidence and prevalence of IBD has increased in Hispanics and Asians; both groups are more likely to have UC than CD. IBD is also more common in Ashkenazi Jews. Although IBD rates among African Americans approximates that of Caucasians, there are differences between racial and ethnic groups in IBD family history, disease location, and extraintestinal manifestations.[4,5] The prevalence of IBD peaks in two age groups: primarily the third decade, with a smaller peak in the seventh decade. In adults, the prevalence of CD is higher among women (odds ratio [OR] 1.18; 95% confidence interval [CI] 1.14–1.23), but equal in both genders for UC (OR 1.00; 95% CI 0.97–1.03).[6] Epidemiologic associations that CD and UC share include higher rates of disease in northern climates and in well-developed areas of the world.[7] Cigarette smoking increases the risk of CD development and recurrence, but decreases the risk of developing UC.[8] Breast feeding may be protective against both CD and UC, and appendectomy appears protective against UC.[9,10] Triggering factors that may play a role via breeching the gut mucosal barrier include diet, perinatal and childhood enteritides, measles infection or vaccination, mycobacterial infection, oral contraceptives, nonsteroidal anti-inflammatory drugs, and "stress" or psychopathology. The latter, while not considered causal, can exacerbate symptoms.[1,11–13]

## PATHOPHYSIOLOGY

Pathologic features of CD and UC are well known, with CD being characterized as having discontinuous "skip lesions" of transmural bowel wall inflammation that can progress to fibrosis, strictures, and fistulas. Although these lesions can occur anywhere along the gastrointestinal tract, they typically occur within the ileum. By contrast, UC involves inflammation of the bowel wall mucosa and submucosa only, and always involves the rectum in untreated disease. Although lesions can extend as far as the cecum, unlike with CD they do so in a continuous pattern. In UC, one may occasionally encounter an isolated area of cecal-periappendiceal orifice inflammation in addition to the characteristic distal colonic inflammation. Aphthous ulcers of any part of the gastrointestinal (GI) tract may be seen in either disease. The classic feature of CD on tissue biopsy is granulomatous inflammation, although granulomas are present in less than 30% of CD biopsy material, whereas both CD and UC manifest acute and chronic inflammation with crypt distortion and abscess formation along with a plasmacytic infiltrate of the lamina propria. Because both forms of IBD comprise a spectrum of mild to marked inflammatory changes and have overlapping signs, symptoms, and laboratory findings, it is sometimes difficult to distinguish CD from UC despite extensive workup; these cases are termed indeterminant colitis.

The development of IBD involves the interaction of at least 3 elements: genetic predisposition, environmental trigger(s), and dysregulation of the immune response. The most persuasive evidence for heritable risk of IBD comes from twin studies. Orholm and colleagues[14] reported a proband-wise concordance rate among monozygotic twin pairs of 58.3% for CD, and 18.2% for UC, with a concordance rate among dizygotic pairs of 0% for CD and 4.5% for UC. However, while positive family history remains the strongest predictor of risk, depending on ethnicity, it occurs in up to 20% of cases.[4] Hence, despite the fact that genetic factors are important, more so in CD than UC, it is evident that environmental factors also play a key role.

Genome-wide association studies have revealed more than 40 susceptibility loci for IBD, some associated specifically with either CD or UC and others associated with both.[15] Prominent among these findings are the IBD1 gene encoding the protein NOD2 (also called CARD15) in CD, OCTN1/2 within the IBD5 locus in CD and UC, ATG16L in CD, IRGM1 in CD, and IL23R in CD and UC.[16] Major histocompatibility complex (MHC) class II associations with UC have also been made, primarily with HLA-DR1.[17]

Defects in NOD2 or OCTN1/2 affect the ability of the host to localize and eradicate bacteria that gain access to gut tissue. By failing to dispose of such an environmental trigger, either an aberrant inflammatory response ensues or the persistence of antigen stimulates an adaptive immune response. ATG16L and IRGM1 are associated with autophagy. Mutations in these genes result in autophagy failure, thereby promoting inflammation. Mutations of IL23R affect the interleukin (IL)-12/23 pathway of inflammation. The significance of understanding these and related pathways is that they may serve as targets for future therapies.

Although several possible environmental triggers are noted, it is also clear that bacteria play a key role as a trigger of IBD. The role of microbial flora in the induction and persistence of disease has been repeatedly demonstrated in murine models of IBD. Although no evidence points to a specific inciting organism, it is noted that patients with IBD fail to show tolerance to their own flora.[16]

Intestinal epithelia and inflammatory cells within the lamina propria provide an innate immune defense for the gastrointestinal tract. Failure of tolerance may result from dysfunction at the epithelial border (eg, disrupted mucus layer, defective tight junctions). This dysfunction can activate innate immune cells, causing them to secrete various cytokines and chemokines. Activated antigen-presenting cells (APCs) present these antigens to naïve CD4$^+$ cells in secondary lymphoid organs (eg, Peyer patches), which modulates the differentiation of CD4$^+$ T cell subgroups (eg, T-helper [Th] 1, 2, 17, and T-regulatory [Treg] cells). These CD4$^+$ subgroups then home in on intestinal lamina propria where they exert their effector functions.

Differing populations of CD4$^+$ subgroups are associated with CD, and UC, probably accounting for differences in disease expression. In CD, there is increased Th1 secretion of interferon (IFN)-$\gamma$ and tumor necrosis factor (TNF)-$\alpha$, and Th17 secretion of IL-17. These factors promote intracellular killing, and induce tissue macrophages to release tissue-altering enzymes (eg, matrix metalloproteinases, collagenases). The CD4$^+$ Th17 cells express the IL23R complex, which consists of the IL-23 receptor, and the IL-12 receptor B1. IL-23 is secreted by APCs, and contributes to Th17 cell proliferation and survival. Binding of IL-23 with its receptor complex activates the Janus-associated kinase signal transducers and activators of transcription (JAK2/STAT3) pathway, which regulates transcriptional activation. In UC, there is increased IL-17 along with Th2 secretions of IL-4, IL-5, and IL-13. A different T-cell subset may also be activated producing IL-13 as well as IFN-$\gamma$, resulting in epithelial dysfunction, antibody production, and immune complex formation, which triggers complement activation and mast cell degranulation. In general, intestinal leukocytes are found in high numbers in IBD. A process that contributes to this cellular migration is upregulation of adhesion molecules on vascular endothelium, leading to increased cellular adherence and recruitment.[16,17]

The normal immunologic state of the GI tract is one of suppression. Regulatory cells are responsible for this suppression, and in IBD Treg cells seem to play the major role. Treg1 cells secrete IL-10, a potent immunosuppressive cytokine that may be responsible for suppressing responses to commensal flora. Defects in Tregs may allow for the perpetuation of active inflammation.[16,17]

## CLINICAL PRESENTATION

Clinical symptoms vary depending on the anatomic location and severity of active disease. Both CD and UC may present with abdominal pain, usually chronic and intermittent, associated with diarrhea or irregular bowel movements. Diarrhea is typical with colonic inflammation in CD or UC, but some patients describe "constipation," which may occur in small bowel CD (partial bowel obstruction) or active UC (dyschezia). Hematochezia and tenesmus are more common in UC and may also be associated with perianal CD. Constitutional symptoms, such as mild fever, fatigue, arthralgias, and weight loss, often accompany acute flares of both diseases but are more commonly seen with CD. Oral aphthous ulcers are also more commonly associated with CD but may also be seen with UC; nausea and bloating may accompany either. Extraintestinal manifestations may be seen with or without intestinal symptom flares: skin conditions such as erythema nodosum and pyoderma gangrenosum; ocular diseases such as episcleritis, uveitis, and iritis; and arthropathies such as sacroiliitis and ankylosing spondylitis.

Physical examination is most often normal during periods of disease quiescence, but during flares associated with diarrhea may be remarkable for weight loss; providers must keep in mind, however, that even morbid obesity does not rule out IBD. In fact, in a recent study obesity was predictive of more aggressive disease.[18] Other positive findings on examination may include mild fever, abdominal tenderness, and palpable warmth, most often correlating with the location of inflammation (eg, right lower quadrant with terminal ileitis, left lower quadrant with left-sided colitis). Rebound tenderness and involuntary guarding, while not specific to IBD, herald fulminant disease with suspicion of intestinal perforation. In CD involving the terminal ileum, a right lower quadrant inflammatory mass may be palpable. Rectal examination may reveal perianal tenderness, with abscess, fistula, and/or soft tissue masses in CD. Occult blood-positive stool may be present in both CD and UC regardless of location, but gross hematochezia is most often associated with distal colitis/proctitis. If the patient is anemic, a systolic murmur and conjunctival pallor may be noted. Tachycardia and dry mucus membranes may signify dehydration and fulminant disease; in patients with prolonged or significant diarrhea, peripheral edema may indicate significant malabsorption with hypoalbuminemia.

## DIAGNOSTIC TESTING

Goals of diagnostic testing in IBD include establishing the diagnosis, defining the extent and severity of disease (direct treatment and predict prognosis), monitoring the efficacy of treatment, and preventing complications.

The differential diagnosis of IBD is extensive, and is outlined in **Table 1**. Because IBD manifests a broad spectrum of severity, not all patients present with all symptoms during an acute flare. In general, IBD should be in the differential diagnosis for any patient with abdominal discomfort and altered bowel habits, especially with "red-flag" symptoms such as rectal bleeding and unintentional weight loss. Although tissue biopsy is essential to the diagnosis, no single sign, symptom, or test confirms the presence of IBD with 100% specificity. The diagnosis of IBD is made by consideration of the patient's medical and family history, findings on physical examination, and supportive results on diagnostic testing. To complicate the initial diagnosis as well as confirmation of disease flares, IBD patients may also have concomitant conditions that are part of the differential diagnosis, such as irritable bowel syndrome (IBS), lactose intolerance, or infectious colitis (**Figs. 1–3**).

**Table 1**
**Differential diagnosis of abdominal pain, diarrhea, and rectal bleeding**

| | |
|---|---|
| Infections | Iatrogenic/Inadvertent |
| • Bacterial: *Campylobacter, Salmonella, Shigella, Yersinia, Escherichia coli* 0157:H7, tuberculosis | • NSAID colitis/enteritis |
| | • Radiation proctocolitis |
| | • Antibiotic-associated colitis |
| • Parasitic: *Entamoeba, Giardia, Cryptosporidium, Strongyloides* | • Short bowel syndrome post resection |
| | • Laxative abuse (including herbal supplements such as aloe vera) |
| • Viral: CMV, HSV | • Overconsumption of nonabsorbed sugar |
| • STDs (proctitis): Gonorrhea, Chlamydia, Syphilis | substitutes (eg, sorbitol, xylitol, sucralose) |
| Functional | Diseases of Malabsorption |
| • Irritable bowel syndrome with hemorrhoids, anal fissures | • Pancreatic insufficiency |
| | • Celiac disease |
| • Benign solitary rectal ulcer | • Small intestinal bacterial overgrowth |
| | • Lactose/fructose/sucrose intolerance |
| Inflammatory | Endocrine/Neuroendocrine |
| • Microscopic/lymphocytic/collagenous colitis | • Hyperthyroidism |
| | • Diabetic autonomic neuropathy |
| • Behçet disease | • Hypoadrenalism |
| • Subacute appendicitis | |
| • Subacute diverticulitis | |
| Vascular | Gynecologic |
| • Ischemic colitis | • Colonic endometriosis |
| • Gastrointestinal angiodysplasias | |
| Neoplasia | |
| • Colon cancer | |
| • Anal cancer | |
| • Neuroendocrine tumors (eg, carcinoid) | |
| • Small bowel lymphoma | |
| • Pancreatic cancer | |

*Abbreviations:* CMV, cytomegalovirus; HSV, herpes simplex virus; NSAID, nonsteroidal anti-inflammatory drug; STD, sexually transmitted disease.

## Laboratory Studies

Complete blood count may reveal anemia suggesting iron deficiency (ie, microcytosis with increased red cell distribution width and thrombocytosis) in both CD and UC, or vitamin B12/folic acid deficiency (ie, macrocytosis) in CD.[19] Follow-up iron studies and

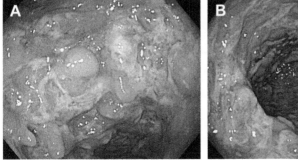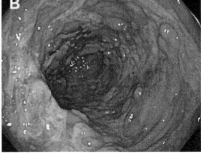

**Fig. 1.** (*A, B*) 38 year old man with Crohn's disease, showing colonic ulcers and pseudopolyposis. (*Courtesy of* K. Trivedi, MD.)

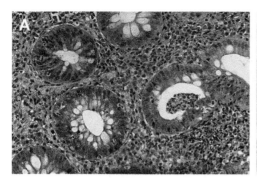
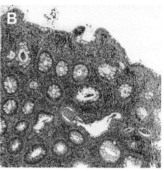

**Fig. 2.** (*A, B*) The photomicrographs are biopsies of a 27 year old woman with Ulcerative Colitis showing chronic inflammation and crypt abscess (light microscopy, hematoxylin and eosin stain, original magnification ×40 and ×400). (*Courtesy of* Benjamin Victor, MD, PhD.)

serum B12/folic acid levels will confirm. Mild leukocytosis is possible during disease flares and in patients on steroids; if significant leukocytosis is seen, infection must be ruled out. Erythrocyte sedimentation rate (ESR) by Westergren method or C-reactive protein (CRP) is used to confirm the presence of an inflammatory process and to monitor the response to treatment, although in some patients symptoms do not

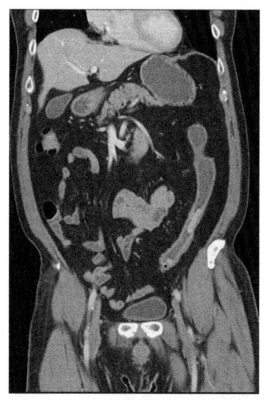

**Fig. 3.** The CT scan is a 30 year old man with Crohn's disease, showing an obstructing inflammatory mass in the descending colon along with the lack of haustra that is classic for IBD. (*Courtesy of* Kay Yan, MD.)

correlate with ESR/CRP levels. It must be noted that patients with active IBD may show a disproportionately elevated cardio-CRP (high-sensitivity CRP), which may falsely elevate their estimated cardiac risk.

Blood chemistries are generally normal but can show elevated liver enzymes if the patient has concomitant biliary disease, as well as low prealbumin/albumin, calcium, and magnesium during periods of malabsorption. If the patient is dehydrated after prolonged diarrhea, elevated blood urea nitrogen and creatinine with or without electrolyte disturbances may also be present.

Stool studies are essential in any patient with chronic diarrhea. Direct smears may reveal red blood cells, white blood cells, and Charcot-Leyden crystals. Recently the fecal lactoferrin test, which indicates the presence of white blood cells, has been used to help distinguish IBD from IBS with a sensitivity of 67%, a specificity of 96%, and a positive predictive value of 87%.[20] It is important to check stool culture for common bacterial pathogens and parasites, as well as *Clostridium difficile* toxin, in patients with diarrhea prior to invasive procedures (ie, colonoscopy) because the presence of infectious colitis increases the risk of procedural complications, namely perforation.

Other tests that may be helpful for differential diagnosis include thyroid stimulating hormone to screen for thyroid disease, tissue transglutaminase plus total IgA level to screen for celiac disease, and lipase with qualitative fecal fat to screen for pancreatic insufficiency (in small bowel CD with malabsorption, fecal fat may be positive).

Once the diagnosis is confirmed, routine blood counts and chemistries are followed to monitor stability, for example, of anemia due to blood loss with flares, and neutropenia, common with many medications used. Ongoing laboratory monitoring in CD, which may impede small bowel absorption, should include iron, ferritin, folic acid, vitamin B12, and calcium. Vitamin D levels should also be checked; low levels of vitamin D are commonly found in patients with CD, and the risk of relapse after attaining remission is higher in patients who remain deficient.[21]

IBD serologic markers (antibodies) may help to differentiate CD from UC and offer prognostic information on disease severity in CD. These markers should not be used to make an initial diagnosis of IBD; a recent study of over 300 pediatric patients determined that one of the proprietary IBD serologic panels (Prometheus) had lower predictive values than routine laboratory tests in making the diagnosis.[22]

Characteristic antibodies present in IBD patients specifically include perinuclear antineutrophil antibody (pANCA) in UC, and anti–*Saccharomyces cerevisiae* antibody (ASCA) in CD. Other antibodies included in the IBD serologic panel include *Escherichia coli* outer membrane porin (OmpC) and flagellin (CBir1). Results are reported as likelihoods for IBD, CD, and UC, which, along with other clinical data, can help to distinguish CD from UC in so-called indeterminant colitis cases. This panel may also be used to predict prognosis; patients who have high ASCA levels are at greater risk of developing fibrostenosing and internal-penetrating disease, and are up to 8 times more likely to undergo surgery within 3 years of diagnosis.[23]

The only genetic test approved for use in clinical care of IBD patients is a baseline thiopurine S-methyltransferase (TPMT) enzyme level drawn prior to prescribing the thiopurine analogues, 6-mercaptopurine (6-MP; Purinethol) and azathioprine (AZA; Imuran). Some patients do not have enzyme levels sufficient to metabolize these drugs and can develop hepatotoxicity; it is considered standard of care to confirm sufficient levels before starting these medications.

Tests for hepatitis B surface antigen and a tuberculin skin test is necessary before initiating therapy with any of the anti-TNF agents, which can reactivate latent infections (see the section Treatment).

### Endoscopy/Biopsy

It is important to remember that the diagnosis of IBD is made by considering the entire clinical and diagnostic picture. A patient suspected of having IBD should undergo both direct mucosal visualization and biopsy of the bowel via endoscopy, though it is not uncommon to encounter "nonspecific" findings on either. Endoscopic appearance of the mucosa is directly proportional to disease severity and predictive of future course; deep ulcers in CD and severe inflammation in UC predicts an increased risk of eventual surgery.[24] Classic "skip" lesions may be noted on endoscopy, suggesting CD over UC; distinct "left-sided disease" only suggests UC over CD. Tissue biopsy helps confirm the chronic nature of the inflammation and the degree of mucosal involvement and may herald classic findings such as granulomas and crypt abscesses. Colonoscopy is the diagnostic test of choice, allowing for complete visualization and biopsy of the entire colon as well as the terminal ileum. Colonoscopy is also utilized to screen for dysplasia and colon cancer, and to monitor for mucosal healing and disease remission after treatment. Patients who are acutely flaring should not undergo colonoscopy if at all avoidable, because of the increased risk of colonic perforation.

Flexible sigmoidoscopy may be performed when symptoms are predominantly anorectal, for partial visualization and tissue biopsy in patients who are unable to tolerate a full colonoscopy bowel preparation, or in patients who have had significant prior colonic resection.

Esophagogastroduodenoscopy may be needed in patients with upper GI symptoms such as nausea, early satiety, and acid reflux; it is also helpful for suspected duodenal/ proximal jejunal disease, and is useful in biopsy for celiac disease, tropical sprue, and parasitic infection.

Wireless capsule endoscopy (WCE) is highly sensitive in detecting small bowel CD and may be indicated in patients with suggestive symptoms or nutritional deficiencies, however, proximal small bowel lesions are present in only 5% of patients with CD. To reduce the risk of capsule retention (3%),[25] small bowel radiography is recommended prior to performance to rule out obvious strictures. Double balloon, or "push" enteroscopy, typically performed only at tertiary centers, is used for interventional small bowel procedures, for example, to biopsy mucosal abnormalities found on WCE.

### Imaging

Small bowel series (radiography) is helpful in screening for obvious small bowel involvement (inflammation, stricture) in a patient with colonoscopic findings consistent with CD; it is also useful pre-WCE, as already mentioned. Computed tomography (CT) of the abdomen and pelvis, which should always be ordered with contrast unless contraindicated, is helpful in localizing the inflammation, ruling out other inflammatory processes such as appendicitis and diverticulitis, and looking for abscess, fistula, or mass lesion. CT or magnetic resonance (MR) enterography provides clearer visualization of the small bowel and is sometimes recommended in patients with CD to evaluate the extent of their disease, as well as in UC patients considering colectomy, to help rule out any possibility of small bowel disease (which may indicate an actual diagnosis of CD and preclude colectomy). Aside from the avoidance of radiation exposure, an additional benefit of MR over CT is the ability to distinguish inflammatory from fibrotic strictures, helping to determine whether surgical treatment (fibrotic) as opposed to aggressive medical therapy (inflammatory) is indicated.[26] Finally, ultrasonography may be helpful in ruling out appendicitis, ovarian cysts, and ectopic pregnancy.

## TREATMENT

Over the past 50 years, an increasing number of therapies have become available for the treatment of IBD. Current management of IBD is dependent on 3 main approaches: lifestyle modifications, medical therapy, and surgery.

### Lifestyle Modifications

Smoking has been shown to be a risk factor for developing CD, unlike its protective effect for UC. A meta-analysis by Mahid and colleagues[8] suggested that ongoing smoking transferred a 42% risk reduction for having UC and that smoking was associated with having a 61% increased risk of having CD (OR 1.61). Despite several theories, it is not clear why smoking affects UC and CD differently.[27] Diet as a cause or as a treatment of IBD is a controversial topic; evidence for a causative role of diet in the development of IBD is mixed and fraught with methodological limitations.[28] Some data suggest that a diet high in sugars, fat, and meat intake may increase the risk of IBD. In some small studies, increased consumption of sweets has been associated with developing UC, whereas increased consumption of fats was associated with an increased risk of developing CD.[29] With regard to treatment, a low-residue diet is routinely recommended during acute flares to help minimize diarrhea. There may be a role for enteral nutrition in the maintenance of adult CD, but studies suggesting this were small.[30] Omega-3 fatty acids have also been studied in the treatment of CD, due to their anti-inflammatory properties, but a recent Cochrane review on the subject did not reveal any convincing evidence to routinely recommend their use.[31] Lactose intolerance is a very common cause of gastrointestinal symptoms in the general population, and is even more common in patients with IBD. One study reported a prevalence in CD of 40%, compared with 29.2% in controls considered "low ethnic risk" for lactose malabsorption.[32] It is reasonable to recommend a lactose-free diet during flares symptomatic of diarrhea and bloating.

### Medical Therapy

Medical treatment of IBD is a rapidly evolving field, especially with the introduction of biological agents. Major goals of therapy are the control of symptoms, induction of remission, healing of endoscopic lesions, and prevention of complications.

5-aminosalicylates (5-ASA) are considered to be the first-line treatment for the induction of remission and long-term maintenance therapy in UC. The many oral forms of 5-ASA are prodrugs that are converted into their active form based on pH, the presence of colonic flora, and time (**Table 2**).[33] Inducing remission in mild UC requires lower doses of oral 5-ASA than in moderate disease (mesalamine equivalent of 2.4 g/d for mild disease, 4.8 g/d for moderate disease). The oral 5-ASA formulations achieve similar remission rates, although sulfasalazine, the least expensive agent in this class, is also the least tolerable, due to its sulfa moiety.[34] Although it is believed that the different 5-ASA formulations perform similarly for maintaining remission, a Cochrane systematic review reveals that sulfasalazine may be superior than newer formulations.[35] Topical 5-ASA therapies such as mesalamine enemas (Rowasa) and suppositories (Canasa) are not only helpful in the treatment of acute left-sided UC, but combination therapy with oral 5-ASAs can induce remission better than oral therapy alone.[36] At present, despite common practice, there is no strong evidence to support the use of 5-ASAs in the induction or maintenance of remission in CD; their effective role is limited to newly diagnosed patients with mild colonic disease.[37]

Although the newer 5-ASAs are well tolerated, there are several possible 5-ASA side effects. Sulfasalazine has been associated with headaches, nausea, rashes, and

**Table 2**
**Oral 5-aminosalicylate formulations**

| Drug | Brand Name, Unit Strength | Delivery Target |
|------|---------------------------|-----------------|
| Mesalamine | Asacol, 400 mg | Colon, terminal ileum |
| Mesalamine | Asacol HD, 800 mg | Colon, terminal ileum |
| Mesalamine | Lialda, 1200 mg | Colon, terminal ileum |
| Mesalamine | Apriso, 0.375 mg | Colon, terminal ileum |
| Mesalamine | Pentasa, 250, 500, 1000 mg | Colon, ileum, duodenum |
| Olsalazine | Dipentum, 250 mg | Colon |
| Sulfasalazine | Azulfidine, 500 mg | Colon |
| Sulfasalazine | Azulfidine EN-tabs, 500 mg | Colon |
| Balsalazide | Colazal, 750 mg | Colon |

*Data from* Hou JK, El-Serag H, Thirumurthi S. Distribution and manifestations of inflammatory bowel disease in Asians, Hispanics, and African Americans: a systematic review. Am J Gastroenterol 2009;104(8):2100–9.

reversible infertility in men. Sulfasalazine can also impair folate absorption, thus folic acid supplementation is necessary when prescribing this medication. Other 5-ASA products may cause headache, diarrhea, and malaise. Less common side effects include pancreatitis, pneumonitis, pericarditis, worsening of colitis, diarrhea, interstitial nephritis, proteinuria, and thrombocytopenia.

Corticosteroids are used in induction of remission in patients with moderate to severe UC who have failed first-line 5-ASA therapy. These agents are also used for induction of remission in CD. Topical corticosteroid therapy in the form of enemas (eg, Cortenema), foams (eg, Proctofoam), and suppositories (eg, Proctocort) has been shown to be inferior to topical 5-ASA agents in the management of active UC, but the combination may be more effective than either alone. Evidence suggests that steroids are associated with higher rates of infection and poorer longer-term IBD outcomes. In addition, the known adverse effects of steroids, namely weight gain, impaired glucose tolerance, mood swings, insomnia, osteoporosis, and adrenal suppression, make them inappropriate to use for long-term maintenance. Thus steroid use should be minimized by providing patient education to improve compliance with maintenance medications. When used for flares, steroids should be managed by providers experienced in treating IBD. Approximately one-third of UC patients will require corticosteroid therapy at some point during their disease course.[38] If a patient has moderately active UC, oral prednisone therapy at 20 to 40 mg/d with a slow taper over several weeks can be effective. If the patient fails oral therapy and/or has severe disease, then hospital admission for intravenous corticosteroids (ie, methylprednisolone 40–60 mg/d) may be warranted. Provided that other infections such as *C difficile* and cytomegalovirus (CMV) are ruled out, it is generally accepted that failure of medical therapy is defined as lack of improvement after 7 to 10 days of intravenous corticosteroids; this is an indication for proctocolectomy.[39]

Unlike mild to moderate UC, there is a role for oral corticosteroids in mild to moderate CD. Budesonide (Entocort), an oral glucocorticoid derivative of which only 10% to 15% is systemically delivered because of extensive first-pass metabolism, is effective in inducing remission in ileocolonic CD at a dose of 9 mg/d, but is not effective in maintaining CD remission at lower doses.[40]

Immunomodulators comprise two general classes: thiopurine derivatives and methotrexate (MTX). Thiopurines come in two formulations: 6-MP (Purinethol) and AZA (Imuran), which is converted into 6-MP by nonenzymatic means. Thiopurines have been shown to maintain remission of mild to moderate CD. These agents are conventionally used in steroid-dependent and/or 5-ASA refractory UC, though the data for this indication are conflicting. The dosing is typically 1 to 1.5 mg/kg/d for 6-MP and 2 to 2.5 mg/kg/d for AZA. Thiopurines can take 12 to 16 weeks to begin having a clinical effect, thus they are often paired with corticosteroids, 5-ASAs, or biological medications (see later discussion) to maintain remission until the thiopurine becomes active. Given the lag between initiating thiopurine therapy and seeing clinical results, thiopurines are not routinely effective for the induction of remission in IBD.

Adverse effects of immunomodulators include bone marrow suppression (neutropenia), hepatotoxicity (transaminitis), and pancreatitis. These effects are usually asymptomatic and are discovered by diligent laboratory monitoring; they are reversed by reducing the dose or, if necessary, withdrawing the drug. Treatment with thiopurines can predispose to the development of opportunistic infections such as CMV, disseminated varicella virus, and herpes simplex virus, among others. Thiopurines also increase the baseline lymphoma risk in IBD, which is already elevated compared with non-IBD patients, from 1.9 per 10,000 to 4 per 10,000.[41]

Approximately 1 out of 300 individuals lack the activity of TPMT, an important enzyme in thiopurine metabolism. Thiopurine administration to these individuals can lead to severe bone marrow suppression and agranulocytosis. Thus, it is the standard of care to check baseline TPMT levels before initiating therapy. Moreover, complete blood counts and liver enzymes should be obtained every 1 to 3 months while on therapy to monitor for bone marrow suppression and hepatotoxicity.

MTX is a steroid-sparing immunomodulator which is effective in the induction and maintenance of remission of CD. MTX does not have a role in the treatment of UC. MTX has several side effects, including nausea, vomiting, leukopenia, hepatic fibrosis and, rarely, hypersensitivity pneumonitis.[38] MTX is usually delivered parenterally either by weekly intramuscular or subcutaneous injection, though some IBD experts give MTX orally.

Biological agents used in the treatment of IBD are targeted against cytokines involved in the inflammatory cascade (see the section Pathophysiology). The two main targets have thus far been TNF and adhesion proteins for inflammatory cell translocation.

Three anti-TNF medications, infliximab, adalimumab, and certolizumab, have been approved for treatment of IBD. Prior to initiation of anti-TNF therapy, patients need to be screened for latent tuberculosis infection, hepatitis B and C, human immunodeficiency virus, and, depending on the patient's exposure risk, coccidiomycosis and histoplasmosis.

Infliximab (Remicade) is a chimeric (human-mouse) monoclonal antibody against tumor necrosis factor; it was the first anti-TNF approved for the induction and maintenance of remission in refractory and fistulizing CD, and for the induction and maintenance of remission in severe UC. Infliximab is also indicated for the treatment of extraintestinal manifestations of IBD, including ankylosing spondylitis, pyoderma gangrenosum, and chronic uveitis.[42] Patients starting treatment begin with an induction dose of 5 mg/kg intravenously at weeks 0, 2, and 6, with maintenance infusions every 8 weeks. In partial responders, the dose can be increased to 10 mg/kg. The development of human antibodies to infliximab (human antichimeric antibodies) is thought to be the mechanism behind loss of response.

Adalimumab (Humira) is a human monoclonal anti-TNF IgG1, self-administered subcutaneously every 2 weeks. It is approved for induction and maintenance of remission in CD but does not currently have approval from the Food and Drug Administration for treatment of UC. Commercially available assays to measure antibody levels are not available.

Certolizumab pegol (Cimzia) is a pegylated human Fab fragment that binds TNF. It is indicated for the induction and maintenance of remission in moderate to severe CD, and is administered every 4 weeks by subcutaneous injection.

Natalizumab (Tysabri) is a recent addition to the biological armamentarium for treating IBD. It is an inhibitor of the α4 ligand that prevents leukocyte translocation. Natalizumab was initially introduced for the treatment of multiple sclerosis, but is now an agent that has been approved to treat CD refractory to anti-TNF therapy.[42] Natalizumab use has been associated with progressive multifocal leukoencephalopathy, a rare demyelinating disease caused by the JC virus (formerly known as papovavirus).

Anti-TNF therapy increases the risk of infection. Anti-TNF agents are often paired with other immunosuppressive medications such as steroids and thiopurine derivatives, which confers an additive infection risk. In addition to systemic infection, other possible side effects include infusion or injection site reactions, serum sickness, lupus-like reactions, formation of antinuclear and anti–double-stranded DNA antibodies, demyelinating neuropathy, and congestive heart failure. Anti-TNF therapy can also increase the risk of developing non-Hodgkin lymphoma, which is further increased with concurrent anti-TNF and thiopurine therapy.[43] Another serious risk is hepatosplenic T-cell lymphoma, a rare but universally fatal disease, which has been associated with concomitant anti-TNF and thiopurine use in young men with IBD (18 cases from 1998 to 2008) and with thiopurine use alone (10 cases).[44] Unfortunately, studies suggest that only approximately one-third of patients who start anti-TNF therapy for IBD are in clinical or endoscopic remission after 1 year.[38] There has not yet been a head-to-head study comparing the aforementioned anti-TNF agents in the treatment of IBD.

Cyclosporine is a calcineurin inhibitor that inhibits T-cell signaling pathways. Although it is commonly used in posttransplant patients, there appears to be role for cyclosporine in the treatment of severe, steroid-refractory UC patients who face impending colectomy. Intravenous cyclosporine can induce remission in approximately 80% of these patients, who can then be transitioned to oral cyclosporine, along with corticosteroids and a maintenance agent, usually 6-MP or AZA. Despite this therapy, approximately 60% of cyclosporine-treated UC patients will need total proctocolectomy after 1 year.[38] Side effects of cyclosporine include hypertension, seizures, and nephrotoxicity. Because cyclosporine treatment in UC is usually combined with corticosteroids and 6-MP or AZA, these patients are at a high risk of infection, especially Pneumocystis jiroveci (formerly carinii), thus prophylaxis is required. Cyclosporine treatment is best reserved for tertiary care centers. There is no role for cyclosporine in the treatment of CD.

Antibiotics are used in the treatment of perianal disease and fistulas in CD and in the treatment of C difficile infection in IBD. There is limited evidence to suggest that antibiotics against anaerobic bacteria (ie, metronidazole) may have a role as bridging therapy to thiopurines in a subset of the CD population.[45] In addition to commonly known antibiotic side effects, chronic antibiotic use can predispose to C difficile infection in a patient population that already has increased susceptibility. Given all these factors and the lack of strong clinical evidence, there is no current role for the routine use of antibiotics as maintenance therapy in CD or UC.

Probiotics are live microbes (bacteria and yeast) that are consumed for their beneficial effect on the host. Despite the current popularity of probiotics as a supplement, there is a paucity of evidence to support routine use of probiotics in IBD.[45] Small trials have demonstrated the efficacy of the probiotic formulation VSL#3 (which contains 3 species of *Bifidobacterium*, 4 species of *Lactobacillus*, and *Streptococcus salvarius*) in the prevention and treatment of pouchitis. A European consensus statement suggests that the bacterium *E coli* Nissl 1917 could be used as an alternative to mesalamine in UC treatment.[46] Further controlled studies are needed to evaluate the role probiotics may have in managing IBD. Although they may be beneficial in preventing *C difficile* colitis and appear to be safe in most patients, fatal cases of fungemia have been reported with the use of *Saccharomyces* supplements in immunocompromised patients.[47]

Alternative therapies abound in the treatment of chronic diseases, and IBD is no exception. Both off-label medical and CAM (Complementary and Alternative) therapies may be used, the details of which are beyond the scope of this review. Examples of medical therapies include tacrolimus, thalidomide, leukopheresis, and helminth therapy. CAM therapies, such as herbs and dietary supplements, have at best limited evidence for their use. Some patients report benefits beyond symptom control, but it is important to remember that some of these therapies can cause significant harm (eg, daily use of turmeric capsules leading to the development of peptic ulcer disease). Because IBD is a lifelong disease with flares that may take many weeks to resolve, patients may feel compelled to try alternative remedies that promise a "cure" and thus increase their sense of control over their disease. The support of an empathetic primary care provider teamed with an experienced gastroenterologist offers the best chance of long-term remission and prevention of complications.

### Surgical and Endoscopic Management

Approximately 25% to 35% of UC patients will require surgery for their disease, typically total proctocolectomy.[48] Indications are severe, fulminant, steroid-refractory disease, the presence of dysplasia on targeted or random biopsies, and the detection of colorectal cancer. The most common surgical intervention for UC patients is total proctocolectomy with either an end-ileostomy or with an ileal-pouch anal anastomosis (IPAA). IPAAs are usually created as part of a 2-stage or 3-stage surgical procedure. Although this procedure avoids the need for an ileostomy and preserves continence, patients with an IPAA can expect to have a median of 6 bowel movements per day with 1 to 2 nocturnal bowel movements. Between 20% and 40% of patients who undergo an IPAA will suffer from inflammation of the ileal pouch, termed pouchitis, at some point during their disease course. This condition can usually be managed by antibiotics (oral and intrapouch) and probiotics. Five-year pouch failure rates are about 8%.[48]

Approximately 80% of CD patients undergo surgery at some point during their disease course. As CD can affect the entire gastrointestinal tract, a variety of surgical approaches may be employed. Intestinal obstruction caused by small bowel strictures is a complication of transmural inflammation. If medical therapy fails to improve obstructive symptoms, segmental resection is required. Unfortunately, CD tends to recur at the site of surgery, so repeat surgeries are often needed.

Surgical intervention is also often required for the management of fistulas, which can involve the bowel and any other visceral organ. The most common fistula is an enteroenteric fistula, which may be asymptomatic depending on the amount of bowel bypassed by the fistulous tract. Other common fistulas requiring surgical management include enterocutaneous, enterovesicular, and in women, enterovaginal fistula. In addition to the risk of a need for repeat surgeries, resection can also lead to short-gut syndrome and malabsorption, depending on the segment and length of bowel removed.

Abscesses (intra-abdominal, perirectal) are common, affecting approximately one-quarter of those with CD.[48] Very small abscesses of less than 1 cm can be managed with antibiotics, but larger ones require surgical evaluation and drainage.

Perianal disease is one of the most difficult aspects of CD to treat; these patients tend to have more aggressive disease overall. In addition to treatment with anti-TNF agents (primarily infliximab), 6-MP or AZA, and antibiotics, surgical management may be required. This procedure could include rectal/perianal examination under anesthesia to explore and expose fistulous tracts, with seton placement to keep fistulas open to be drained while the patient is undergoing medical treatment.

Prevention of postoperative CD recurrence is an important goal in management. Evidence suggests that disease severity prior to surgery is a predictor of recurrence. High-risk postsurgical patients may need to start or continue anti-TNF or immunomodulator therapy. In others, endoscopic or radiographic visualization of the surgical anastomosis 3 to 6 months after surgery may help determine whether to recommence medical treatment.

### Health Maintenance

There are several health maintenance considerations about which primary care providers should be aware when it comes to the ongoing care of IBD patients.

#### Osteopenia and osteoporosis

IBD patients are at risk of osteopenia and osteoporosis, with some studies estimating a prevalence as high as 70%.[49] This risk is attributable to several mechanisms, including antecedent corticosteroid use, vitamin D and calcium malabsorption, and the osteoporotic consequences of chronic inflammation. Current guidelines from the American Gastroenterological Association (AGA) recommend that the following high-risk IBD patients should be screened for osteoporosis: those with a history of vertebral fractures, postmenopausal females, males older than 50 years, those on chronic corticosteroid therapy, or those with hypogonadism.[50] Patients with evidence of osteopenia should be checked for vitamin D deficiency and treated accordingly (800 IU daily for vitamin D insufficiency; 50,000 IU weekly for 8 weeks then 800–1000 IU daily for deficiency). Patients with osteoporosis should begin treatment with a bisphosphonate and calcium supplementation.

#### Nutritional deficiency

Patients with IBD often have iron deficiency due to blood loss and chronic inflammation; iron studies (including percent iron saturation) should be checked and repleted. Folate and vitamin B12 levels are also important to assess, especially in patients with anemia. Sulfasalazine impairs folate absorption, thus patients on this drug should receive daily supplementation. Patients with ileocolonic or gastric CD may also suffer from vitamin B12 deficiency; serum levels should be checked and appropriate supplementation given. Lastly, patients with active IBD may be malnourished; increasing caloric intake and consultation with a registered dietitian may be helpful.

#### Colorectal cancer screening

The cumulative probability for developing colorectal cancer (CRC) in UC has been estimated to be as high as 8% at 20 years and 18% at 30 years,[51] but newer evidence suggests the that the number may be lower, at less than 0.2% per year. In Crohn colitis, there is a fourfold increase in CRC risk compared with the general population. There is some evidence to suggest that surveillance colonoscopy may lead to earlier detection of CRC and detection of CRC at earlier stages, but this may be due to lead-time bias.[52] Although there are no large trials that demonstrate a survival benefit from increased surveillance in IBD, indirect evidence of benefit has led the major gastroenterological societies to recommend regular annual surveillance with colonoscopy in those who have had pancolonic UC and Crohn colitis for 8 or more years. In those with left-sided IBD (disease distal to the splenic flexure), annual CRC screening with colonoscopy should begin 10 to 15 years after initial diagnosis. The role of chemoprevention of CRC in patients with IBD is controversial; emerging evidence suggests that 5-ASAs may have a role in decreasing the risk of CRC in UC, but further studies are needed.

### Vaccinations

IBD patients are often on immunosuppressive medications and thus are at higher risk for infection. Unfortunately, a sizable percentage of IBD patients have not been immunized against vaccine-preventable infections.[53] IBD patients should routinely be vaccinated for the following if they are not yet immune: hepatitis A, hepatitis B, influenza, tetanus, streptococcal pneumonia (*Pneumococcus*), diphtheria, pertussis, and varicella. *Meningococcus* and human papilloma virus vaccines should be administered to target populations (adolescents and young women, respectively). It is important to administer vaccinations prior to the administration of immunomodulators, anti-TNF therapy, or steroids, because of the decreased immune response while on these agents, although it has been found that the QuantiFERON TB test is not affected by immunomodulator therapy.[54]

### Pregnancy, fertility, and women's health

Fertility is decreased for both men and women with IBD. In men, ongoing therapy with immunomodulators (MTX, 6-MP) decreases fertility rates. This situation is reversible with cessation of therapy. For women, fertility is decreased with ongoing MTX therapy and in those with a history of pelvic surgery. Women attempting to get pregnant should not be on MTX, as it is an abortifacient and teratogen; two types of birth control should be used by any woman of reproductive age on this medication. Annual gynecologic examinations are especially important in women with IBD, as they are at increased risk for cervical cancer.

Women with IBD tend to improve clinically during pregnancy; however, CD increases the risk for preterm birth.[55] It is important to maintain a supportive and openly communicative physician-patient relationship with IBD patients who are contemplating pregnancy. Continued use of other agents during pregnancy, particularly the immunomodulators, is controversial; though they are category C, it is generally agreed that the benefit of continued use in patients who are well controlled on their current regimen outweighs the risk of disease flare on discontinuation. Individualized planning and close coordination of care between the patient's primary provider, a high-risk obstetrician, and an expert gastroenterologist is imperative for a successful pregnancy and healthy delivery.

### SUMMARY

IBD is a chronic disease with a substantial impact on quality of life. The care of IBD is challenging as the diagnosis is often delayed, and there are a multitude of treatment options to consider. Many of the medications for CD and UC are immunosuppressive, thus vigilant follow-up and laboratory monitoring is required to prevent and/or minimize complications. The severity and progression of disease is variable, most often manifesting a relapsing/remitting pattern over the patient's life span, and may require both medical and surgical intervention. There are important health maintenance considerations for these patients, including the provision of vaccinations and screening for osteoporosis, colon cancer, and vitamin deficiencies. Patient education and close coordination between primary care providers and consultants is critical in achieving positive outcomes in these often complicated patients.

---

**Key Points for Primary Care**

*Morbidity/mortality and overall health care costs in IBD can be reduced by primary care providers who offer:*

- Timely consideration of IBD in the differential diagnosis with early referral to a gastroenterologist experienced in managing this disease

- Patient education[a] on prognosis and the importance of long-term compliance with medications, labs, and follow-up visits

- Continuity of care and psychosocial support while coordinating essential multidisciplinary care and referrals

- Diligent adherence to health maintenance guidelines, particularly nutritional status and high-risk colon cancer screening

[a] For more information, contact and refer patients to the Crohn's and Colitis Foundation of America (CCFA) at www.ccfa.org.

---

## REFERENCES

1. Loftus EV. Clinical epidemiology of inflammatory bowel disease: incidence, prevalence, and environmental influences. Gastroenterology 2004;126(6):1504–17.
2. U.S. Census Bureau. U.S. POPClock projection. Available at: http://www.census.gov/population/www/popclockus.html. Accessed June 15, 2010.
3. Statistics Canada. Canada's population clock. Available at: http://www.statcan.gc.ca/pub/82-003-x/pop/pop-h-clock-eng.htm. Accessed June 15, 2010.
4. Hou JK, El-Serag H, Thirumurthi S. Distribution and manifestations of inflammatory bowel disease in Asians, Hispanics, and African Americans: a systematic review. Am J Gastroenterol 2009;104(8):2100–9.
5. Lynch HT, Brand RE, Locker GY. Inflammatory bowel disease in Ashkenazi Jews: implications for familial colorectal cancer. Fam Cancer 2004;3(3–4):229–32.
6. Kappelman MD, Rifas-Shiman SL, Kleinman K, et al. The prevalence and geographic distribution of Crohn's disease and ulcerative colitis in the United States. Clin Gastroenterol Hepatol 2007;5(12):1424–9.
7. Sonnenberg A, McCarty DJ, Jacobsen SJ. Geographic variation of inflammatory bowel disease within the United States. Gastroenterology 1991;100(1):143–9.
8. Mahid SS, Minor KS, Soto RE, et al. Smoking and inflammatory bowel disease: a meta-analysis. Mayo Clin Proc 2006;81(11):1462–71.
9. Klement E, Cohen RV, Boxman J, et al. Breastfeeding and risk of inflammatory bowel disease: a systematic review with meta-analysis. Am J Clin Nutr 2004; 80(5):1342–52.
10. Andersson RE, Olaison G, Tysk C, et al. Appendectomy and protection against ulcerative colitis. N Engl J Med 2001;344(11):808–14.
11. Cornish JA, Tan E, Simillis C, et al. The risk of oral contraceptives in the etiology of inflammatory bowel disease: a meta-analysis. Am J Gastroenterol 2008;103(9): 2394–400.
12. Guslandi M. Exacerbation of inflammatory bowel disease by nonsteroidal anti-inflammatory drugs and cyclooxygenase-2 inhibitors: fact or fiction? World J Gastroenterol 2006;12(10):1509–10.
13. Kurina LM, Goldacre MJ, Yeates D, et al. Depression and anxiety in people with inflammatory bowel disease. J Epidemiol Community Health 2001;55(10):716–20.
14. Orholm M, Binder V, Sørensen TIA, et al. Concordance of inflammatory bowel disease among Danish twins. Scand J Gastroenterol 2000;35(10):1075–81.

15. Hakonarson H, Grant SFA. Genome-wide association studies in type 1 diabetes, inflammatory bowel disease and other immune-mediated disorders. Semin Immunol 2009;21(6):355–62.
16. Mayer L. Evolving paradigms in the pathogenesis of IBD. J Gastroenterol 2010; 45(1):9.
17. Abraham C, Cho JH. Mechanisms of disease: inflammatory bowel disease. N Engl J Med 2009;361(21):2066–78.
18. Louis E, Belaiche J, Reenaers C. Do clinical factors help to predict disease course in inflammatory bowel disease? World J Gastroenterol 2010;16(21):2600–3.
19. Yakut M, Ustun Y, Kabacam G, et al. Serum vitamin B12 and folate status in patients with inflammatory bowel disease. Eur J Intern Med 2010;21:320–3.
20. Sidhu R, Wilson P, Wright A, et al. Faecal lactoferrin, a novel test to differentiate between the irritable and inflamed bowel? Aliment Pharmacol Ther 2010;31:1365–70.
21. Jorgensen SP, Agnholt J, Glerup H, et al. Clinical trial: vitamin D3 treatment in Crohn's disease—a randomized double-blind placebo controlled study. Aliment Pharmacol Ther 2010;32:377–83.
22. Benor S, Russell G, Silver M, et al. Shortcomings of the inflammatory bowel disease serology 7 panel. Pediatrics 2010;125(6):1230–6.
23. Dubinsky M. Serologic and laboratory markers in prediction of the disease course in inflammatory bowel disease. World J Gastroenterol 2010;16(21):2604–8.
24. Allez M, Lemann M. Role of endoscopy in predicting the disease course in inflammatory bowel disease. World J Gastroenterol 2010;16:2626–32.
25. Petruzziello C, Onali S, Calabrese E, et al. Wireless capsule endoscopy and proximal small bowel lesions in Crohn's disease. World J Gastroenterol 2010; 16:3299–304.
26. Messaris E, Nikolaos C, Grand D, et al. Role of magnetic resonance enterography in the management of Crohn's disease. Arch Surg 2010;145:471–5.
27. Colombel JF, Watson AJ, Neurath MF. The 10 remaining mysteries of inflammatory bowel disease. Gut 2008;57:429–33.
28. Yamamoto T, Nakahigashi M, Saniabadi AR. Review article: diet and inflammatory bowel disease–epidemiology and treatment. Aliment Pharmacol Ther 2009;30: 99–112.
29. Sakamoto N, Kono S, Wakai K, et al. Dietary risk factors for inflammatory bowel disease: a multicenter case-control study in Japan. Inflamm Bowel Dis 2005;11: 154–63.
30. Akobeng AK, Thomas AG. Enteral nutrition for maintenance of remission in Crohn's disease. Cochrane Database Syst Rev 2007;3:CD005984. Accessed July 31, 2010.
31. Turner D, Zlotkin SH, Shah PS, et al. Omega 3 fatty acids (fish oil) for maintenance of remission in Crohn's disease. Cochrane Database Syst Rev 2009;1:CD006320. Accessed July 31, 2010.
32. Goh J, O'Morain CA. Review article: nutrition and inflammatory bowel disease. Aliment Pharmacol Ther 2003;17:307–20.
33. Baumgart DC, Sandborn WJ. Inflammatory bowel disease: clinical aspects and established and evolving therapies. Lancet 2007;369:1641–57.
34. Sutherland L, Macdonald JK. Oral 5-aminosalicylic acid for induction of remission in ulcerative colitis. Cochrane Database Syst Rev 2006;2:CD000543. Accessed July 31, 2010.
35. Sutherland L, Macdonald JK. Oral 5-aminosalicylic acid for maintenance of remission in ulcerative colitis. Cochrane Database Syst Rev 2006;2:CD000544. Accessed July 31, 2010.

36. Bergman R, Parkes M. Systematic review: the use of mesalazine in inflammatory bowel disease. Aliment Pharmacol Ther 2006;23:841–55.

37. Sparrow M, Irving P, Baidoo L, et al. Current controversies in Crohn's disease: a roundtable discussion of the BRIDGe Group. Gastroenterol Hepatol 2008;4: 713–20.

38. Lichtenstein GR, Abreu MT, Cohen R, et al. American gastroenterological association institute technical review on corticosteroids, immunomodulators, and infliximab in inflammatory bowel disease. Gastroenterology 2006;130:940–87.

39. Roses RE, Rombeau JL. Recent trends in the surgical management of inflammatory bowel disease. World J Gastroenterol 2008;14:408–12.

40. Benchimol EI, Seow CH, Otley AR, et al. Budesonide for maintenance of remission in Crohn's disease. Cochrane Database Syst Rev 2009;1:CD002913. Accessed July 31, 2010.

41. D'Haens G, Rutgeerts P. Immunosuppression-associated lymphoma in IBD. Lancet 2009;374:1572–3.

42. Rutgeerts P, Vermeire S, Van Assche G. Biological therapies for inflammatory bowel diseases. Gastroenterology 2009;136:1182–97.

43. Lakatos PL, Miheller P. Is there an increased risk of lymphoma and malignancies under anti-TNF therapy in IBD? Curr Drug Targets 2010;11:179–86.

44. Mackey AC, Green L, Leptak C, et al. Hepatosplenic T cell lymphoma associated with infliximab use in young patients treated for inflammatory bowel disease: update. J Pediatr Gastroenterol Nutr 2009;48:386–8.

45. Prantera C, Scribano ML. Antibiotics and probiotics in inflammatory bowel disease: why, when, and how. Curr Opin Gastroenterol 2009;25:329–33.

46. Travis SP, Stange EF, Lemann M, et al. European evidence based consensus on the diagnosis and management of Crohn's disease: current management. Gut 2006;55(Suppl 1):i16–35.

47. Herbrecht R, Nivoix Y. *Saccharomyces cerevisiae* fungemia: an adverse effect of *Saccharomyces boulardii* probiotic administration. Clin Infect Dis 2005;40: 1635–7.

48. Hwang JM, Varma MG. Surgery for inflammatory bowel disease. World J Gastroenterol 2008;14:2678–90.

49. Ali T, Lam D, Bronze MS, et al. Osteoporosis in inflammatory bowel disease. Am J Med 2009;122:599–604.

50. Bernstein CN, Leslie WD, Leboff MS. AGA technical review on osteoporosis in gastrointestinal diseases. Gastroenterology 2003;124:795–841.

51. Eaden JA, Abrams KR, Mayberry JF. The risk of colorectal cancer in ulcerative colitis: a meta-analysis. Gut 2001;48:526–35.

52. Mpofu C, Watson AJ, Rhodes JM. Strategies for detecting colon cancer and/or dysplasia in patients with inflammatory bowel disease. Cochrane Database Syst Rev 2004;2:CD000279. Accessed July 31, 2010.

53. Melmed GY, Ippoliti AF, Papadakis KA, et al. Patients with inflammatory bowel disease are at risk for vaccine-preventable illnesses. Am J Gastroenterol 2006; 101:1834–40.

54. Qumseya B, Ananthakrishnan A, Skaros S, et al. QuantiFERON TB gold testing for tuberculosis screening in an inflammatory bowel disease cohort in the United States. Inflamm Bowel Dis 2011;17(1):77–83.

55. Stephansson O, Larsson H, Pederson L, et al. Crohn's disease is a risk factor for preterm birth. Clin Gastroenterol Hepatol 2010;8(6):509–15.

# Irritable Bowel Syndrome

Michael A. Malone, MD

**KEYWORDS**

- Irritable bowel syndrome • Gastrointestinal disorder
- Constipation • Diarrhea

Irritable bowel syndrome (IBS) is a common gastrointestinal disorder that leads to crampy pain, gassiness, bloating, and changes in bowel habits in the absence of any currently identifiable organic disorder. Patients with IBS may be classified by their predominant bowel habit: diarrhea-predominant, constipation-predominant, or IBS with alternating bowel movements.[1]

IBS may also be referred to as a "spastic" or "nervous colon" because it is often associated with stress or anxiety. Although IBS can be frustrating and concerning to patients with this disorder, it does not cause permanent harm to the intestines and does not lead to a serious disease such as cancer. Although treatments exist for its symptoms, there is no known cure.[2]

## EPIDEMIOLOGY

IBS is the most commonly diagnosed gastrointestinal condition and these patients are commonly seen by physicians. For gastrointestinal symptoms or other concerns, patients with IBS have a tendency to visit physicians more frequently than those without IBS.[3] Even though fewer than 20% of patients with IBS actually seek medical treatment, IBS in its various forms constitutes 25% to 50% of all referrals to gastroenterologists[4] IBS also accounts for the second highest cause of work absenteeism after the common cold.[5] The estimated costs related to IBS are as high as $30 billion per year.[6]

The prevalence of IBS in North America, as estimated from population-based studies, is approximately 10% to 20%.[7–12] Studies in Europe have found a similar prevalence of 11.5%.[13] IBS affects men and women, young patients, and elderly people; however, younger patients and women are more likely to be diagnosed. Multiple studies have estimated that there is an overall 2:1 female predominance in North America.[9,14,15]

Risk factors for IBS include a family history of first-degree relatives with IBS, a history of sexual abuse, and a diagnosis of anxiety or depression.[16–20] Although not all

Department of Family Medicine, Penn State College of Medicine, 845 Fishburn Road, Hershey, PA 17033, USA
E-mail address: mmalone@hmc.psu.edu

Prim Care Clin Office Pract 38 (2011) 433–447
doi:10.1016/j.pop.2011.05.003 **primarycare.theclinics.com**
0095-4543/11/$ – see front matter © 2011 Elsevier Inc. All rights reserved.

patients with IBS have a mood or anxiety disorder, a population study of patients with IBS showed that approximately half of these patients had a lifetime prevalence of a mood or anxiety disorder.[21]

## PHYSIOLOGY AND PATHOPHYSIOLOGY

The pathophysiology of IBS remains uncertain, although the cause may differ between individuals with similar symptoms. Although no specific physiologic process is unique to or characterizes IBS, multiple mechanisms are proposed to be involved.[22]

### Altered Gastrointestinal Reactivity (Secretion and Motility)

The symptoms of IBS have traditionally been directed toward colonic motility dysfunction. Altered small bowel motility has been directly correlated with symptoms in IBS.[23] An alteration in the gastrointestinal tract in response to meals in general also seems to be present. Jepsen and colleagues[24] showed a "gastro-colonic" response to test meals or sham feeding in patients with IBS, which resulted in prolonged rectosigmoid motor activity compared with controls.

Transit time and bowel activity are different depending on the type of IBS. Patients with diarrhea-predominant IBS have accelerated or decelerated transit time because of changes in myoelectrical activity in the small bowel. Patients with constipation and abdominal distension as predominant symptoms of IBS have prolonged colonic transit times compared with healthy volunteers and patients with IBS and constipation but without distension.[25]

### Visceral Afferent Hypersensitivity

Enhanced perception of normal motility and visceral pain is a reproducible characteristic in patients with IBS. In one study, rectal distension in patients with IBS produced cerebral cortical activity more than in controls.[26–28] Increased colonic sensitivity was also shown by a study in which balloon distention of the descending colon produced pain at lower volumes in patients with IBS than in controls.[29] Other studies have shown similar increased sensitivity in patients with IBS who complained of bloating and excess gas, but who actually had volumes of gas in the gastrointestinal tract similar to asymptomatic controls.[26,30]

Despite being a reproducible characteristic in some patients with IBS, visceral hyperalgesia is only found in a subset of patients with IBS. As an example, community-based patients who report IBS symptoms but do not seek medical attention do not have visceral hyperalgesia.[31] Whether visceral hypersensitivity is mediated by the local gastrointestinal nervous system, central modulation from the brain, or some combination of the two is still unclear.[32,33] Central nervous system processing of visceral afferent impulses may be important in IBS, and studies show possible influences mediated by N-methyl D-aspartate (NMDA) receptors, serotonin, calcitonin gene-related peptide, substance P, bradykinin, tachykinins, and neurotrophins.[34,35]

### Inflammation in IBS

Conventional wisdom has held that no inflammation occurs in patients with IBS, but that belief may be changing. Recent evidence shows that some patients with IBS have an increased number of inflammatory cells in the colonic and ileal mucosa.[36] Immunohistologic studies have revealed mucosal immune system activation in a subset of patients with IBS, although most patients had diarrhea-predominant IBS.[37,38] Similar observations of gastrointestinal inflammation have been made in patients with presumed postinfectious IBS, suggesting a possible common link.

A study in which full-thickness jejunal biopsies were obtained in 10 patients with severe IBS found an increase in lymphocyte infiltration in the myenteric plexus in 9 patients and neuronal degeneration in 6.[39] Other studies have shown a correlation between abdominal pain in IBS and the presence of activated mast cells in proximity to colonic nerves.[40,41]

The extent to which inflammation might contribute to the pathogenesis of IBS in the general population remains unclear because only a small number and limited subset of patients have been studied.

### Alteration in Fecal Microflora

The bacteria within the gastrointestinal tract wall have a key role in permeability of the intestine and may play a role in IBS. Emerging data suggest that the fecal microbiota in individuals with IBS differ from those in healthy controls, and treatment of patients with probiotics have yielded promising results.[42]

### Postinfectious IBS

IBS may develop after recent infectious enteritis and may occur in as high as 25% of patients after severe acute enteritis.[43]

A systematic review of eight studies estimated a prevalence of postinfectious IBS in 10% of patients with a history of bacterial gastroenteritis compared with approximately 1% of controls.[44]

The cause of persistent or new bowel symptoms after acute infection is uncertain, although several theories have been proposed: one possible explanation is suggested by the association of persistent symptoms with more severe acute illness. The severity of illness may reflect the degree to which the organism invades the mucosa, causing disruption of mucosal nerves, which could lead to irritability.[45,46] Another possible explanation is the development of postinfectious bile acid malabsorption, because some postinfectious IBS responds to cholestyramine.[47,48] Patients treated with antibiotics for enteritis may also develop IBS symptoms related to alteration in colonic flora. Reduced disaccharidase activity with resulting malabsorption of dietary sugars has been observed after enteric infections and may be another mechanism involved in the pathophysiology of postinfectious IBS.[49]

Some controversy, however, surrounds the findings in studies of postinfectious IBS. One potentially important observation is that patients with preexisting IBS may be more likely to present to their physician with bacterial gastroenteritis than those without IBS.[50] Therefore, epidemiologic studies examining the rate of IBS incidence after bacterial gastroenteritis may have overestimated the rate at which new symptoms develop. Furthermore, not all studies have detected an increase in IBS after acute infectious diarrhea.[51]

### Food Allergies

The role of food allergy in IBS is unclear. Although food allergy may have a role in the development of symptoms, no reliable means is available to identify these individuals. Testing for serum immunoglobulins directed at specific dietary antigens has been proposed, but the relationship between results of this testing and improvement of symptoms is not well documented in the medical literature.

### CLINICAL MANIFESTATIONS

Chronic abdominal pain and altered bowel habits remain the nonspecific yet primary characteristics of IBS.[52,53] The severity of the pain may range from mildly irritating to debilitating. Patients with IBS also frequently present with abdominal bloating and increased gas production in the form of flatulence or belching. Approximately one-half of all patients with IBS will complain of mucus discharge with stools.[54]

Patients with diarrhea-predominant IBS may report frequent loose bowel movements that are preceded by lower abdominal cramps and urgency even to the point of fecal incontinence, and that may be followed by a feeling of incomplete evacuation even when the rectum is empty. Constipation may last from days to months, with interludes of diarrhea or normal bowel function. Stools are often hard and may be described as pellet-shaped.

IBS is also associated with upper gastrointestinal symptoms. The prevalence of IBS is higher among patients with dyspepsia than among those without. Upper gastrointestinal symptoms, including gastroesophageal reflux disease (GERD), dysphagia, early satiety, intermittent dyspepsia, nausea, and noncardiac chest pain, are also common in patients with IBS.[52] Between 25% and 50% of patients with IBS complain of dyspepsia, heartburn, nausea, and vomiting.

Patients with IBS often complain of a broad range of nongastrointestinal symptoms. These symptoms include impaired sexual function, dysmenorrhea, dyspareunia, increased urinary frequency or urgency, and fibromyalgia symptoms.[55,56]

### Abdominal Pain

Abdominal pain is a prerequisite clinical feature of IBS. Abdominal pain is highly variable in location and intensity and is often cramp-like. Pain is often exacerbated by eating or emotional stress and is often improved by defecation. Women also often report worsening symptoms during premenstrual periods.[57]

### Altered Bowel Habits

Alteration in the bowel habits is the most consistent feature in IBS. Often constipation occurs with alternating diarrhea. Most patients experience a feeling of incomplete emptying, which leads to repeated attempts at defecation in a short time span. Some patients exhibit constipation-predominant symptoms, others diarrhea-predominant symptoms, and some experience a mixture. Most patients, however, will change subtypes in as little as 1 year.

### Physical Examination

Physical examination findings are highly variable. Patients may have diffuse or focal tenderness to palpation of the abdomen. Rebound tenderness and unintentional abdominal guarding are not typical and should cause a clinician to consider other diagnoses.

### DIAGNOSIS

Given that no clear diagnostic markers exist for IBS, after ruling out other pathologies as directed by history and physical findings, the diagnosis is ultimately based on clinical presentation. A thorough history and physical examination is useful. The presence of blood, fever, or weight loss should make an examiner consider other diagnoses. An important consideration, however, is that IBS must be associated with abdominal discomfort: painless diarrhea or constipation does not fulfill diagnostic criteria for IBS.

### Diagnostic Criteria

The concept of diagnostic criteria for IBS originated in 1978 when Manning and colleagues[54] formulated a symptom complex suggestive of IBS consisting of six criteria. These criteria included pain associated with more frequent bowel movements, onset of pain associated with looser bowel movements, relief of pain with bowel movements, passage of mucus, visible abdominal bloating, and a sense of incomplete emptying. Data have conflicted on the predictive ability of the Manning criteria. The overall sensitivity and specificity of the Manning criteria have been estimated at approximately 78% and 72%, respectively.[58–60]

The American Gastroenterological Association, however, recommends that the diagnosis of IBS should be based on the identification of symptoms summarized by newer criteria created by a consensus panel. In an effort to standardize clinical research protocols, an international working team published a consensus definition in 1992 called the *Rome criteria* (**Box 1**), which was revised most recently in 2006 (Rome III criteria). IBS was defined as recurrent abdominal pain or discomfort associated with altered defecation.[52] The original Rome (Rome I) criteria was reported to have a sensitivity and specificity of 71% and 85%, respectively.[61]

The Rome criteria were developed to improve the homogeneity of patients for clinical investigations into functional gastrointestinal disorders and may not have applicability to clinical practice. These criteria have been criticized for overemphasis on abdominal pain and failure to emphasize postprandial urgency, abdominal pain, or diarrhea.[62] Some investigators continue to use the Manning criteria or a combination of both. Other criteria have been proposed for IBS diagnosis (such as the Kruis criteria) but are rarely used.[63,64]

---

**Box 1**
**Rome Diagnostic Criteria for IBS**

*At least 12 weeks, which need not be consecutive, in the preceding 12 months of abdominal discomfort or pain that has at least 2 of 3 features:*

1. Relieved with defecation

2. Onset associated with a change in frequency of stool

3. Onset associated with a change in form (appearance) of stool

*Symptoms that cumulatively support the diagnosis of IBS:*

1. Abnormal stool frequency (for research purposes, "abnormal" may be defined as greater than three bowel movements per day and fewer than three bowel movements per week)

2. Abnormal stool form (lumpy/hard or loose/water stool)

3. Abnormal stool passage (straining, urgency, or feeling of incomplete evacuation)

4. passage of mucus

5. Bloating or feeling of abdominal distention

The diagnosis of a functional bowel disorder always presumes the absence of a structural or biochemical explanation for the symptoms.[57]

*Four subtypes of IBS were recognized:*

- IBS with constipation (hard or lumpy stools ≥25%; loose or watery stools <25% of bowel movements)

- IBS with diarrhea (loose or water stools ≥25%; hard or lumpy stools <5% of bowel movements)

- Mixed IBS (hard or lumpy stools ≥25%; loose or watery stools ≥25% of bowel movements)

- Unsubtyped IBS (insufficient abnormality of stool consistency to meet the other subtypes)

### Differential Diagnosis

Because abdominal pain, abdominal bloating, and a change in bowel habits are very common gastrointestinal complaints, the list of differential diagnoses is extensive. The quality, location, and timing of the pain as well as associated symptoms can be useful. Differential diagnoses include but are not limited to: hyperthyroidism, hypothyroidism, parathyroid disorders, acute intermittent porphyria, acute lead poisoning, inflammatory bowel disease, parasitic infections, malabsorption, diverticulitis, lactose intolerance, laxative abuse, and celiac sprue, ischemic bowel, pancreatitis, food allergies, endometriosis, abdominal malignancy and biliary disease.

There are several "red flag" signs and symptoms that should occur in IBS and should make one consider an alternative diagnosis. Bleeding without hemorrhoids, nocturnal diarrhea or pain, weight loss, and abnormal blood tests should not occur with IBS.

## DIAGNOSTIC TESTS

The Rome and Manning criteria provide guidelines to identify patients with suspected IBS. Identifying symptoms compatible with IBS and then using judicious diagnostic testing can avoid unnecessary and costly testing. Because specific biomarkers of IBS are not yet available, diagnostic tests are frequently performed to exclude organic diseases.

Multiple diagnostic tests have been recommended for patients with IBS symptoms. However, limited evidence supports routine diagnostic testing in patients without alarm features and in those without diarrhea. Complete blood cell count (CBC), chemistry, thyroid tests, stool examination, ultrasound, hydrogen breath test, erythrocyte sedimentation rate, and C-reactive protein all have very limited accuracy in discriminating IBS from other abdominal pathologies.[3] Nevertheless, some amount of testing is usually performed. In most patients who have symptoms suggestive of IBS based on the Rome III criteria and no alarm symptoms or signs on the history and physical examination, a limited number of diagnostic studies can rule out organic illness. Common tests are CBC, chemistry, stool evaluation, thyroid stimulating hormone, and erythrocyte sedimentation rate or C-reactive protein.

Because of the high predominance of celiac disease in patients with IBS, screening for the disease with serum IgA antibody to tissue transglutaminase or antiendomysial antibody should be considered in any initial evaluation for IBS, but particularly diarrhea-predominant IBS. In a meta-analysis of 14 studies focusing on unselected adults who met diagnostic criteria for IBS, celiac disease was four times as likely as in controls without IBS.[65]

Dietary modifications may be useful for both diagnosis and treatment. For example, improvement with the initiation of a lactose-free diet for 1 week in conjunction with lactase supplements suggests lactose intolerance, although response may be unreliable. If lactose intolerance is suspected hydrogen breath testing can be performed. Having the patient perform a 48-hour fast may also be useful for determining the presence of a secretory cause for diarrhea. Persistent diarrhea after the fast suggests a secretory cause, and a 24-hour stool collection may be useful.[52]

Imaging studies and invasive procedures are usually unnecessary but may be needed depending on suspicion for a specific diagnosis. Tests that may be considered include and upper gastrointestinal barium study, abdominal CT scan, abdominal ultrasonography, barium enema, esophagogastroduodenoscopy, colonoscopy, and flexible sigmoidoscopy.

## MANAGEMENT OF IBS

Because of the variability of IBS, the most successful treatments will be likely be comprehensive and involve multiple strategies, including medication and behavioral therapies. A thorough history is important to determine recent medications, dietary changes, concerns about serious illness, stressors, secondary gain (disability claims, narcotics), or psychiatric comorbidities before developing a therapy plan.[66]

IBS with mild symptoms may respond to dietary changes, such as increasing fluid intake, caffeine avoidance, and avoidance of lactose or fructose. Increasing fiber intake might also help reduce symptoms of both constipation and diarrhea, although a systematic review of fiber for IBS showed no significant benefit.[67]

### Patient Education

Education regarding the proposed mechanisms of IBS helps validate the patient's illness experience and sets the basis for interventions. Patients should be informed of the chronic and benign nature of IBS and that they should have a normal life span.

### Antispasmodics

Antispasmodic agents are the most frequently used pharmacologic agents in the treatment of IBS. Certain antispasmodic drugs may provide short-term relief, but long-term efficacy has not been shown.[9]

The antispasmodic agents include medications that directly affect intestinal smooth muscle relaxation (mebeverine and pinaverine, available in the United Kingdom only) and those that act via their anticholinergic or antimuscarinic properties (dicyclomine and hyoscyamine). Antispasmodics reduce stimulated colonic motor activity and may be beneficial in patients with postprandial abdominal pain, gas, bloating, and fecal urgency.[68]

### Antidiarrheal Agents

Loperamide is the most commonly used antidiarrheal agent and has been shown to be more effective than placebo for treating diarrhea but not for the treatment of global IBS symptoms or abdominal pain. Administration on an as-needed basis is preferred to a regular scheduled dosing regimen in patients with diarrhea. Patients who consistently develop diarrhea after meals may benefit from taking a regular dosing regimen. Loperamide should not be used in patients with constipation and should be used cautiously in those with alternating diarrhea and constipation.

### Cognitive Behavior Therapy

Most treatment trials involving psychological therapies in IBS have featured cognitive behavior therapy (CBT). CBT is a time-limited, structured, problem-focused, and prescriptive therapy. It is based on the assumption that IBS symptoms are learned and reflect maladaptive behaviors. Furthermore, it assumes that modification of behaviors and thinking patterns can correct the symptoms of IBS. The methods include problem-solving strategies for stress, muscle relaxation exercises, and cognitive restructuring to modify faulty appraisals of perceived threats that tend to underlie emotional and physical reactivity. A meta-analysis of 17 studies on CBT for IBS showed a greater than 50% reduction in gastrointestinal symptoms.[69]

### Gut-Directed Hypnotherapy

Gut-directed hypnotherapy (GDH) is a form of hypnosis that is reported to have a beneficial effect on IBS symptoms. It uses hypnotic induction with progressive relaxation and other techniques, followed by imagery directed toward control of gastrointestinal function. Therapy often includes self-hypnosis education, and some evidence suggests that it is effective in improving symptoms.[70]

Despite trials showing efficacy, a 2008 Cochrane review of all randomized and quasi-randomized clinical studies comparing hypnotherapy to no treatment or another treatment noted that previous trials were of poor quality, and no conclusion could be made about the efficacy of GDH. No harmful side effects were reported in any of the trials, and therefore it may still be indicated in patients who are interested.[71]

Besides poor-quality evidence of supportive efficacy, other difficulties are associated with GDH. It is an intensive process, with most programs reporting 6 to 12 sessions lasting 30 to 60 minutes. Therefore, GDH would seem to be best for patients with severe or refractory IBS if it could be offered through home hypnotherapy using audio recordings.[72]

### Antidepressant Drugs

Antidepressants are effective for the treatment of some IBS symptoms. A 2009 meta-analysis that included 13 placebo-controlled trials of antidepressants in 789 adults with IBS concluded that antidepressants were significantly more effective than placebo for the relief of pain and global symptoms. The treatment effects were similar for selective serotonin reuptake inhibitors (SSRIs) and tricyclic antidepressants (TCAs) in this study, although overall fewer data have been published for SSRIs or serotonin norepinephrine reuptake inhibitors than for TCAs.[73]

Antidepressants have analgesic properties independent of their mood-improving effects and may therefore be beneficial in patients with neuropathic pain. The postulated mechanisms of pain modulation with TCAs and SSRIs in IBS is facilitation of endogenous endorphin release, blockade of norepinephrine reuptake leading to enhancement of descending inhibitory pain pathways, and blockade of serotonin. TCAs, via their anticholinergic properties, also slow intestinal transit time, which may provide benefit in diarrhea-predominant IBS.

Improvement in neuropathic pain with TCAs occurs at lower doses than required for treatment of depression. Therefore, low doses should be administered initially and titrated to pain control or tolerance. Because of the delayed onset of action, 3 to 4 weeks of therapy should be attempted before treatment is considered insufficient and the dose increased. TCAs should be used cautiously in patients with constipation. Paroxetine, fluoxetine, sertraline, citalopram, or other SSRI antidepressant medications should be considered in patients with a coexisting depression.

### Antiflatulence Drugs

The management of excessive gas with any treatment is seldom highly efficacious. Avoiding flatogenic foods, exercising, and losing excess weight are safe but unproven remedies. Data regarding simethicone are conflicting. Beano, an over-the-counter oral B-glycosidase solution, may reduce rectal passage of gas but will not decrease bloating and pain.[74,75]

### Serotonin Receptor Agonist and Antagonists

Agonists of the serotonin (5-hydroxytryptamine [5-HT]) receptor have shown some improvement of IBS symptoms but have serious negative side effects.

Zelnorm (Tegaserod) was the first of this drug class approved for IBS treatment. Tegaserod showed some benefit over placebo when used to treat IBS with constipation as a major symptom. However, tegaserod had not been shown to relieve symptoms of abdominal pain, bloating, stool consistency, and straining.[76] Tegaserod was removed from the market in March 2007 because of cardiovascular side effects.[77]

Alosetron (Lotronex), a 5-HT3 agonist, was developed for use in IBS based on its favorable effects on colonic motility and secretion and afferent neural systems. In clinical trials the drug was most effective in women with diarrhea-predominant IBS. However, the drug was associated with ischemic colitis and severe constipation, prompting the U.S. Food and Drug Administration (FDA) to remove it from the United States market. Demand from a subset of patients who had responded to treatment, however, prompted the FDA to allow the drug to return to the market under tight regulation.[78]

### Anticonvulsants

Anticonvulsant medications have been used for the treatment of all types of chronic pain. The anticonvulsant agents gabapentin and pregabalin make theoretical sense for the treatment of neuropathic pain and visceral hypersensitivity in IBS, but few data support their use for IBS, and use is considered off-label.

Gabapentin (Neurontin), which first gained FDA approval in 1994 for epilepsy and received approval for treatment of neuropathic pain in 2002, is the most frequently prescribed anticonvulsant for the treatment of chronic neuropathic pain. Although it has been used for chronic pain syndromes, a large meta-analysis investigating the efficacy of anticonvulsants such as gabapentin for chronic pain syndromes suggested poor treatment results.[79] Gabapentin has been shown to reduce rectal mechanosensitivity and increase rectal compliance in patients with diarrhea-predominant IBS, but few data are available on the clinical effectiveness of gabapentin for IBS.[80]

Pregabalin (Lyrica) was released and marketed as a successor to gabapentin. It was approved by the FDA for the treatment of epilepsy, diabetic neuropathy, and postherpetic neuralgia in June 2005. It was approved for the treatment of fibromyalgia in 2007. Pregabalin is not indicated for treatment of IBS, but in one study of 26 patients with IBS, pregabalin was found to increase sensory distension thresholds to normal levels in patients with rectal hypersensitivity, and to decrease pain and improve rectal compliance.[81]

### Chloride Channel Activators

These medications enhance chloride-rich intestinal fluid secretions without changing sodium and potassium concentrations in the serum. Lubiprostone is a locally acting chloride channel activator and received initial approval from the FDA for treatment of chronic idiopathic constipation but later also received approval for treatment of IBS with constipation in women aged 18 years and older.

Approval of lubiprostone was based on two multicenter placebo-controlled trials involving 1154 adults (92% women) with IBS and constipation who were randomly assigned to lubiprostone (8 μg twice daily) or placebo for 12 weeks.[82] Patients randomized to lubiprostone were significantly more likely to achieve an overall response (18% vs 10%), and serious adverse events were similar to placebo. However, the placebo response was far lower than in most studies of IBS, and why a secretory agent would improve symptoms other than constipation in a disorder such as IBS is not clear. Because efficacy is still questionable and it is an expensive medication, lubiprostone is best reserved for patients with IBS and severe constipation in whom other approaches have been unsuccessful.

## Probiotics

A popular alternative to conventional drug therapies is probiotics, which have been used in several conditions, including IBS. Probiotics are live microbial food supplements. Examples include *Lactobacillus* and *Bifidobacteria*, which are widely used in yogurts and other dairy products. They retain viability during storage and survive passage through the stomach and small bowel. The colonic microflora normally present a barrier to invading organisms, but when the microflora are altered, pathogens may become established.[83]

A recent study involving 362 patients with IBS evaluated the efficacy of *Bifidobacterium infantis*, a bacterium that resists colonization of pathogens in the large bowel. The results of the study showed improvement in abdominal pain, abdominal discomfort, bloating, straining, and feelings of incomplete evacuation, with no significant increase in side effects compared with placebo. However, *B infantis* did not significantly change the stool frequency.[84,85]

Guandalini and colleagues[86] performed a small prospective, multicenter, double-blind, placebo-controlled, crossover trial assessing the efficacy and safety of the probiotic VSL#3 (containing *B infantis*) in children identified as having IBS. Compared with placebo, patients treated with VSL#3 had a significant improvement in the global relief of IBS symptoms, abdominal pain, and bloating. However, no change in stool frequency or pattern was seen, consistent with the aforementioned study.

## Peppermint

Peppermint is rich in menthol, a smooth muscle relaxant that is proposed to reduce the amount of cramping and pain associated with IBS. A review article of 16 clinical trials showed a mean response rate of 58% for peppermint compared with 29% for placebo. The authors concluded that this response makes peppermint a good first-line choice for treatment of IBS, because of the efficacy and low adverse effect profile.[87] Other studies have not duplicated the high response rate. However, a recent meta-analysis of four clinical trials involving 329 patients treated with peppermint oil suggested a significant benefit in overall IBS symptoms.[88]

## Other Treatments

Benzodiazepines are of limited usefulness in IBS because of the risk of drug interactions, habituation, addiction, and rebound withdrawal. Furthermore, benzodiazepines may lower pain thresholds by stimulating gamma aminobutyric acid (GABA), which can lead to a decrease in brain serotonin.

Acupuncture has been used to treat IBS and should be considered for patients who desire complementary and alternative treatments for their IBS. Multiple, mostly poor-quality studies have used acupuncture to treat IBS with mixed results, although no randomized controlled trials have shown beneficial effects in the treatment of IBS. A recent systematic review of the existing literature showed no current evidence either supporting or against the use of acupuncture in the treatment of IBS.[89]

## COMPLICATIONS/ADMISSION CRITERIA/REFERRAL CRITERIA

Pain that is progressive, awakens the patient from sleep or prevents sleep, and is associated with anorexia, malnutrition, or weight loss is extremely rare in IBS unless a concurrent major psychological illness is present. Pain such as this requires a consultation to determine whether another cause is present.

## FIVE KEY POINTS FOR PRIMARY CARE

Abdominal discomfort is a prerequisite for the diagnosis of IBS. Diarrhea and constipation without abdominal discomfort does not meet criteria for IBS.

No specific serologic markers exist for IBS.

IBS is diagnosed clinically based on diagnostic criteria. The Manning and Rome criteria are the most commonly used.

IBS should not cause rectal bleeding (without hemorrhoids), weight loss, anemia, or nocturnal diarrhea that prevents sleep.

IBS is a complex syndrome that has multiple possible causative mechanisms.

Counseling patients about the possible mechanisms and the chronic and benign nature of IBS is the first step in the treatment of this condition. Given the variability of IBS, the most successful treatment will be comprehensive and involve multiple strategies.

## REFERENCES

1. Tillisch K, Labus JS, Naliboff BD, et al. Characterization of the alternating bowel habit subtype in patients with irritable bowel syndrome. Am J Gastroenterol 2005; 100(4):896–904.
2. American Gastroenterological Association. Available at: http://www.gastro.org/patient-center/digestive-conditions/irritable-bowel-syndrome. Accessed July 1, 2010.
3. Park JH, Byeon JS, Shin WG, et al. Diagnosis of irritable bowel syndrome: a systematic review. Korean J Gastroenterol 2010;55(5):308–15 [in Korean].
4. Everhart JE. Renault PF. Irritable bowel syndrome in office-based practice in the United States. Gastroenterology 1991;100(4):998–1005.
5. Schuster MM. Diagnostic evaluation of the irritable bowel syndrome. Gastroenterol Clin North Am 1991;20:269.
6. Sandler RS, Everhart JE, Donowitz M, et al. The burden of selected digestive diseases in the United States. Gastroenterology 2002;122:1500.
7. Talley NJ, Zinsmeister AR, Van Dyke C, et al. Epidemiology of colonic symptoms and the irritable bowel syndrome. Gastroenterology 1991;101:927.
8. Drossman DA, Li Z, Andruzzi E, et al. U.S. householder survey of functional gastrointestinal disorders. Prevalence, sociodemography and health impact. Dig Dis Sci 1993;38:1569.
9. American College of Gastroenterology Task Force of Irritable Bowel Syndrome. An evidence-based position statement on the management of irritable bowel syndrome. Am J Gastroenterol 2009;104(Suppl 1):S1.
10. Hahn BA, Saunders WB, Maier WC. Differences between individuals with self-reported irritable bowel syndrome (IBS) and IBS-like symptoms. Dig Dis Sci 1997;42:2585.
11. Saito YA, Locke GR, Talley NJ, et al. A comparison of the Rome and Manning criteria for case identification in epidemiological investigations of irritable bowel syndrome. Am J Gastroenterol 2000;95:2816.
12. Thompson WG, Irvine EJ, Pare P, et al. Functional gastrointestinal disorders in Canada: first population-based survey using Rome II criteria with suggestions for improving the questionnaire. Dig Dis Sci 2002;47:225.
13. Hungin AP, Whorwell PJ, Tack J, et al. The prevalence, patterns and impact of irritable bowel syndrome: an international survey of 40 000 subjects. Aliment Pharmacol Ther 2003;17:643.
14. Chial H, Camilleri M. Gender differences in irritable bowel syndrome. J Gender Specif Med 2002;5:37–45.

15. Chang L, Heitkemper M. Gender differences in irritable bowel syndrome. Gastroenterology 2002;123:1686–701.
16. Locke GR III, Zinsmeister AR, Talley NJ, et al. Familial association in adults with functional gastrointestinal disorders. Mayo Clin Proc 2000;75:907–12.
17. Levy RL, Jones KR, Whitehead WE, et al. Irritable bowel syndrome in twins: heredity and social learning both contribute to etiology. Gastroenterology 2001; 121:799–804.
18. Morris-Yates A, Talley NJ, Boyce PM, et al. Evidence of a genetic contribution to functional bowel disorder. Am J Gastroenterol 1998;93:1311–7.
19. Delvaux M, Denis P, Allemand H. Sexual abuse is more frequently reported by IBS patients than by patients with organic digestive diseases or controls: results of a multicentre inquiry: French Club of Digestive. Eur J Gastroenterol Hepatol 1997;9:345–52.
20. Gwee KA, Leong YL, Graham C, et al. The role of psychological and biological factors in postinfective gut dysfunction. Gut 1999;44:400–6.
21. Mykletun A, Jacka F, Williams L, et al. Prevalence of mood and anxiety disorder in self reported irritable bowel syndrome. An epidemiological population based study of women. BMC Gastroenterol 2010;10:88.
22. American Gastroenterological Association. American Gastroenterological Association Medical position statement, irritable bowel syndrome. Available at: http://www.gastrojournal.org/article/S0016-5085(02)00480-8/fulltext#section. Accessed September 1, 2010.
23. Kellow JE, Phillips SF. Altered small bowel motility in irritable bowel syndrome is correlated with symptoms. Gastroenterology 1987;92:1885–93.
24. Jepsen JM, Skoubo-Kristensen E, Elsborg L. Rectosigmoid motility response to sham feeding in irritable bowel syndrome: evidence of a cephalic phase. Scand J Gastroenterol 1989;24:53.
25. Agrawal A, Houghton LA, Reilly B, et al. Bloating and distension in irritable bowel syndrome: the role of gastrointestinal transit. Am J Gastroenterol 2009;104:1998.
26. Lawal A, Kern M, Sidu H, et al. Novel evidence for hypersensitivity of visceral sensory neural circuitry in irritable bowel syndrome patients. Gastroenterology 2006;130(1):26–33.
27. Mayer EA, Gebhart GF. Basic and clinical aspects of visceral hyperalgesia. Gastroenterology 1994;107:271–93.
28. Mertz H, Naliboff B, Munakata J. Altered rectal perception is a biological marker of patients with irritable bowel syndrome. Gastroenterology 1995;109:40–52.
29. Dorn SD, Palsson OS, Thiwan SI, et al. Increased colonic pain sensitivity in irritable bowel syndrome is the result of an increased tendency to report pain rather than increased neurosensory sensitivity. Gut 2007;56:1202.
30. Lasser RB, Bond JH, Levitt MD. The role of intestinal gas in functional abdominal pain. N Engl J Med 1975;293(11):524–6.
31. Zighelboim J, Talley NJ, Phillips SF, et al. Visceral perception in irritable bowel syndrome: rectal and gastric responses to distension and serotonin type 3 antagonism. Dig Dis Sci 1995;40:819.
32. Silverman DH, Munakata J, Ennes H, et al. Regional cerebral activity in normal and pathological perception of visceral pain. Gastroenterology 1997;112:64.
33. Mertz H, Morgan V, Tanner G, et al. Regional cerebral activation in irritable bowel syndrome and control subjects with painful and nonpainful rectal distention. Gastroenterology 2000;118:842.
34. Bueno L, Fioramonti J, Garcia-Villar R. Pathobiology of visceral pain: molecular mechanisms and therapeutic implications. III. Visceral afferent pathways:

a source of new therapeutic targets for abdominal pain. Am J Physiol Gastrointest Liver Physiol 2000;278:G670.

35. Willert RP, Woolf CJ, Hobson AR, et al. The development and maintenance of human visceral pain hypersensitivity is dependent on the N-methyl-D-aspartate receptor. Gastroenterology 2004;126:683.

36. Barbara G, DeGiorgio R, Cremon C, et al. A role for inflammation in irritable bowel syndrome? Gut 2002;51:41–4.

37. Chadwick VS, Chen W, Shu D, et al. Activation of the mucosal immune system in irritable bowel syndrome. Gastroenterology 2002;122:1778.

38. Liebregts T, Adam B, Bredack C, et al. Immune activation in patients with irritable bowel syndrome. Gastroenterology 2007;132:913.

39. Tornblom H, Lindberg G, Nyberg B, et al. Full-thickness biopsy of the jejunum reveals inflammation and enteric neuropathy in irritable bowel syndrome. Gastro-enterology 2002;123:1972.

40. Barbara G, Stanghellini V, De Giorgio R, et al. Activated mast cells in proximity to colonic nerves correlate with abdominal pain in irritable bowel syndrome. Gastro-enterology 2004;126:693.

41. Guilarte M, Santos J, de Torres I, et al. Diarrhoea-predominant IBS patients show mast cell activation and hyperplasia in the jejunum. Gut 2007;56:203.

42. Kassinen A, Krogius-Kurikka L, Makivuokko H, et al. The fecal microbiota of irri-table bowel syndrome patients differs significantly from that of healthy subjects. Gastroenterology 2007;133:24.

43. Thabane M, Kottachchi DT, Marshall JK. Systematic review and meta-analysis: the incidence and prognosis of post-infectious irritable bowel syndrome. Aliment Pharmacol Ther 2007;26:535–44.

44. Halvorson HA, Schlett CD, Riddle MS. Postinfectious irritable bowel syndrome– a meta-analysis. Am J Gastroenterol 2006;101:1894.

45. Everest PH, Goossens H, Butzler JP, et al. Differentiated Caco-2 cells as a model for enteric invasion by Campylobacter jejuni and E coli. J Med Microbiol 1992;37:319.

46. Swain MG, Blennerhassett PA, Collins SM. Impaired sympathetic nerve function in the inflamed rat intestine. Gastroenterology 1991;100:675.

47. Niaz SK, Sandrasegaran K, Renny FH, et al. Postinfective diarrhoea and bile acid malabsorption. J R Coll Physicians Lond 1997;31:53.

48. Sinha L, Liston R, Testa HJ, et al. Idiopathic bile acid malabsorption: qualitative and quantitative clinical features and response to cholestyramine. Aliment Phar-macol Ther 1998;12:839.

49. Muldoon C, Maguire P, Gleeson F. Onset of sucrase-isomaltase deficiency in late adulthood. Am J Gastroenterol 1999;94:2298.

50. Parry SD, Stansfield R, Jelley D, et al. Is irritable bowel syndrome more common in patients presenting with bacterial gastroenteritis? A community-based, case-control study. Am J Gastroenterol 2003;98:327.

51. Ilnyckyj A, Balachandra B, Elliott L, et al. Post-traveler's diarrhea irritable bowel syndrome: a prospective study. Am J Gastroenterol 2003;98:596.

52. Longstreth GF, Thompson WG, Chey WD, et al. Functional bowel disorders. Gastroenterology 2006;130:1480.

53. Swarbrick ET, Bat L, Hegarty JE, et al. Site of pain from the irritable bowel. Lancet 1980;2:443.

54. Manning AP, Thompson WG, Heaton KW, et al. Towards a positive diagnosis of the irritable bowel. Br Med J 1978;2:653.

55. Whorwell PJ, McCallum M, Creed FH, et al. Non-colonic features of irritable bowel syndrome. Gut 1986;27:37.

56. Hershfield NB. Nongastrointestinal symptoms of irritable bowel syndrome: an office-based clinical survey. Can J Gastroenterol 2005;19:231.
57. Drossman DA, Camilleri M, Mayer EA, et al. AGA technical review on irritable bowel syndrome. Gastroenterology 2002;123:2108.
58. Talley NJ, Phillips SF, Melton LJ, et al. Diagnostic value of the Manning criteria in irritable bowel syndrome. Gut 1990;31:77.
59. Smith RC, Greenbaum DS, Vancouver JB, et al. Gender differences in Manning criteria in the irritable bowel syndrome. Gastroenterology 1991;100:591.
60. Taub E, Cuevas JL, Cook EW III, et al. Irritable bowel syndrome defined by factor analysis: gender and race comparisons. Dig Dis Sci 1995;40:2647.
61. Tibble JA, Sigthorsson G, Foster R, et al. Use of surrogate markers of inflammation and Rome criteria to distinguish organic from nonorganic intestinal disease. Gastroenterology 2002;123(2):450–60.
62. Camilleri M, Choi MG, et al. Review article: irritable bowel syndrome. Aliment Pharmacol Ther 1997;11:3.
63. Kruis W, Thieme C, Weinzierl M, et al. A diagnostic score for the irritable bowel syndrome. Its value in the exclusion of organic disease. Gastroenterology 1984;87:1.
64. Frigerio G, Beretta A, Orsenigo G, et al. Irritable bowel syndrome: still far from a positive diagnosis. Dig Dis Sci 1992;37:164.
65. Ford AC, Chey WD, Talley NJ, et al. Yield of diagnostic tests for celiac disease in individuals with symptoms suggestive of irritable bowel syndrome: systematic review and meta-analysis. Arch Intern Med 2009;169:651.
66. Cash BD, Schoenfeld P, Chey WD. The utility of diagnostic tests in irritable bowel syndrome patients: a systematic review. Am J Gastroenterol 2002;97:2812.
67. Brandt LJ, Bjorkman D, Fennerty MB, et al. Systematic review on the management of irritable bowel syndrome in North America. Am J Gastroenterol 2002; 97(11 Suppl):S7–26.
68. Lynn RB, Friedman LS. Irritable bowel syndrome. N Engl J Med 1993;329:1940.
69. Lackner JM, Jaccard J, Krasner SS, et al. How does cognitive behavior therapy for IBS work? A mediational analysis of a randomized clinical trial. Gastroenterology 2007;133(2):433–44.
70. Houghton LA, Heyman DJ, Whorewell PJ. Symptomatology, quality of life and economic features of IBS: the effect of hypnotherapy. Aliment Pharmacol Ther 1996;10(1):91–5.
71. Webb AN, Kukuruzovic RH, Catto-Smith AG, et al. Hypnotherapy for treatment of irritable bowel syndrome. Cochrane Database Syst Rev 2007;4:CD005110.
72. Wald A, Rakel D. Behavioral and complementary approaches for the treatment of irritable bowel syndrome. Nutr Clin Pract 2008;23:284.
73. Ford AC, Talley NJ, Schoenfeld PS, et al. Efficacy of antidepressants and psychological therapies in irritable bowel syndrome: systematic review and meta-analysis. Gut 2009;58:367.
74. Talley NJ. Evaluation of drug treatment for irritable bowel syndrome. Br J Clin Pharmacol 2003;56:362.
75. Fauci AS, Braunwald E, Kasper DL, et al, editors. Harrison's principles of internal medicine. 17th edition. McGraw-Hill publishing; 2008.
76. Evans BW, Clark WK, Moore DJ, et al. Tegaserod for the treatment of irritable bowel syndrome and chronic constipation. Cochrane Database Syst Rev 2007; 4:CD003960.
77. Scott LJ, Perry CM. Tegaserod. Drugs 1999;58:491.

78. Gershon MD. Serotonin and its implication for the management of irritable bowel syndrome. Rev Gastroenterol Disord 2003;3(Suppl 2):S25.
79. Wiffen P, Collins S, McQuay H, et al. Anticonvulsant drugs for acute and chronic pain. Cochrane Database Syst Rev 2000;2:CD001133.
80. Lee KJ, Kim JH, Cho SW. Gabapentin reduces rectal mechanosensitivity and increases rectal compliance in patients with diarrhoea-predominant irritable bowel syndrome. Aliment Pharmacol Ther 2005;22(10):981–8.
81. Houghton LA, Fell C, Whorwell PJ, et al. Effect of a second-generation alpha2delta ligand (pregabalin) on visceral sensation in hypersensitive patients with irritable bowel syndrome. Gut 2007;56:1218–25.
82. Drossman DA, Chey WD, Johanson JF, et al. Clinical trial: lubiprostone in patients with constipation-associated irritable bowel syndrome–results of two randomized, placebo-controlled studies. Aliment Pharmacol Ther 2009;29:329.
83. Macfarlane GT, Cummings JH. Probiotics and prebiotics: can regulating the activities of intestinal bacteria benefit health? BMJ 1999;318(7189):999–1003.
84. Yamazaki S, Kamimura H, Momose H, et al. Protective effect of bifidobacterium monoassociation against lethal activity of E coli. Bifidobacteria Microflora 1982; 1:55–60.
85. Whorwell PJ, Altringer L, Morel J, et al. Efficacy of an encapsulated probiotic Bifidobacterium infantis 35624 in women with irritable bowel syndrome. Gastroenterology 2007;132(2):813–6.
86. Guandalini S, Magazzù G, Chiaro A, et al. VSL#3 improves symptoms in children with IBS: a multicenter, randomized, placebo controlled, double blind, crossover study. J Pediatr Gastroenterol Nutr 2010;51(1):24–30.
87. Grigoleit HG, Grigoleit P. Peppermint oil in irritable bowel syndrome. Phytomedicine 2005;12(8):601–8.
88. Ford AC, Talley NJ, Spiegel BM, et al. The effect of fiber, antispasmodics, and peppermint oil in IBS. Systematic review and meta-analysis. BMJ 2008;337: 1388–92.
89. Lim B, Manheimer E, Lao L, et al. Acupuncture for treatment of irritable bowel syndrome. Cochrane Database Syst Rev 2006;4:CD005111.

# Screening for Cancerous and Precancerous Conditions of the Colon

Manjula Julka, MD*, Manjula Cherukuri, MD, Rahele Lameh, MD

**KEYWORDS**

- Colorectal cancer • Polyps • Screening • Colonoscopy
- Fecal immunochemical tests

## EPIDEMIOLOGY

Colorectal cancer (CRC) causes significant mortality and morbidity in the United States. It is the third most commonly diagnosed cancer and the second leading cause of cancer-related deaths in both men and women. The lifetime risk to be diagnosed with CRC is 5.5% in men and 5.1% in women. Of the new cases 20% to 25% occur in individuals with positive family history or predisposing illness and 75% are sporadic.[1] As shown in **Table 1**, the incidence and mortality are higher in African Americans. Overall, the incidence and mortality are 35% higher in men than in women.[1]

## RISK FACTORS

Incidence and death rate of CRC increase with age. Almost 91% of new cases and 94% of deaths occur in individuals 50 years and older.[1] So, age older than 50 years is the predominant risk factor. However, there are other risk factors that increase the likelihood of CRC in patients, which include positive personal history or family history of CRC or adenoma polyps, inherited CRC syndromes (ie, familial adenomatous polyposis (FAP), hereditary nonpolyposis colorectal cancer [HNPCC], and inflammatory bowel disease [IBD]).

The authors have nothing to disclose.
Department of Family and Community Medicine, University of Texas Southwestern Medical Center at Dallas, 6263 Harry Hines Boulevard, Clinical Building 1, Forest Park Road Suite#651, Dallas, TX 75390-9165, USA
* Corresponding author.
*E-mail address:* Manjula.Julka@UTSouthwestern.edu

Prim Care Clin Office Pract 38 (2011) 449–468
doi:10.1016/j.pop.2011.05.009
0095-4543/11/$ – see front matter. Published by Elsevier Inc.

| Table 1 CRC incidence and mortality[a] by race/ethnicity and sex, 2001 to 2005 | | | | |
|---|---|---|---|---|
| | Incidence | | Mortality | |
| Race | Men | Women | Men | Women |
| African American | 71.2 | 54.5 | 31.8 | 22.4 |
| White | 58.9 | 43.2 | 22.1 | 15.3 |
| Asian American/Pacific Islander | 48.0 | 35.4 | 14.4 | 10.2 |
| Hispanic | 47.3 | 32.8 | 16.5 | 10.8 |
| American Indian/Alaska Native | 46.0 | 41.2 | 20.5 | 14.2 |
| All persons | 59.2 | 43.8 | 22.7 | 15.9 |

[a] Per 100,000, age-adjusted to the 2000 US Standard Population. Incidence data based on the Contract Health Service Delivery Area.

*Data from* Surveillance, Epidemiology, and End Results (SEER) Program.

## Personal History

### History of CRC

Personal history of CRC increases the chance of recurrent polyps or cancer elsewhere in the colon and rectum even if the first malignancy is completely removed. In patients undergoing resection of single CRC, the risk of recurrence of primary cancer in the first 5 years postoperatively is 1.5% to 3%. The risk of recurrence is even higher if the patient is younger than 60 years.[1]

### History of adenomatous polyps

All individuals with a history of adenomatous polyps are at risk for development of additional adenomas. More than 95% of CRCs in the United States arise from adenomatous polyps. Risk of malignancy transformation depends on the size, number, and histology of the polyps. The risk of malignancy increases if the polyps are larger or if more than 1 is present.[2] For example, more than 1% of adenomatous polyps less than 1 cm in size are malignant, whereas 40% of adenomas greater than 2 cm are malignant. On the other hand, the risk of malignancy is about 8 to 10 times higher for villous and tubulovillous adenomas than for tubular adenomas.[3]

## Family History

People who have first-degree family members with CRC are at increased risk of developing it when compared with the general population. About 20% of all individuals with CRC have a positive family history in a close relative.[1] The family history can be sporadic CRC or inherited CRC syndrome.

### Sporadic CRC

Sporadic colon cancers account for about 80% of CRCs and the rest are attributed to inherited syndromes.[4] An individual with 1 first-degree family member (parents, sibling, offspring) with CRC has a 2-fold to 3-fold increased risk of developing the disease compared with people who do not have the history.[1,5] An individual with 2 first-degree relatives with CRC or a single first-degree relative diagnosed with CRC before age 50 years has a 3-fold to 6-fold increased risk of CRC development. Two second-degree relatives with CRC increase an individual's risk for CRC development by 1-fold to 2-fold.[6,7]

*Inherited syndromes*

About 5% to 30% of patients with CRC have an inherited genetic alteration that causes the cancer. Out of those, 1% to 5% have known genetic defects.[5] Inherited CRC syndromes are described later.

**FAP** FAP is autosomal dominant caused by mutation in the adenomatous polyposis coli (APC) gene. APC is a tumor suppressor gene on chromosome 5q21. Its prevalence in the population is 2 to 3/100,000.[5] FAP is characterized by multiple (>100) adenomatous polyps throughout the colon developing after the first decade of life, but the age of developing colon adenomas is different. For example, by age 10 years only 15% of FAP gene carriers have adenomas; by age 20 years, the possibility increases to 75%; and by age 30 years, 90% have colon polyps.[8] Patients usually present after puberty, generally by age 25 years, and if colostomy has not been performed, then CRC develops in most of these patients before they are aged 40 years.[9] Other possible clinical features of FAP are polyps in the upper gastrointestinal (GI) tract, and extraintestinal manifestations.[8] A variant syndrome of FAP is attenuated FAP, which is characterized with fewer polyps (usually <100) and late onset of colon polyps, but gene mutation is still APC.[5]

**HNPCC** HNPCC is also called Lynch syndrome. It is autosomal dominant caused by mutation in 1 of several mismatch repair (MMR) genes. These individuals are usually diagnosed with CRC at the average age of 44 years versus 64 years in sporadic CRC.[8] In Lynch syndrome, CRC is usually present on the right side (proximal to the splenic flexure) versus sporadic CRC, which happens most likely in the left colon. HNPCC can be diagnosed based on Amsterdam II criteria[5]:

Amsterdam criteria II[8]:

1. There should be at least 3 relatives with a Lynch syndrome-associated cancer (CRC or cancer of the endometrium, small bowel, ureter, or renal pelvis).
2. One should be a first-degree relative of the other 2.
3. At least 2 successive generations should be affected.
4. At least 1 should be diagnosed before age 50 years.
5. FAP should be excluded in the CRC cases.
6. Tumors should be verified by pathologic examination.

**Turcot syndrome** Turcot syndrome is a disease that can be a variant of FAP or HNPCC. It is characterized with colon polyps and tumors in the central nervous system, primarily medulloblastomas, and gliomas. It has been shown that if the brain tumors are cerebellar medulloblastomas the condition is likely a variant of FAP. If the brain tumors are indolent glioblastoma multiforme, then the condition may be a variant of HNPCC. This syndrome can be also associated with duodenal periampullary adenomas, nonadenomatous gastric polyps, desmoid tumors, and osteomas.[5]

**Gardner syndrome** Gardner syndrome is an autosomal dominant disorder that is probably a variant of FAP. It is characterized by triad of bone tumors (ie, osteoma), soft tissue tumors (ie, desmoids tumors), and GI tract polyps (including upper and lower GI tract).[5]

**Familial juvenile polyposis** Familial juvenile polyposis (FJP) is an autosomal dominant disease with a prevalence of approximately 1/100,000. Individuals with FJP have a 60% lifetime risk of CRC. The mutation occurs in 3 genes: the SMAD 4 or MADH4 gene, the BMPR-1A gene, and the PTEN genes.[3] The polyps are usually hamartomatous and have a high risk of bleeding; they are mostly diagnosed in childhood (4–14 years of age).[3]

**Peutz-Jeghers syndrome**  Peutz-Jeghers syndrome (PJS) is autosomal dominant and the prevalence is about 1/200,000. Lifetime risk of CRC in these individuals is 40%. The mutation occurs in a gene encoding a serine threonine kinase (LKBI) located on chromosome 19.[5] It is characterized by multiple GI polyps, which are usually hamartomatous, and they may undergo malignant transformation. Growing of the polyps at an early age (between 10 and 30 years) can cause obstruction (intussusceptions or occlusion) of the lumen by the polyp.[10] There is also risk of other GI and nongastrointestinal cancers in PJS, which include cancers of the biliary tree, gallbladder, and esophagus; uterine, bilateral breast, cervical, and ovarian cancers in women; and Sertoli cell testicular tumors in men.[2,11–16]

**Cowden syndrome**  Cowden syndrome is also called multiple hamartomas syndrome and is another autosomal dominant disease, with a prevalence of 1/200,000. The mutation occurs in chromosome 10.[5] Polyps can occur in the colon, small intestine, stomach, and also the esophagus. Malignant potential is low but occurs with adenomatous changes in hamartomatous polyps. There is an increased incidence of breast and thyroid carcinoma (**Table 2**).[17]

### IBD

The risk of adenocarcinoma of the colon begins to increase 7 to 10 years after disease onset in patients with ulcerative colitis and Crohn disease. The cumulative risk approaches 5% to 10% after 20 years and 20% after 30 years. Chronic treatment with 5-aminosalicylic acid agents and folate is associated with a lower risk of cancer in patients with ulcerative colitis.[18] In individuals with IBD, the mucosa undergoes dysplasia and proceeds through a series of mutations that can result in colon cancer.

### Physical activity

Studies indicate that regular physical activity is associated with a lower risk of CRC. The American Cancer Society (ACS) recommends at least a moderate level of activity, which is 30 minutes or more for 5 days or more per week, although high-level exercise (as much as 45–60 minutes) is more favorable and decreases the risk of CRC in men and women by 50%.[1]

### Overweight, obesity, and diabetes

Obesity and overweight put individuals at higher risk of developing CRC. Abdominal obesity is more important than overall obesity. Diabetes mellitus type 2 has been shown to be associated with higher risk of CRC.[1]

### Diet

There is enough evidence to support a positive relationship between consumption of high amounts of processed and red meat with CRC risk. On the other hand, high garlic consumption may reduce the risk, but there is no certain association between a diet high in fiber, fruits, and vegetables and risk of CRC. Vitamin D may reduce the risk of CRC, and consumption of milk and calcium also decreases the risk.[1]

### Smoking and alcohol

Although consistent evidence supports that smoking increases the rate of aggressive adenomatous polyps, only some studies support the increased risk of developing CRC in chronic tobacco smoking. The International Agency for Research on Cancer and the Surgeon General do not recognize smoking as a cause of CRC. Moderate

**Table 2**
Inherited syndromes related to colorectal cancer

| Syndrome | Common Site of Polyps | Histology | Malignancy Risk | Extracolonic Lesions |
|---|---|---|---|---|
| FAP | Colon | Adenomatous | Common | Congenital hypertrophy of retinal pigment epithelium (CHRPE)<br>Osteomas<br>Epidermoid cysts<br>Desmoid formation<br>Thyroid tumors<br>Small bowel cancer<br>Hepatoblastoma<br>Brain tumors particularly medulloblastoma |
| HNPCC (Lynch syndrome) | Right side of colon | Adenomatous | Common | Endometrial carcinoma<br>Ovarian cancer<br>Stomach cancer<br>Small bowel cancer<br>Pancreas cancer<br>Hepatobiliary system cancer<br>Renal pelvis cancer<br>Ureter cancer |
| Turcot syndrome | Colon | Adenomatous | Common | Brain tumors |
| Gardner syndrome | Colon and small intestine | Adenomatous | Common | Osteomas<br>Fibromas<br>Lipomas<br>Epidermoid cysts<br>Ampullary cancers<br>CHRPE |
| PJS | Colon and small intestine, stomach | Hamartomatous | Rare | Mucocutaneous pigmentation<br>Gallbladder and biliary tree cancer<br>Esophagus cancer<br>Tumors of the ovary, breast, pancreas, endometrium, and testicular cancer |
| Cowden syndrome | Colon and small intestine, stomach and esophagus | Hamartomatous | Rare | Breast cancer<br>Thyroid cancer |
| FJP | Colon and small intestine, stomach | Hamartomatous rarely progressing to adenoma | Common | Various congenital abnormalities |

use of alcohol has been known to be a risk of developing CRC. The definition of moderate drinking is 30 g or about 2 drinks per day.[1]

### Medication supplement

The ACS currently does not recommend any medication or dietary supplement to prevent CRC because of lack of evidence about dosage, side effects, and effectiveness. Good evidence suggests that regular use of aspirin (ASA) and nonsteroidal anti-inflammatory drugs (NSAIDs) lowers the risk of CRC, but because of potential side effects including GI side effects for NSAIDs and ASA and also coronary artery disease (CAD) risk for cyclooxygenase 2 inhibitors, the ACS does not support use for prevention. Postmenopausal hormonal replacement therapy decreases the risk of CRC, but increases the risk of breast cancer and CAD. Supplemental calcium decreases risk of precancerous polyps and CRC (**Table 3**).[1]

## MOLECULAR GENETICS

Sporadic colon cancers account for about 80% of CRCs and the rest are attributed to inherited syndromes.[4] There is a multistep process in the transformation of normal colonic mucosa to life-threatening CRC.[9] There are at least 3 different steps that make this transformation, including chromosomal instability, microsatellite instability (MSI), and CpG island methylation[4]: In the chromosomal instability pathway, the mutation involves the tumor suppressor gene APC, which is located on chromosome 5, and also mutation on the k-ras protooncogene. Then other genetic changes happen, which include changes in the DCC gene on 18q and mutation on tumor suppressor gene p35 on chromosome 17p.[4]

The main target in the MSI pathway is the DNA MMR genes. Alterations in these genes occur in inherited form (HNPCC syndrome/Warthin-Lynch syndrome), and silencing of 1 of the genes, which is called hMLH1, occurs sporadically by methylation.[4] In the CpG island methylation pathway the method is epigenetic hypermethylation of DNA, which causes the suppression of gene expression by methylation in gene promoters. All of these events affect expression of important regulatory proteins controlling cell morphology, growth, and adhesion.[4]

## PATHOPHYSIOLOGY OF COLORECTAL ADENOCARCINOMA

Most CRCs are adenocarcinomas and about two-thirds of them occur in the rectum, rectosigmoid, or sigmoid.[19,20] More than 95% of CRCs in the United States arise from adenomatous polyps.

| Table 3<br>Incidence of CRC | |
| --- | --- |
| **Risk Factor** | **Incidence (%)** |
| General population | 5 |
| Personal history | |
|   CRC | 15–20 |
|   Adenomatous polyps | Variable |
| IBD | 15–40 |
| HNPCC | 70–80 |
| FAP | >95 |

## Colon Polyps

### Definition

A polyp is a protrusion from the colonic mucosal surface that carries a small risk of transformation to malignancy (<1%).[21] Its prevalence is high and increases with age. More than 30% of autopsies performed in people older than 60 years show polyps.[22] It has been shown that larger colonic polyps tend to be more distal, although they can be found throughout the colon and rectum.[5]

### Polyp types

Histologically, there are 3 major groups of polyps: neoplastic (adenomatous), nonneoplastic polyps (hyperplastic polyps, hamartomas, lymphoid aggregates), and inflammatory polyps.[22]

**Neoplastic polyps (adenomatous)** Adenomatous polyps are the most common type of polyps found in the colon (60%–70%).[23] It has been shown that more than 95% of adenocarcinomas of the colon are from neoplastic adenomatous polyps. The risk of malignancy correlates with size and histology of the polyp.[22] Of all adenomatous polyps, 70% to 85% are classified as tubular (0%–25%, villous tissue), 10% to 25% are tubulovillous (25%–75%, villous tissue), and less than 5% are villous adenomas (75%–100%, villous tissue).[22] Polyps greater than 1 cm, which contain more than 25% villous component, or have high-grade dysplasia are usually categorized as advanced neoplasms and are associated with an increased cancer risk.[21] Based on clinical observation most of the small tubular adenomas (<1 cm) remain the same or may even retract with time.[22] It has been shown that removing the adenomatous polyps at the time of colonoscopy decreases the incidence of CRC by 76% to 90%.[17]

**Nonneoplastic polyps** Hyperplasic polyps are the most common nonneoplastic polyps in the colon. They are usually small, about 0.5 cm in size, and mainly in the rectosigmoid area.[21] The hyperplastic polyps are not generally associated with CRC, but there some may be associated with premalignancy.[24] Features of high-risk hyperplastic polyps that increase risk of malignant transformation are: greater than 1 cm in size, located on the right colon, and mixed histology of hyperplastic-adenomatous type, and number more than 20 in the whole colon; also a positive family history of hyperplastic polyposis syndrome or colon cancer increases the risk of malignant transformation.[24]

**Submucosal polyps** Submucosal polyps are classified as lymphoid polyps, lipomas, metastatic cancer (eg, melanoma), and rectosigmoid carcinoid tumors, leiomyomas, neurofibromas, fibromas, hemangiomas, Kaposi sarcoma, and endometriosis. Lymphoid polyps are a result of hyperplasia of normal underlying lymphoid tissue. They most commonly occur in the rectum and in the second and fifth decades of life. Lipomas usually occur in the proximal colon (close to the ileocecal valve) as a yellow single polyp.

## COLONIC ADENOCARCINOMA: HISTOPATHOLOGY

Adenocarcinomas account for about 90% to 95% of all CRCs. They often arise from malignant transformation of adenomatous polyps to invasive adenocarcinoma. Cancer transformation usually starts as an intramucosal epithelial lesion in the adenomatous glands or polyps, and then invades surrounding tissues such as lymph nodes, adjacent organs, and other distant organs, particularly the liver (**Fig. 1**).[25]

Grading:
- Well differentiated
- Moderately differentiated
- Poorly differentiated
  - ○ Possible severe genetic mutation
  - ○ 20% of CRCs are poorly differentiated
  - ○ Poor prognosis
- Undifferentiated.

Higher tumor grade has lower prognostic value

- Low-grade tumors: grades 1 and 2
- High-grade tumors: grades 3 and 4.

---

***Colon Cancer Survival Rates with the New American Joint Committee on Cancer Staging Sixth Edition***

Stages as defined by the *American Joint Committee on Cancer (AJCC) Staging Systems Fifth and Sixth Editions.*

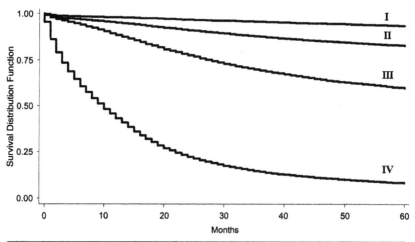

| Stage | 0 mo | | 30 mo | | | 60 mo | | |
|---|---|---|---|---|---|---|---|---|
| | Survival (%) | N | Survival (%) | N | P | Survival (%) | N | P |
| I | 100 | 14500 | 96.1 | 8591 | — | 93.2 | 4515 | — |
| II | 100 | 34361 | 89.2 | 19492 | <.0001 | 82.5 | 10105 | <.0001 |
| III | 100 | 26949 | 72.7 | 12192 | <.0001 | 59.5 | 5514 | <.0001 |
| IV | 100 | 20802 | 17.3 | 1832 | <.0001 | 8.1 | 432 | <.0001 |

**Fig. 1.** Five-year survival by *American Joint Committee on Cancer Fifth Edition System Stages I to IV. (Data from* O'Connell JB, Maggard MA, Ko CY. Colon cancer survival rates with the new American Joint Committee on Cancer sixth edition staging. J Natl Cancer Inst 2004; 96(19):1420–5.)

| Staging System | T Stage | N Stage | M Stage |
| --- | --- | --- | --- |
| *AJCC Fifth Edition* | | | |
| I | T1 or T2 | N0 | M0 |
| II | T3 or T4 | N0 | M0 |
| III | Any T | N1 | M0 |
| IV | Any T | Any N | M1 |
| *AJCC Sixth Edition* | | | |
| I | T1 or T2 | N0 | M0 |
| IIa | T3 | N0 | M0 |
| IIb | T4 | N0 | M0 |
| IIIa | T1 or T2 | N1 | M0 |
| IIIb | T3 or T4 | N1 | M0 |
| IIIc | Any T | N2 | M0 |
| IV | Any T | Any N | M1 |

*Abbreviations:* M0, no distant metastasis; M1, distant metastasis; N0, no regional lymph node metastasis; N1, metastasis to 1 to 3 regional lymph nodes; N2, metastasis to 4 or more regional lymph nodes; T1, tumor invades submucosa; T2, tumor invades muscularis propria; T3, tumor invades through the muscularis propria into the subserosa or into nonperitonealized pericolic tissues; T4, tumor directly invades other organs or structures or perforates visceral peritoneum.

*Data from* O'Connell JB, Maggard MA, Ko CY. Colon cancer survival rates with the new American Joint Committee on Cancer sixth edition staging. J Natl Cancer Inst 2004;96(19):1420–5.

## SCREENING MODALITIES

Multiple investigative options are available for screening, to detect either early stage disease or precancerous adenomas. Optical colonoscopy, flexible sigmoidoscopy, guaiac-based fecal occult blood tests (gFOBTs), and double-contrast barium enema (DCBE) have been the screening tests of choice for several years. Newer choices available for physicians to offer to their patients include computed tomographic colonography (CTC), fecal immunochemical tests (FITs), and tests for stool DNA.

No single test is considered by any recommending organization to have an undeniable advantage.

Whereas stool-based tests improve disease prognosis by detecting early stage cancers, endoscopic or radiologic tests that structurally examine the bowel mucosa prevent cancer by detecting precancerous polyps that can be removed at the time of the test. It is preferred that an informed decision is made by the patient with the help of their clinician about the type of screening test based on the patient's personal preferences.

### Fecal Occult Blood Tests

Colorectal adenomas and cancers may bleed intermittently. Detection of blood in the stool can lead to an evaluation that identifies and removes preneoplastic lesions. There are several surveillance techniques for performing fecal occult blood tests (FOBTs), as described in the following sections.

### gFOBTs

gFOBTs are inexpensive, readily available, and have been widely used. This test is performed by smearing a stool sample on guaiac-impregnated card and adding hydrogen peroxide drops to the sample. Blood in the stool is detected when the card turns blue by way of a pseudoperoxidase enzymatic reaction with hemoglobin. Although several guaiac reagents were used in the past, sensitive gFOBT (eg,

Hemoccult SENSA, Beckman Coulter, Inc) is recommended secondary to increased sensitivity.[26] Benefits of gFOBT for detection of colorectal neoplasm have been studied extensively. The Minnesota Colon Cancer Randomized Control Study followed the participants for 18 years and found annual or biennial screening with gFOBT to have significantly reduced incidence of CRC.[27] A 2007 Cochrane review that followed more than 320,000 participants for 8 to 18 years showed that screening with gFOBT reduced risk of CRC mortality by possibly avoiding 1 in 6 CRC deaths.[28] The effectiveness of FOBTs depends on the amount of blood loss, amount of hemoglobin degradation (decreased sensitivity caused by storage or action of fecal flora), and interfering substances that may either enhance or inhibit oxidation of the developing solution. It is reported that approximately 2 mL of blood in the stool is necessary to produce a positive result in gFOBT. Location of a colonic lesion may also affect detection of blood in the stool. Proximal colon lesions are known to have greater blood loss. False-negative test results can occur if gFOBT is performed when the colorectal lesion (polyp/adenoma/neoplasia) is not bleeding.[29]

Providers may choose not to restrict diet with the exception of vitamin C in large amounts during gFOBT, based on a meta-analysis that showed no difference in positivity rates with restriction of diet.[30] False-negative results are possible with consumption of large amounts of vitamin C (>250 mg/day) during the gFOBT.[31] Single digital gFOBT is not a recommended mode of CRC screening. Sensitivity is enhanced with sampling of multiple stool specimens.[32] Three successive stool specimens (applying 2 samples for each card per specimen) is the recommended method of performing gFOBT.

### FITs

Newer FITs have been developed to address most of the deficits of traditional gFOBTs. In FIT, an intact globin portion of human hemoglobin is detected using a reaction that uses monoclonal or polyclonal antibodies. If blood is present in the stool specimen, the labeled antibody attaches to its antigens (globin protein), creating a positive test result. No dietary modification or medication restrictions are required during FIT because this test does not react with nonhuman hemoglobin or vegetable peroxidase. FIT is also more specific for lower GI bleeding from the colon and rectum because FIT detects the globin portion of hemoglobin, which does not survive passage through the upper GI tract.[33] Several studies examined potential benefit of FIT over traditional gFOBT and reported FIT to have more sensitivity and specificity compared with traditional gFOBT in detecting CRC, particularly advanced adenomas and rectal cancers.[34] Fecal samples should be sent for laboratory evaluation in less than 5 days. Delay between fecal sampling and delivery at the laboratory of 5 days or more produces false-negative results for detecting advanced adenomas and possibly stage 1 CRC.[35] Although immunochemical tests are more expensive compared with traditional gFOBT, FIT might still be cost-effective secondary to its increased specificity and sensitivity, resulting in fewer colonoscopies for false-positive results.

Although FIT has advantages over gFOBT, both tests have similar goals. Some adenomas may bleed infrequently, making the potential for CRC prevention through adenoma detection and removal lower with FIT and all FOBT methods compared with endoscopic screening modalities.

### Fecal DNA tests

Fecal DNA tests detect abnormal DNA shed in the feces of people with colorectal neoplasm. Newer fecal DNA tests are being developed to detect precancerous and early stage neoplasms, which bleed infrequently but shed abnormal DNA continuously. One study compared stool DNA testing with traditional gFOBT for CRC screening in 2507 adults aged 50 years. A follow-up colonoscopy is performed in all participants. Even although both tests missed many advanced polyps and cancers detected by colonoscopy, the stool DNA test was shown to be more sensitive compared with traditional gFOBT in detecting colorectal neoplastic lesions.[36] Specimens to test for abnormal stool DNA should include an entire bowel movement with a minimum weight of 30 g of stool, delivered to the laboratory with an ice pack. The test is expensive compared with traditional gFOBT. Limited data on screening populations result in difficulty determining effective screening intervals using this procedure.

### Flexible Sigmoidoscopy

A flexible sigmoidoscope is 60-cm long and is an effective tool that can be used by an experienced clinician to accurately evaluate the distal colon and perform a biopsy or remove a lesion if it is identified during the procedure. Decrease in CRC-related mortality by flexible sigmoidoscopy screening was noted in a randomized trial of 55,736 patients aged 55 to 64 years in which subjects were randomized to no screening versus 1-time flexible sigmoidoscopy screening with or without a single round of FOBT.[37]

Several cohort and case-control studies have reported a 60% to 85% reduction in mortality from distal cancer. Selby and colleagues[38] reported that screening proctosigmoidoscopy in a large health maintenance organization reduced mortality from large bowel cancer by approximately 60%. Newcomb and colleagues[39] reported a significant reduction in mortality from cancers within the reach of the sigmoidoscope. Minimal patient preparation is needed compared with colonoscopy, and sedation is not necessary. The major complication of sigmoidoscopy is perforation. The risk of perforation increases in women and older patients but the risk is less compared with colonoscopy.[40] The primary disadvantage of flexible sigmoidoscopy is that it is unable to detect lesions that are beyond the reach of the instrument. Approximately 40% of all CRCs arise proximal to the splenic flexure and approximately 75% of these individuals do not have a neoplasm distal to the splenic flexure. The flexible sigmoidoscopic examination is therefore normal in approximately 30% of patients with CRC.[41] This risk is higher in women secondary to increased frequency of proximal colon lesions.[42] Follow-up colonoscopy may be beneficial if a large adenoma (>1.0 cm) or a tubulovillous/villous adenoma or multiple adenomas are detected in sigmoidoscopy.[43]

### Optical Colonoscopy

Colonoscopy has been increasingly advocated as a CRC screening strategy because of the possibility of visualizing the entire colon mucosa and removing or performing a biopsy of any identified lesions during the procedure. CRC incidence and mortality have been lowered by screening colonoscopy in several case-control and cohort studies in average-risk adults.[44,45] Colonoscopy was also shown to have a higher sensitivity compared with sigmoidoscopy, especially in detecting proximal colon adenomatous polyps.[46]

The US National Polyp Study provides significant supportive evidence that colonoscopic polypectomy provides an effective secondary prevention of CRC.[47] A population-based retrospective analysis of 35,975 people showed that negative colonoscopy is associated with decreased incidence of CRC for the next 10 years.[48] Meticulous bowel preparation is necessary before the procedure for successful visualization of the entire mucosa during colonoscopy. Patients must be given detailed written instructions on bowel preparation before the procedure according to their learning needs. Colonoscopy is expensive and the patient requires sedation during the procedure. Major complications with colonoscopy are bleeding and perforation. Several factors have been shown to increase the incidence of complications with the procedure including increasing age, association of comorbidities, performance of polypectomy during the procedure, and decreased expertise of the performer.[49,50]

### Virtual Colonoscopy (CTC)

Virtual colonoscopy obtains several, thin-slice computerized tomographic figures of the bowel mucosa in 2 and 3 dimensions for interpretation. Although CTC has decreased efficacy in detecting smaller lesions (2–10 mm), it has been shown to have an equivalent efficacy to optical colonoscopy for the detection of colorectal lesions larger than 10 mm in asymptomatic average-risk adults.[51,52] Meticulous bowel preparation similar to that needed for optical colonoscopy is needed before the procedure. The advantages of CTC over optical colonoscopy are that it is noninvasive and no sedation is needed, so the patient can return to their daily activities after the procedure. The major disadvantage of virtual colonoscopy is that abnormal results need to be followed up by optical colonoscopy for removal, biopsy, and tissue identification.

### DCBE

A DCBE is a procedure in which radiographs of the entire colon are taken after coating the colonic mucosa with an enema of barium and inserting air through the rectum to distend the colon. Use of this test as an optional CRC surveillance technique is based on the reported sensitivity of 80% to 95% and specificity of approximately 90% in identifying lesions. However, studies have reported that DCBE misses more than 20% of adenomas compared with colonoscopy.[53] In the National Polyp Study, barium enema was reported to miss approximately 50% of adenomas larger than 1 cm.[54] Meticulous bowel preparation similar to that needed for optical colonoscopy is needed before the procedure. The advantages of DCBE over optical colonoscopy are that it is noninvasive and no sedation is needed. Besides low sensitivity, a major disadvantage of DCBE is the need for follow-up colonoscopy to remove or perform a biopsy of any lesions detected during DCBE (**Table 4**).

## SCREENING RECOMMENDATIONS

The optimal strategy for CRC screening continues to be evaluated. Based on the available data, practice guidelines have been developed by several organizations. The US Preventive Services Task Force (USPSTF), Multi-Society Task Force, and American College of Gastroenterology are among several organizations that have developed recommendations for screening, taking into account several factors, including cost-effectiveness and test sensitivity. An overview of recommended guidelines is outlined in the following sections.

### Recommendations for Individuals at Average Risk for CRC

Average-risk patients are 50 years and older with no risk factors for CRC other than their age.

## USPSTF GUIDELINES

These guidelines, based on a systematic literature review, found 3 screening strategies using high-sensitivity FOBT, flexible sigmoidoscopy, or colonoscopy to have equivalent efficacy.

**Table 4**
**Screening modalities advantages and disadvantages**

| Screening Modality | Advantages | Disadvantages |
|---|---|---|
| gFOBT | Easily available, affordable and accessible<br>Patient can collect samples at home with no complications | Test detects polyps or cancers only if they are bleeding<br>False-positive results are possible with FOBT<br>Positive results have to be followed by a confirmatory test like colonoscopy |
| FSIG | Minimal preparation of colon and fewer complications compared with colonoscopy<br>Mortality is decreased by detecting or removing cancers in rectum and distal colon<br>May be performed by a trained primary care physician in office without need for sedation | Colonic lesions present beyond the reach of sigmoidoscope (beyond splenic flexure) will be missed resulting in false-negative report<br>Colonic perforation may result in some patients with increasing age<br>Depending on lesion noted further evaluation of proximal colon with colonoscopy may be needed |
| Colonoscopy | Allows inspection of entire colon and rectum<br>Lesions can be identified and biopsied/removed during the procedure | Meticulous bowel cleansing is needed before the procedure<br>Expensive<br>Sedation is necessary<br>Increased risk of complications like bowel perforation, bleeding |
| DCBE | No sedation is needed<br>Entire colon and rectum can be examined<br>Minimal complications | False-positive and false-negative results are possible<br>No removal or biopsy of lesion is possible if detected during the test<br>Positive results have to be followed by a confirmatory test like colonoscopy |
| FIT | More specific than gFOBT<br>Needs fewer samples (1 or 2 compared with 3 with gFOBT) | Expensive |
| CTC | Noninvasive<br>Entire colon can be examined | Expensive<br>Meticulous bowel cleansing is necessary<br>Optical colonoscopy may be needed after CTC to perform a biopsy or remove the detected lesion |

*Abbreviation:* PCP, primary care physician.

The USPSTF guidelines for average-risk adults aged 50 to 75 years are:

- Annual sensitive FOBT
- Combination of sigmoidoscopy every 5 years, with interval sensitive FOBT every 3 years
- A colonoscopy every 10 years. The Task Force found inadequate evidence to recommend for or against CTC and fecal DNA testing. The USPSTF advises against screening between ages of 76 and 85 years unless there is evidence to

support the need for screening, taking in to consideration previous screening results, existing comorbidities, and individual life expectancy before screening. USPSTF guidelines recommend against screening adults older than 85 years.

## ACS, US MULTI-SOCIETY TASK FORCE ON COLORECTAL CANCER, AND THE AMERICAN COLLEGE OF RADIOLOGY GUIDELINES

Guidelines by a consortium of the ACS, the US Multi-Society Task Force on Colorectal Cancer (MSTF) and the American College of Radiology (ACR) stress prevention as the primary goal of CRC screening, rather than early detection. These guidelines also prefer the tests that are accurate at a single point in time (eg, colonoscopy) rather than screening with repeated testing (eg, annual FOBT). The ACS-MSTF makes a distinction between tests that can identify cancers at an early stage (eg, FOBT) and tests that can also identify precancerous lesions like polyps, leading to cancer prevention (eg, colonoscopy, DCBE, or CTC). These guidelines encourage physicians to educate patients to make an informed choice of their preferred test to improve the probability of occurrence of screening.

The ACS-MSTF recommends initiating screening for CRC in all average-risk individuals aged 50 years and older and stopping screening when life expectancy is less than 10 years. Screening options for prevention and early detection includes tests that visualize the colonic mucosa structurally and can detect early stage colon cancer as well as precancerous lesions:

- A colonoscopy every 10 years
- Flexible sigmoidoscopy every 5 years (procedure must be able to visualize a minimum of 40 cm of bowel)
- Screening every 5 years with CTC; follow-up optical colonoscopy for polypectomy is recommended for patients with a polyp larger than 6 mm
- DCBE every 5 years; if a polyp 6 mm or larger is detected by DCBE, follow-up colonoscopy and polypectomy are recommended.

All these procedures must be performed by specially trained clinicians applying state-of-the-art techniques to improve the quality of CRC screening.

Screening options for early detection only include noninvasive laboratory tests that primarily identify early cancer but have less potential to prevent cancer because they cannot detect precancerous lesions and lesions that do not bleed. If any of the following tests are abnormal, colonoscopy is needed.

- Annual high-sensitivity FOBT
- Annual FIT
- Fecal DNA testing, frequency uncertain.

## AMERICAN COLLEGE OF GASTROENTEROLOGY GUIDELINES

The American College of Gastroenterology (ACG) recommends initiating CRC screening at age 50 years for all average-risk patients except for African Americans. The ACG recommends initiating screening at age 45 years for African Americans because of the high frequency of CRC and a larger incidence of proximal or right-sided colonic lesions in this population. ACG recommends a preferred approach, prioritizing selection of preventive and early detection CRC screening tests listed in the ACS-MSTF guidelines.

Colonoscopy every 10 years is recommended as a preferred test for prevention and early detection.

Annual high-sensitivity FIT is recommended as a preferred test for early detection. If FIT results are abnormal, further investigation is required by a colonoscopy. The ACG recommends offering the screening options to detect early cancer if the patient declines colonoscopy and other alternative CRC prevention tests. The ACG does not recommend a barium enema for CRC screening (**Table 5**).

## Recommendations for Individuals at Increased Risk for CRC

Recommendations for adults at increased and high risk were last updated in 2001, and in 2006, the ACS and the US MSTF issued a joint guideline update for postpolypectomy and post-CRC resection surveillance.

**Table 5**
**Recommended screening strategy for CRC screening in average-risk adults**

| Organization | Age | Recommended Modalities and Intervals |
|---|---|---|
| USPSTF | Start at age 50 y<br>Not recommended between 76 and 85 y unless benefit is greater than risk<br>Stop at the age of 85 y | Annual high-sensitivity FOBT<br>Sigmoidoscopy every 5 y with FOBT every 3 y<br>Colonoscopy every 10 y |
| ACS-MSTF | Start at age 50 y and stop when risk greater than benefit | Preferred<br> Preventive tests:[a]<br>  1. Colonoscopy every 10 y<br>  2. CTC every 5 y<br>  3. Sigmoidoscopy every 5 y<br>  4. DCBE every 5 y<br>Alternative<br> Detection tests:[b]<br>  1. FOBT every year<br>  2. FIT every year<br>  3. Stool DNA (frequency unknown) |
| ACG | Start at age 50 y except in African Americans start at age 45 y | Preventive tests<br> Preferred: Colonoscopy every 10 y<br> Alternate: Sigmoidoscopy every 5 y<br> CTC every 5 y<br>Detection tests:<br> Preferred: FIT every year<br> Alternate: Hemoccult SENSA every year or fecal DNA every 3 y |

5 points for PCP
1. CRC is the second leading cause of cancer-related death in both men and women in the United States
2. Guidelines recommend initiating CRC screening in average-risk patients at age 50 years, but in African Americans at age 45 years
3. It is preferred that an informed decision is made by the patient with the help of their clinician about the type of screening test based on the patient's personal preferences
4. Patients with personal history of chronic ulcerative colitis and Crohn colitis have significant cancer risk 8 years after the onset of pancolitis or 12 to 15 years after the onset of left-sided colitis. Colonoscopy every 1 to 2 years should be performed, with biopsies for dysplasia
5. Counseling to consider genetic testing and early screening recommendations for those with personal or family history of FAP or HNPCC

*Abbreviation:* PCP, primary care physician.
[a] Tests that visualize the colonic mucosa structurally and can detect early stage colon cancer as well as precancerous lesions.
[b] Noninvasive laboratory tests that primarily identify early cancer but have less potential to prevent cancer because they cannot detect precancerous lesions and lesions that do not bleed.

## PATIENTS WITH A FAMILY HISTORY

An individual with CRC or adenomatous polyp in a first-degree relative younger than 60 years or in 2 or more first-degree relatives at any age should have a colonoscopy starting at age 40 years or 10 years before the youngest case in the immediate family and it should be repeated every 5 years. For an individual with CRC or adenomatous polyps in a first-degree relative aged 60 years or older or in 2 second-degree relatives at any age, colonoscopy should begin at age 40 years and at a screening interval based on average-risk individuals.

## PATIENTS WITH HISTORY OF POLYPS AT PREVIOUS COLONOSCOPY

Patients with small rectal hyperplastic polyps should have colonoscopy or other screening options at intervals recommended for average-risk individuals.

- Those with 1 or 2 small tubular adenomas with low-grade dysplasia are recommended to have colonoscopy 3 years after the initial polypectomy. The precise timing within this interval should be based on other clinical factors (such as previous colonoscopy findings, family history, and the preferences of the patient and judgment of the physician).
- Patients with 3 to 10 adenomas or 1 adenoma larger than 1 cm or any adenoma with villous features or high-grade dysplasia should have colonoscopy 3 years after the initial polypectomy. Adenomas must have been completely removed. If the follow-up colonoscopy is normal or shows only 1 or 2 small, tubular adenomas with low-grade dysplasia, then the interval for the subsequent examination should be 5 years.
- A history of more than 10 adenomas on a single examination needs consideration of the possibility of an underlying familial syndrome. Colonoscopy is recommended less than 3 years after the initial polypectomy.
- Patients with sessile adenomas that are removed piecemeal require colonoscopy at 2 to 6 months to verify complete removal. Once complete removal has been established, subsequent surveillance needs to be individualized based on the endoscopist's judgment. Completeness of removal should be based on both endoscopic and pathologic assessments.

## PATIENTS WITH HISTORY OF CRC

Patients with colon and rectal cancer should undergo colonoscopy 3 to 6 months after cancer resection, if no unresectable metastases are found during surgery; alternatively, colonoscopy can be performed intraoperatively in nonobstructive tumors. Patients undergoing curative resection for colon or rectal cancer should have a colonoscopy 1 year after the resection. If the examination performed at 1 year is normal, then the interval before the next subsequent examination should be 5 years. After the examination at 1 year, the intervals before subsequent examinations may be shortened if there is evidence of HNPCC or if adenoma findings warrant earlier colonoscopy. Periodic examination of the rectum for the purpose of identifying local recurrence, usually performed at 3-month to 6-month intervals for the first 2 or 3 years, may be considered after low-anterior resection of rectal cancer.

## RECOMMENDATIONS FOR INDIVIDUALS AT HIGH RISK FOR CRC
### FAP

Individuals with genetic diagnosis of FAP or suspected FAP without genetic testing evidence are recommended to begin screening at age 10 to 12 years with annual

**Table 6**
**Screening modalities for average-risk adults at age 50 years or older (age ≥45 years in African Americans)**

| Modality | Recommendation |
|---|---|
| High-sensitivity gFOBT | USPSTF: annually<br>ACS-MSTF, ACG: annually as an alternative option for patients (see **Table 2** for preferred recommended screening modality) |
| Flexible sigmoidoscopy | USPSTF, ACS-MSTF, ACG: every 5 y |
| Colonoscopy | USPSTF, ACS-MSTF, ACG: every 10 y |
| DCBE | USPSTF: not recommended<br>ACS-MSTF: every 5 y (see **Table 2** for preferred screening modality)<br>ACG: not recommended |
| FIT | USPSTF: annually<br>ACS-MSTF, ACG: annually (see **Table 2** for preferred screening modality) |
| Stool DNA | USPSTF: no recommendation<br>ACS-MSTF: frequency unknown (see **Table 2** for preferred recommended screening modality)<br>ACG: every 3 y (see **Table 2** for preferred recommended screening modality) |
| CTC | USPSTF: no recommendation<br>ACS-MSTF, ACG: every 5 y (see **Table 2** for preferred recommended screening modality) |

flexible sigmoidoscopy to determine if the individual is expressing the genetic abnormality and counseling to consider genetic testing. If the genetic test is positive, colectomy should be considered.

### HNPCC or Lynch Syndrome

Individuals with genetic or clinical diagnosis of HNPCC or those at increased risk of HNPCC should begin screening either at age 20 to 25 years or 10 years before the youngest case in the immediate family. The test of choice is colonoscopy, which should be repeated every 1 to 2 years. Counseling to consider genetic testing is important and should be offered to first-degree relatives of persons with a known inherited MMR gene mutation. It should also be offered when the family mutation is not already known, but 1 of the first 3 of the modified Bethesda criteria is present.

**Maximizing the impact of screening**

Several factors play an important role in improving CRC screening rates and quality including

- Adequate training of clinicians in screening techniques
- Physician advice to patient
- Patient and clinician reminders
- Patient education programs to aid the patient in decision process
- Appropriate monitoring and follow-up
- Outreach activities to enhance awareness of the importance of CRC screening

### IBD

In patients with history of chronic ulcerative colitis, and Crohn colitis, their cancer risk begins to be significant 8 years after the onset of pancolitis or 12 to 15 years after the onset of left-sided colitis. So, colonoscopy every 1 to 2 years should be performed with biopsies for dysplasia. These patients are best referred to a center with experience in the surveillance and management of IBD (**Table 6**).

### REFERENCES

1. Colorectal facts and figures 2008–2010, American Cancer Society. Available at: http://www.cancer.org/acs/groups/content/@nho/documents/document/f861708 finalforwebpdf.pdf. Accessed May 28, 2011.
2. Rebsdorf Pedersen I, Hartvigsen A, Fischer Hansen B, et al. Management of Peutz-Jeghers syndrome. Experience with patients from the Danish Polyposis Register. Int J Colorectal Dis 1994;9:177.
3. Grotsky HW, Rickert RR, Smith WD, et al. Familial juvenile polyposis coli. A clinical and pathologic study of large kindred. Gastroenterology 1982;82:494.
4. Thomas MB, Hoff PM, Wolff RA. Colorectal cancer. In: Kantarjian HM, Wolff RA, Koller CA, editors. MD Anderson Manual of Medical Oncology. Part VI. Gasterointestinal carcinomas. Chapter 16. Available at: http://www.accessmedicine.com/content.aspx?aID=2790218. Accessed May 28, 2011.
5. Winawer SJ, Sherlock P. Colorectal cancer screening. Best Pract Res Clin Gastroenterol 2007;21(6):1031–48.
6. Fuchs CS, Giovannucci EL, Colditz GA, et al. A prospective study of family history and the risk of colorectal cancer. N Engl J Med 1994;331:1669–74.
7. Rex DK. Colorectal disorders. In: Benjamin S, editor. Educational review manual in gastroenterology. New York: Castle Connolly Graduate Medical Publishing; 2000. p. 1–31.
8. National Cancer Institute, US National Institute of Health. Genetic of colorectal cancer (PDQ), Major genetic syndromes. Available at: www.cancer.gov. Accessed July 11, 2010.
9. Mayer R. Neoplastic disorders, oncology and hematology, gastrointestinal tract cancer. Harrison's Principles of Internal Medicine 16/e. McGraw-Hill: Education Customer Services.
10. Utsunomiya J, Gocho H, Miyanaga T, et al. Peutz-Jeghers syndrome: its natural course and management. Johns Hopkins Med J 1975;136:71.
11. Giardiello FM, Brensinger JD, Tersmette AC, et al. Very high risk of cancer in familial Peutz-Jeghers syndrome. Gastroenterology 2000;119:1447.
12. Boardman LA, Thibodeau SN, Schaid DJ, et al. Increased risk for cancer in patients with the Peutz-Jeghers syndrome. Ann Intern Med 1998;128:896.
13. Boardman LA, Pittelkow MR, Couch FJ, et al. Association of Peutz-Jeghers-like mucocutaneous pigmentation with breast and gynecologic carcinomas in women. Medicine (Baltimore) 2000;79:293.
14. Srivatsa PJ, Keeney GL, Podratz KC. Disseminated cervical adenoma malignum and bilateral ovarian sex cord tumors with annular tubules associated with Peutz-Jeghers syndrome. Gynecol Oncol 1994;53:256.
15. Trau H, Schewach-Millet M, Fisher BK, et al. Peutz-Jeghers syndrome and bilateral breast cancer. Cancer 1982;50:788.
16. Wilson DM, Pitts WC, Hintz RL, et al. Testicular tumors with Peutz-Jeghers syndrome. Cancer 1986;57:2238.

17. Chen YM, Ott DJ, Wu WC, et al. Cowden's disease: a case report and literature review. Gastrointest Radiol 1987;12(4):325–9.
18. Cornett PA, Dea TO. Current medical diagnosis and treatment. 14th Edition. McGraw-Hill Companies, Inc; 2010. Chapter 39.
19. Bruckner HW, Pitrelli J, and Merrick M. A24990. Adenocarcinoma of the colon and rectum. Cancer of the colon and rectum Available at: www.ncbi.nlm.nih.gov. Accessed July 11, 2010.
20. Skibber JM, Minsky B, Hoff PM. Cancer of the colon. In: DeVita VT Jr, Hellman S, Rosenberg SA, editors. Principles and practice of oncology. 6th edition. Philadelphia: Lippincott-Raven; 2001. p. 1144–96. From the Textbook of medical oncology, Part VI. Gastrointestinal carcinomas, Chapter 16. Colorectal cancer.
21. Enders GH, El-Deiry WS. E-medicine: GI and colon section; colonic polyps. Disclosures Updated. Available at: http://www.medicine.medscape.com/article/172674-overview. Accessed December 15, 2009.
22. Bond JH. Polyp guideline: diagnosis, treatment, and surveillance for patients with colorectal polyps. Practice parameters committee of the american college of gastroenterology. Am J Gastroenterol 2000;95(11):3053–63.
23. Heitman SJ, Ronksley PE, Hilsden RJ, et al. Prevalence of adenomas and colorectal cancer in average risk individuals: a systematic review and meta-analysis. Clin Gastroenterol Hepatol 2009;7:1272.
24. Cappell MS. Pathophysiology, clinical presentation, and management of colon cancer. Gastroenterol Clin North Am 2008;37(1):1–24.
25. O'Connell JB, Maggard MA, Ko CY. Colon cancer survival rates with the new American Joint Committee on Cancer sixth edition staging. J Natl Cancer Inst 2004;96(19):1420–5.
26. Allison JE. A comparison of fecal occult-blood tests for colorectal-cancer screening. N Engl J Med 1996;334(3):155–9.
27. Mandel JS, Church TR, Bond JH, et al. The effect of fecal occult-blood screening on the incidence of colorectal cancer. N Engl J Med 2000;343(22):1603–7.
28. Hewitson P, Glasziou P, Irwig L, et al. Screening for colorectal cancer using the faecal occult blood test, Hemoccult. Cochrane Database Syst Rev 2007;1: CD001216.
29. Griffith CD. False-negative results of Hemoccult test in colorectal cancer. Br Med J (Clin Res Ed) 1981;283(6289):472.
30. Pignone M. Meta-analysis of dietary restriction during fecal occult blood testing. Eff Clin Pract 2001;4(4):150–6.
31. Helen F. Researchers suggest relaxation of food guidelines before colon cancer test. Lancet 2001;358(9282):645.
32. Collins JF, Veterans Affairs Cooperative Study #380 Group. Accuracy of screening for fecal occult blood on a single stool sample obtained by digital rectal examination: a comparison with recommended sampling practice. Ann Intern Med 2005;142(2):81–5.
33. Rockey DC, Auslander A, Greenberg PD. Detection of upper gastrointestinal blood with fecal occult blood tests. Am J Gastroenterol 1999;94:344–50.
34. Guittet L. Comparison of a guaiac and an immunochemical faecal occult blood test for the detection of colonic lesions according to lesion type and location. Br J Cancer 2009;100(8):1230–5.
35. van Rossum LG. False negative fecal occult blood tests due to delayed sample return in colorectal cancer screening. Int J Cancer 2009;125(4):746–50.
36. Imperiale TF. Fecal DNA versus fecal occult blood for colorectal-cancer screening in an average-risk population. N Engl J Med 2004;351(26):2704–14.

37. Hoff G. Risk of colorectal cancer seven years after flexible sigmoidoscopy screening. BMJ 2009;338:b1846.
38. Selby JV, Friedman GD, Quesenberry CP, et al. A case-control study of screening sigmoidoscopy and mortality from colorectal cancer. N Engl J Med 1992;326:653.
39. Newcomb PA, Norfleet RG, Storer BE, et al. Screening sigmoidoscopy and colorectal cancer mortality. J Natl Cancer Inst 1992;84(20):1572–5.
40. Anderson ML. Endoscopic perforation of the colon: lessons from a 10-year study. Am J Gastroenterol 2000;95(12):3418–22.
41. Waye JD, Lewis BS, Frankel A, et al. Small colon polyps. Am J Gastroenterol 1988;83:110, 116, 120, 128.
42. Schoenfeld P. Colonoscopic screening of average-risk women for colorectal neoplasia. N Engl J Med 2005;352(20):2061–8.
43. Atkin WS. Long-term risk of colorectal cancer after excision of rectosigmoid adenomas. N Engl J Med 1992;326(10):658–62.
44. Kahi CJ. Effect of screening colonoscopy on colorectal cancer incidence and mortality. Clin Gastroenterol Hepatol 2009;7(7):770–5 [quiz: 711].
45. Baxter NN. Association of colonoscopy and death from colorectal cancer. Ann Intern Med 2009;150(1):1–8.
46. Lieberman DA. Screening for colon malignancy with colonoscopy. Am J Gastroenterol 1991;86(8):946–51.
47. Winawer SJ, Zauber AG, Ho MN, et al; The National Polyp Study Workgroup. Prevention of colorectal cancer by colonoscopic polypectomy. N Engl J Med 1993;329(27):1977–81.
48. Singh H, Turner D, Xue L, et al. Risk of developing colorectal cancer following a negative colonoscopy examination: evidence for a 10-year interval between colonoscopies. JAMA 2006;295(20):2366–73.
49. Rabeneck L. Bleeding and perforation after outpatient colonoscopy and their risk factors in usual clinical practice. Gastroenterology 2008;135(6):1899–906, e1.
50. Warren JL. Adverse events after outpatient colonoscopy in the Medicare population. Ann Intern Med 2009;150(12):849–57, W152.
51. Pickhardt PJ. Computed tomographic virtual colonoscopy to screen for colorectal neoplasia in asymptomatic adults. N Engl J Med 2003;349(23):2191–200.
52. Johnson CD. Accuracy of CT colonography for detection of large adenomas and cancers. N Engl J Med 2008;359(12):1207–17.
53. Toma J. Rates of new or missed colorectal cancer after barium enema and their risk factors: a population-based study. Am J Gastroenterol 2008;103(12):3142–8.
54. Winawer SJ. A comparison of colonoscopy and double-contrast barium enema for surveillance after polypectomy. National Polyp Study Work Group. N Engl J Med 2000;342(24):1766–72.

# Diagnostic Approach to the Patient with Jaundice

James Winger, MD, CAQ*, Aaron Michelfelder, MD

KEYWORDS

• Jaundice • Bilirubin • Liver disease • Cholestasis

Jaundice is a yellow staining of skin, sclera, and mucous membranes caused by the bile pigment bilirubin, and is a common presentation of hepatobiliary disease.[1] Serum bilirubin levels are reflective of the heme load imparted to the circulation via destruction of erythrocytes or hematoma reabsorption, the ability of the hepatocyte to absorb and process bilirubin, and the normal functioning of the biliary drainage system that transports bile to the duodenum. Disruption of any of these stages may produce hyperbilirubinemia and a clinical picture of jaundice. Hyperbilirubinemia may be characterized as either unconjugated or conjugated, depending on which fraction of bilirubin is predominant. Together with historical features and findings on examination, patterns of bilirubin fractionation suggest pathologic categories to health care providers and thus this is where the workup of the jaundiced adult patient begins.[2]

## HEME METABOLISM, BILIRUBIN FORMATION, AND EXCRETION

Heme is liberated during the destruction of senescent erythrocytes by monocytic macrophages in the spleen and bone marrow, as well as Kupffer cells within the liver. An additional 20% of the daily production results from breakdown of heme proteins such as cytochrome P450 isoenzymes, myoglobin, and others.[3] Heme oxygenase is the enzyme responsible for catabolism of the heme molecule. This enzyme is phylogenetically ancient and is highly conserved from algae to humans,[4] likely because of its anti-inflammatory, anti-apoptotic, and anti-proliferative actions. Enzymatic cleavage of heme at the $\alpha$ carbon bridge yields biliverdin, which is rapidly converted to bilirubin by biliverdin reductase, as well as ferrous iron ($Fe^{2+}$) and carbon monoxide (CO).[5] This action produces nearly 300 mg of bilirubin daily in healthy individuals.[6]

Unconjugated bilirubin (UCB) is a biplanar tetrapyrrole consisting of 2 rigid, planar dipyrrole units at approximately a 90 degree angle to each other.[7] In the plasma, the molecule exists as a pair of optical enantiomers. This tertiary structure leads to

Department of Family Medicine, Loyola Stritch School of Medicine, 2160 South First Avenue, Building 54, Room 260, Maywood, IL 60153, USA
* Corresponding author.
E-mail address: jwinger@lumc.edu

Prim Care Clin Office Pract 38 (2011) 469–482
doi:10.1016/j.pop.2011.05.004
0095-4543/11/$ – see front matter © 2011 Elsevier Inc. All rights reserved.

primarycare.theclinics.com

its poor aqueous solubility and it is tightly bound to albumin in the circulation.[7,8] Albumin-bound serum UCB is a powerful free-radical scavenger, with antioxidant as well as cytoprotective properties.[8-12]

The splenic vein transports UCB-rich blood to the portal circulation. After entering the hepatic sinusoid, bilirubin dissociates from albumin in the space of Disse.[13] Hepatocellular uptake of bilirubin is mediated by active transport membrane proteins as well as facilitated diffusion via chemical and electrochemical gradients.[7] Organic anion transport proteins (OATPs) on the basolateral surface of hepatocytes are presumed to facilitate transmembrane passage.[14] Cytosolic bilirubin is bound to one of two stabilizing proteins and is transported to the endoplasmic reticulum, where it is conjugated with a glucuronic acid by a UDP-glucuronyl transferase (UGT), which confers greater aqueous solubility on the compound molecule via a conformational change and exposure of multiple hydroxyl groups.[15] The conjugated bilirubin is subsequently actively exported via an ATP-dependent mechanism through the canalicular membrane of hepatocyte and into the bile.[16] Canalicular multispecific organic anion transporter (cMOAT) proteins are responsible for transcanalicular membrane transport. In the biliary tree, bilirubin is bound primarily to biliary mixed micelles. These drain down the biliary tree and are stored between meals in the gallbladder.

In the intestinal lumen, deconjugation and further reduction occur via intestinal and bacterial enzymes, respectively. This produces unconjugated bilirubin as well as urobilinogens and the former may then be reabsorbed by enterocytes and return to the liver via the enterohepatic circulation.[3]

## DIAGNOSTIC APPROACH TO HYPERBILIRUBINEMIA
### History and Physical Examination

A carefully performed history and physical examination usually indicate whether jaundice is hepatobiliary in origin or secondary to another disease process, such as hemolysis or overwhelming infection.[17] The clinical evaluation is unlikely to miss significant jaundice-producing disease.[18] As with most illness, a thorough history will suggest a differential diagnosis. Jaundiced patients may present with myriad chief concerns. Patients with acute illness, which is frequently infection, may present with fever, chills, abdominal pain, or influenza-like symptoms. A diagnosis of acute viral hepatitis is suggested by a compatible medical history of typical prodromal symptoms in a patient who has jaundice with fever and tender hepatomegaly. Those patients with noninfectious causes of jaundice may note weight loss, pruritus, or simply color change of their skin, mucous membranes, or sclera. The patient's history may also hold clues suggesting alcoholic hepatitis as well as drug-induced or toxin-induced hepatocellular injury.[17] Rarely, patients present with jaundice as well as extrahepatic manifestation of liver disease, such as polyarthralgias or pyoderma gangrenosum.[2]

The diagnosis of jaundice caused by extrahepatic biliary obstruction can be made with 90% accuracy from results of only the medical history, physical examination, and routine laboratory tests.[18] The physical examination should focus on general nutritional status as well as signs of liver disease, such as spider angiomata, gynecomastia, testicular atrophy, and palmar erythema.[2] Acute onset of right upper quadrant abdominal pain, fever, nausea and vomiting are typical of choledocholithiasis, and may be accompanied by a classic description of biliary colic. Cholangitis may be described by these same symptoms in addition to hypotension and mental status changes, known as Reynolds pentad. Inspiratory arrest upon deep palpation of the right upper quadrant (Murphy sign) is consistent with cholecystitis. A palpable, nontender gallbladder may indicate malignant obstruction, especially when combined with painless jaundice.[17]

### Laboratory Evaluation

The goal of serum testing in a jaundiced patient is to determine the pattern of disease process (prehepatic, hepatocellular, obstructive) that may be causing hyperbilirubinemia: determinations of relative erythrocyte number/hemoglobin mass and indications of hepatocellular synthetic function, dysfunction and levels and fractions of serum bilirubin are used to classify these patterns.[19] Initial testing should include a complete blood count (CBC), direct and total bilirubin fractionation, aspartate aminotransferase (AST), alanine aminotransferase (ALT), γ-glutamyl transpeptidase (GGT), alkaline phosphatase, albumin, total protein, and prothrombin time.[2,20,21]

A review of these common and useful serum tests in the setting of jaundice will permit more judicious and appropriate use of testing, as well as a deeper understanding of the significance of abnormal results. A CBC is useful in detecting decreased hemoglobin mass. In addition, a peripheral blood smear may show schistocytes, which indicate intravascular hemolysis. Tests of hepatocyte integrity include the aminotransferases ALT and AST. These hepatocellular enzymes participate in production and interconversion of amino acids as well as gluconeogenesis.[21] ALT is more specific for liver parenchymal damage, as it is found primarily in the liver. AST is also found in skeletal and cardiac muscle, kidneys, brain, and other tissues. The sensitivity of elevated transaminases indicating hepatocellular damage may be limited in chronic liver disease when the amount of uninjured liver parenchyma is limited. GGT is found in hepatocytes and biliary epithelial cells.[22] It may be used in a similar manner as the hepatocellular transaminases; however, its utility is limited owing to poor specificity. Elevated levels may be present in pancreatic disease, myocardial infarction, renal failure, chronic obstructive pulmonary disease, diabetes, and alcoholism.[23]

Alkaline phosphatase originates primarily in liver as well as bone tissue, and different isoenzymes predominate depending on the tissue of origin.[24] It is also expressed constitutively in tissues such as kidney, intestine, placenta, and leukocytes. Elevation may be physiologic or pathologic.[21] Alkaline phosphatase is present in the bile canalicular membrane, and thus in liver disease is a marker for cholestasis; as bile obstruction progresses, levels of this enzyme rise to several times greater than normal.[25]

Although commonly referred to as "liver function tests," the previously mentioned serum enzymes are more specifically markers for liver dysfunction, as they have little reflection on the synthetic or metabolic functions of the hepatocyte.[20] Examples of serum tests that do reflect this synthetic function include albumin, total protein, prothrombin time, and international normalized ratio (INR).[26] The liver is the production site of serum albumin and approximately 10 g is synthesized and secreted daily; thus, decreased levels of albumin may be reflective of decreased liver function. Albumin levels decrease when cirrhosis occurs and have prognostic values in these patients.[21] Clotting factors I, II, V, VII, and X are also produced in the liver and decreased levels and prolonged INR may reflect this decreased function. It is clear, however, that a decrease in albumin and prolongation of INR must be considered in the total context of the patient, as neither is specific for liver pathology and may be altered in such disease states as nephrotic syndrome, protein-losing enteropathy, vitamin K deficiency, malnutrition, and other disease states.[27]

### Radiographic Evaluation

A rational imaging strategy for the jaundiced patient reflects the fact that imaging is important only in those patients hypothesized to have obstructive jaundice.[28] Methods currently used in the evaluation of the jaundiced patient include ultrasound (US), computed tomography (CT), radionuclide cholescintigraphy (CS), and magnetic resonance imaging (MRI). US is the least-invasive and lowest-cost imaging technique available for radiographic evaluation of obstructive jaundice.[28] With a sensitivity of approximately 55% to 95% and specificity of 71% to 96%, US can detect the dilated biliary ducts indicative of extrahepatic biliary obstruction.[29] However, US is less able to accurately diagnose the site and cause of obstruction than other modalities. CT demonstrates a sensitivity of 74% to 96% and specificity of 90% to 94% in determining the presence of biliary obstruction, and demonstrates an increased ability to indicate the site and cause of obstruction.[30] Because CS is unreliable in differentiating intrahepatic cholestasis from obstructive jaundice, its use is no longer routinely advocated in the evaluation of jaundice.[29] Plain MRI demonstrates similar advantages to CT, without the risks of radiation. MR cholangiopancreatography (MRCP) has been shown to be useful in depicting the complex anatomy of the biliary and pancreatic ductal trees. MRCP is the most sensitive of noninvasive methods for the detection of ductal calculi.[31]

## INTERVENTIONAL PROCEDURES

When noninterventional methods fail to sufficiently diagnose the cause and/or site of biliary obstruction, interventional procedures may be used. Transhepatic cholangiopancreatography (PTC) allows detailed visualization of the intrahepatic and extrahepatic biliary tree.[28] The complication rate is 3% to 5% and the procedure is more expensive than either CT or US. Endoscopic retrograde cholangiopancreatography (ERCP) has replaced PTC in most institutions for the evaluation of obstructive jaundice.[32] Its complication rate is lower or equal to that of PTC and it provides a greater range and ease of therapeutic options for relief of obstruction, including internal biliary stent placement.[33] Finally, liver biopsy provides information on the architecture of the liver and is used mostly for determining prognosis.[2]

The American College of Radiology has developed recommendations regarding the appropriateness of imaging tests in the setting of likely obstructive jaundice.[28] These depend largely on the pretest probabilities of a patient having mechanical obstruction, of that obstruction being malignant in nature, and of the likelihood of attempted resection should a malignancy be discovered. With a high likelihood of benign biliary obstruction with no risk factors for sclerosing cholangitis, screening with noninvasive imaging (US, CT, MR) is indicated. In patients with acute presentation of jaundice and fever, or patients with a high likelihood of sclerosing cholangitis (eg, patients with inflammatory bowel disease), direct cholangiopancreatography with ERCP is primarily indicated; PTC is an alternative if ERCP is technically infeasible or not available. If ERCP is unsuccessful or inadequate, MRCP is the most sensitive modality to detect the presence of biliary ductal calculi.[33]

Patients with a high likelihood of malignant biliary obstruction may present with insidious development of jaundice and constitutional symptoms. Initial approach in this category of patients depends extensively on the philosophy of the surgeon, as imaging strategies are primarily descriptions of the obstructing mass and its surrounding anatomy. Perioperative staging is required at institutions where curative resection is attempted, although instances in which resection is not attempted may require palliative stent placement with ERCP.

Patients with a low likelihood of mechanical biliary obstruction require either CT or US as a first-line test owing to their lowered cost, low complication rates, and patient convenience. Ultrasonography is less expensive, but CT results in fewer unsatisfactory studies. In the clinical situation of indeterminate likelihood of obstruction, the workup should be geared toward the dominant symptom and may encompass any number of several modalities.

## LIVER BIOPSY

Percutaneous liver biopsy carries a small but real risk of further injury and therefore it is crucial that the information gleaned from tissue diagnosis alters the patient's treatment or gives information about prognosis that is more important than the inherent risk.[34] Studies have indicated that histologic findings after biopsy may alter care in only a third of cases.[35]

Following the previously described evaluation pathway, a clinical picture of conjugated (direct) hyperbilirubinemia, unconjugated (indirect) hyperbilirubinemia, or normal bilirubin levels will be revealed. Specific entities producing each of these clinical scenarios are described in the following sections.

## UNCONJUGATED HYPERBILIRUBINEMIA

In general, disease states that cause unconjugated hyperbilirubinemia are those that (1) increase erythrocyte destruction or turnover, (2) impair uptake of bilirubin into the hepatocyte, or (3) feature impaired hepatic bilirubin conjugation (**Box 1**). As this article focuses on adult medicine, pediatric conditions, such as neonatal jaundice and severe genetic hyperbilirubinemias with presentation early in life such as Crigler-Najjar disease are discussed elsewhere.

Conditions that produce increased hemolysis owing to constitutive changes in the erythrocyte, such as glucose-6-phosphate dehydrogenase deficiency or hereditary spherocytosis, may produce a rapid, large load of unconjugated bilirubin that may briefly overwhelm hepatic conjugation abilities, producing a transient jaundice.[36] Hemolytic jaundice, hematoma resorption jaundice, or that produced after blood transfusion is caused by a similar mechanism. Conditions, such as thalassemias or cobalamin, folate, and iron deficiency, producing ineffective erythropoiesis may predispose erythrocytes to early destruction and thus increase serum unconjugated bilirubin.

Hepatic uptake of unconjugated bilirubin may be impaired in several disease states, such as congestive heart failure, sepsis, and administration of contrast agents or certain drugs (rifampicin, rifamycin, probenecid, and others). OATP transmembrane

---

**Box 1**
**Causes of unconjugated hyperbilirubinemia**

Gilbert syndrome

Neonatal jaundice

Hemolysis

Blood transfusion (hemolysis)

Resorption of a large hematoma

Shunt hyperbilirubinemia

Crigler-Najjar syndrome

Ineffective erythropoiesis

*Data from* Green RM, Flam S. AGA technical review on the evaluation of liver chemistry tests. Gastroenterology 2002;123:1367–84.

organic anion shuttling has been demonstrated to be decreased in lipo-polysaccharide-treated animals, indicating a likely mechanism for sepsis-related decreased hepatocyte bilirubin uptake.[14]

Asymptomatic screening of healthy populations for abnormalities in serum bilirubin will reveal approximately 5% of individuals with elevated isolated unconjugated bilirubin characteristic of Gilbert syndrome.[37] This syndrome is a result of a polymorphism in the bilirubin UGT gene, resulting in decreased protein expression and enzyme activity and subsequent impaired ability to conjugate bilirubin. Given its high prevalence and benign nature, this condition is best viewed as a variant of normal, rather than a disease state, and in fact, the antioxidant benefits of mildly elevated bilirubin may have cardio-protective effects.[38] In asymptomatic individuals with incidentally discovered mildly elevated unconjugated hyperbilirubinemia (<4 mg/dL), confirmation of normal serum liver chemistries is usually sufficient to diagnose this common condition.[39]

## CHOLESTATIC SYNDROMES

A patient with a cholestatic liver biochemical profile is usually suffering from 1 of 2 categories of pathology: disease of the liver parenchyma or biliary obstruction (intra-hepatic or extrahepatic).[40] The clinical evaluation in these cases should focus on distinguishing between hepatocellular, intrahepatic, and extrahepatic causes of liver disease (**Table 1**).

## INTRAHEPATIC CHOLESTATIC CONDITIONS PRODUCING CONJUGATED HYPERBILIRUBINEMIA

Cholestatic conditions are characterized by impaired hepatobiliary production and excretion of bile, thus leading to bile components entering the circulation. Drugs,

| Table 1 Differential diagnosis of cholestatic liver disease | |
|---|---|
| **Intrahepatic Cholestasis** | **Extrahepatic Biliary Obstruction** |
| Primary biliary cirrhosis | Intraductal obstruction/abnormalities |
| Primary sclerosing cholangitis | Gallstones |
| Drug toxicity | Surgical strictures |
| Hepatocellular diseases | Infections |
|   Alcoholic hepatitis |   HIV/AIDS (*Cryptosporidium*, CMV) |
|   Viral hepatitis (B, C) | Malignancy |
|   Autoimmune hepatitis | Malformation (atresia) |
| Sarcoidosis | Cholangiocarcinoma |
| Postoperative state | Extrinsic compression |
| Parenteral nutrition | Malignancy (pancreatic, metastasis) |
| Idiopathic adult ductopenia | Pancreatitis |
| Dubin-Johnson syndrome | Lymphoma |
| Rotor syndrome | |
| Recurrent (benign) intrahepatic cholestasis | |
| Cholestatic jaundice of pregnancy | |

*Abbreviations:* AIDS, acquired immunodeficiency syndrome; CMV, cytomegalovirus; HIV, human immunodeficiency virus.

*Data from* Pasha TM, Lindor KD. Diagnosis and therapy of cholestatic liver disease. Med Clin North Am 1996;80(5):995–1019.

toxins, autoimmune conditions, hepatocellular diseases, and other conditions can cause cholestasis. Cholestatic pathology may be divided into classes of hepatocellular, small ductal, and large ductal for classification and description purposes. Approximately 5% of all cells in the liver are cholangiocytes: ciliated cells lining the biliary duct system. Integrated prosecretory and antisecretory signals govern the transport of bile acids to the canaliculus in a regulated manner. Cholangiocytes lining larger ducts are primarily involved in secretion, whereas those in smaller ducts are related to proliferation and inflammatory response; it is these latter cells that begin and maintain the process of hepatic fibrosis. Here several cholestatic conditions that produce conjugated hyperbilirubinemia are reviewed.

Alcohol must always be considered when the etiology of cholestasis is evaluated. This syndrome is characterized by marked, tender hepatomegaly and biochemical evidence of hepatocellular failure, along with a supportive history of ethanol ingestion and possibly fever owing to the systemic inflammatory response syndrome mediated by Kupffer cell activation. Jaundice may be present in 38% to 100% of patients with alcoholic liver disease, regardless of liver histology.[41] Ethanol metabolism in susceptible patients produces reactive oxygen species that result in apoptosis or necrosis and hepatocellular death. Autoantibodies to neoantigens composed of ethanol metabolites conjugated to cellular proteins provide targets for immune system response. Thus, immunologic and nonimmunologic pathology induces injury in alcoholic cholestasis.[42]

Dubin-Johnson and Rotor syndromes are the familial conjugated hyperbilirubinemias, and patients follow a relatively benign course with no decrease in life expectancy. Dubin-Johnson syndrome is caused by a recessive defect in a cMOAT protein responsible for conjugated bilirubin efflux from the hepatocyte into the canaliculus.[43] Rotor syndrome is associated with impaired hepatocyte bilirubin storage capacity. Both produce an isolated hyperbilirubinemia without alterations in other hepatic enzymes. Identification, but not differentiation, of these mostly benign syndromes is important for the purposes of prognosis and avoidance of expensive and invasive testing.

A severe cholestatic syndrome may accompany the acute phase of viral hepatitis, usually caused by the hepatitides A, C, or E, although Epstein-Barr virus and others have been reported to cause such a clinical presentation.[44–47] Acute hepatitis C infection usually causes jaundice in only 10% to 20% of patients; however, in intravenous drug users it may be as high as 70%.[45]

Decompensated liver cirrhosis owing to alcohol or hepatitis C may account for a cholestatic syndrome characterized by jaundice, ascites, variceal hemorrhage, and encephalopathy.[48]

Wilson disease is characterized by copper deposition into the liver parenchyma, hepatocellular dysfunction, and jaundice.[49] Rarely, other infiltrative disease of the hepatic parenchyma, such as sarcoidosis, amyloidosis, α1 antitrypsin deficiency, lymphoma, hepatocellular carcinoma or metastatic malignancy, tuberculosis or fungal infection, may cause mild elevations in bilirubin and a cholestatic syndrome.[50,51]

Given the liver's role in drug metabolism, toxicity is a common cause of acute hepatocellular injury and may be caused by myriad different compounds (**Box 2**) and in fact may cause several different scenarios of hepatic injury and dysfunction. Only a select few drugs causing liver injury have a predictable, dose-dependent toxic mechanism of action, the most commonly recognizable being acetaminophen.[52] Among patients with drug-induced liver injury (DILI), 10% exhibit jaundice.[53] Even patients with clinically significant liver injury and jaundice have a generally favorable prognosis; one

| Box 2 |
| Medications that can cause elevations of the serum bilirubin |
| Anabolic steroids |
| Gold salts |
| Allopurinol |
| Imipramine |
| Amoxicillin-clavulanic acid |
| Indinavir |
| Captopril |
| Iprindole |
| Carbamazepine |
| Nevirapine |
| Chlorpropamide |
| Methyltestosterone |
| Cyproheptadine |
| Methylenedioxymethamphetamine (MDMA) |
| Diltiazem |
| Oxaprozin |
| Erythromycin |
| Pizotyline |
| Estrogens |
| Quinidine |
| Floxuridine |
| Tolbutamide |
| Flucloxacillin |
| Total parenteral hyperalimentation |
| Fluphenazine |
| Trimethoprim-sulfamethoxazole |

*Data from* Green RM, Flam S. AGA technical review on the evaluation of liver chemistry tests. Gastroenterology 2002;123:1367–84.

series of 784 patients with DILI demonstrated that 90.8% of patients with jaundice recovered.[54]

On the contrary, Hy's rule indicates that the combination of nonobstructive hyperbilirubinemia and signs of significant hepatocellular injury, as represented by an ALT rise to greater than or equal to 3 times the upper limit of normal (ULN) and a serum bilirubin greater than or equal to 2 times the ULN, carries a poor prognosis and results in a mortality rate of 10% to 50%.[55] DILI accounts for only 5% to 10% of hospitalized patients with jaundice, so this is not an overwhelmingly common cause of jaundice, although it is the most common cause of fulminant hepatic failure in the United States and Europe.[52]

Postoperative cholestatic jaundice is a common hepatocellular complication of many types of surgery. Cardiogenic, noncardiogenic shock and respiratory failure are common causes of hepatocellular necrosis in this setting.[56]

Total parenteral nutrition (TPN) is associated with cholestasis via an unclear mechanism. This picture is more common in younger patients, whereas in adults, a steatohepatitis usually occurs. Given that TPN is administered in individuals who are already quite sick, it may be clinically difficult to distinguish TPN-related cholestasis from that caused by other syndromes, such as sepsis. Both taurine deficiency and lithocholic acid concentrations have been associated with cholestasis caused by TPN.[57]

Primary biliary cirrhosis (PBC) is a common cholestatic disease with an autoimmune etiology. An antimitochondrial antibody produces a specific nonsuppurative small-duct cholangitis that, if left untreated, progresses to cirrhosis, portal hypertension, and liver failure.[40] It is commonly seen in association with other autoimmune disorders, and as expected, exhibits a female preponderance.

Primary sclerosing cholangitis (PSC) is a chronic inflammatory large duct cholangiopathy characterized by a male patient predominance. It is seen frequently in patients with coexistent colitis, and is most commonly diagnosed via asymptomatic targeted surveillance in these same patients.[40] Pathologically, it is characterized by fibro-obliterative cholangitis, and ductal proliferation in some areas and ductopenia in others. Its natural history is one of recurrent cholangitis, progressive liver cirrhosis, portal hypertension, and liver failure, occasionally complicated by hepatic or colorectal malignancy.[58,59]

## EVALUATION OF INTRAHEPATIC CHOLESTATIC LIVER DISEASE WITH HYPERBILIRUBINEMIA

After confirmation of cholestatic conjugated hyperbilirubinemia via bilirubin fractionation and liver chemistry review, imaging of the liver and perihepatic structures is necessary. How this is best accomplished is somewhat dependent on clinical presentation, but CT and US are the modalities of choice. Frequently, US will be the initial study, because of its lack of exposure to ionizing radiation and its lower cost. Upon imaging, if ductal dilation is noted, biliary drainage and/or biopsy is indicated. If, however, initial imaging studies are normal, cholangiography via ERCP or PTC is the next step. ERCP is preferred owing to the ability to visualize the duodenum and the hepatopancreatic ampulla, as well as perform tissue biopsy. Specific testing may become appropriate as the workup continues (for example, serum and urine copper), but should be directed only by prior results.

## EXTRAHEPATIC OR OBSTRUCTIVE CONDITIONS PRODUCING CONJUGATED HYPERBILIRUBINEMIA

Extrahepatic cholestasis may be caused by a number of conditions. Most commonly, an obstruction to the intrahepatic or distal biliary tree increases intraluminal pressure and, as a result, bile salt efflux from the hepatocyte is impaired. A rational manner of considering these causes divides neoplastic from non-neoplastic and the latter further into congenital, inflammatory and infectious, postsurgical, and stone-related.[60]

Cholangiocarcinoma is a malignant neoplasm of the distal biliary tract. Prognosis is dismal owing to the difficulty in tumor detection methods and frequent advanced stage at time of presentation. These malignancies are associated with conditions that injure or chronically inflame bile duct epithelium, leading to increased mitotic activity in the cholangiocyte and increased likelihood of mutation and malignant transformation. These conditions include PSC, choledochal cysts, various infections (*Salmonella typhi,*

*Clonorchis sinensis, Opisthorchis viverrini*, hepatitis C) or chemical irritation (smoking, dioxin).[61] The imaging modality of choice for early evaluation of cholangiocarcinoma is ultrasonography, whereas the detailed images provided by contrast-enhanced CT provide invaluable information for planning management considerations. Palliation may be achieved via biliary stent placement as well as other interventions.[62]

Hepatocellular carcinoma (HCC) may cause jaundice via 2 distinct mechanisms: parenchymal infiltration causing hepatocellular insufficiency and direct biliary tree obstruction.[63] HCC is associated strongly with hepatitis B and C and more than 80% of HCC is found in cirrhotic livers. In jaundiced patients, parenchymal infiltrative disease has a significantly worse prognosis, whereas that of obstructive disease is similar to those patients without jaundice.

Pancreatic adenocarcinoma is the fourth leading cause of cancer-related death in the United States.[60,64] These cancers of the ductal epithelium are relatively asymptomatic or exhibit only nonspecific symptoms until large enough to produce a local mass effect, commonly producing a progressive jaundice by externally obstructing the common bile duct. Therefore, most cancers are advanced at diagnosis. Courvoisier sign is a distended, palpable, nontender gallbladder in a jaundiced patient and may be 90% specific but only 55% sensitive for malignant bile duct obstruction.[64] Currently, the US Preventive Services Task Force (USPSTF) does not recommend screening average-risk, asymptomatic patients with ultrasonography or serologic markers for hepatic, biliary, or pancreatic neoplasms.[64]

## NON-NEOPLASTIC EXTRAHEPATIC OBSTRUCTION

Acute pancreatitis is an inflammation of pancreatic parenchyma likely caused by activation of pancreatic pro-enzymes and leading to autodigestion and inflammation of the gland.[65] The incidence of common bile duct stricture in chronic pancreatitis is approximately 9%, which can lead to biliary obstruction.[64–66]

Choledochojejunostomy is a feature of several operations, including the Whipple and Bilroth procedures. Postoperative complications include anastamotic stricture that may increase intraductal biliary pressure and subsequent obstruction. After orthotopic liver transplantation, biliary tract disease is the second-most common complication and occurs in 25% of cases.[67] Among these, bile duct strictures at anastomotic sites are the most common and are likely caused by iatrogenic trauma and subsequent scar formation. A similar pathogenesis is responsible for the strictures seen in 0.6% of patients who have undergone cholecystectomy.[68]

Stone-related complications are common causes of biliary obstruction and subsequent jaundice. Choledocholithiasis is the most common cause of biliary obstruction, and may lead to jaundice.[69,70] The Mirizzi syndrome is a form of obstructive jaundice caused by a stone impacted in the neck of the cystic duct that locally compresses the hepatic duct. This is a complication of fewer than 1% of patients with symptomatic gallstones.[71]

Congenital causes of bile duct stricture are exceedingly rare and comprise such entities as choledochal webs and cysts.[60]

## EVALUATION OF EXTRAHEPATIC OR OBSTRUCTIVE DISEASE WITH HYPERBILIRUBINEMIA

The evaluation of extrahepatic obstruction is highly dependent on the expertise of the treating physicians and surgeons as well as the resources available at the treating institution. If initial US suggests dilated biliary ducts and obstruction, significant likelihood of malignant obstruction exists, and resection is planned, then perioperative staging with CT may be appropriate. Cholangiogram should be considered if the aforementioned studies remain insufficient for diagnosis. However, if resection is not planned, then palliation with ERCP and possible stent placement may be a next appropriate step.[28]

## FIVE KEY POINTS FOR PRIMARY CARE

1. Jaundice is caused by many disease processes ranging from benign to life threatening.
2. History and physical examination remain important tools in evaluating etiology of jaundice.
3. The conjugation state of bilirubin, along with other laboratory tests judiciously ordered, can guide the provider toward category of illness.
4. Hyperbilirubinemia may be categorized as to its etiology: unconjugated/prehepatic, intrahepatic, or extrahepatic/obstructive (see **Box 1**; **Table 1**).
5. Referral should be considered when likelihood of malignancy, chronic autoimmune condition, or need for intervention exists.

## REFERENCES

1. Hazin R, Abu-Rajab Tamimi TI, Abuzetun JY, et al. Recognizing and treating cutaneous signs of liver disease. Cleve Clin J Med 2009;76(10):599–606.
2. Roche SP, Kobos R. Jaundice in the adult patient. Am Fam Physician 2004;69(2): 299–304.
3. Fevery J. Bilirubin in clinical practice: a review. Liver Int 2008;28(5):592–605.
4. Morse D, Choi AM. Heme oxygenase-1: from bench to bedside. Am J Respir Crit Care Med 2005;172(6):660–70.
5. Otterbein LE, Soares MP, Yamashita K, et al. Heme oxygenase-1: unleashing the protective properties of heme. Trends Immunol 2003;24(8):449–55.
6. Stocker R, Yamamoto Y, McDonagh AF, et al. Bilirubin is an antioxidant of possible physiological importance. Science 1987;235:1043–6.
7. Ostrow JD, Mukerjee P, Tiribelli C. Structure and binding of unconjugated bilirubin: relevance for physiological and pathophysiological function. J Lipid Res 1994;35(10):1715–37.
8. Stocker R, Glazer AN, Ames BN. Antioxidant activity of albumin-bound bilirubin. Proc Natl Acad Sci U S A 1987;84:5918–22.
9. Mancuso C, Pani G, Calabrese V. Bilirubin: an endogenous scavenger of nitric oxide and reactive nitrogen species. Redox Rep 2006;11(5):207–13.
10. McGeary RP, Szyczew AJ, Toth I. Biological properties and therapeutic potential of bilirubin. Mini Rev Med Chem 2003;3(3):253–6.
11. Stocker R. Antioxidant activities of bile pigments. Antioxid Redox Signal 2004; 6(5):841–9.
12. Tomaro ML, Batlle AM. Bilirubin: its role in cytoprotection against oxidative stress. Int J Biochem Cell Biol 2002;34(3):216–20.
13. Kamisako T, Kobayashi Y, Takeuchi K, et al. Recent advances in bilirubin metabolism research: the molecular mechanism of hepatocyte bilirubin transport and its clinical relevance. J Gastroenterol 2000;35(9):659–64.
14. Chand N, Sanyal AJ. Sepsis-induced cholestasis. Hepatology 2007;45(1): 230–41.
15. Shibahara S, Kitamuro T, Takahashi K. Heme degradation and human disease: diversity is the soul of life. Antioxid Redox Signal 2002;4(4):593–602.

16. Boyer JL. New perspectives for the treatment of cholestasis: lessons from basic science applied clinically. J Hepatol 2007;46(3):365–71.
17. Frank BB. Clinical evaluation of jaundice. A guideline of the Patient Care Committee of the American Gastroenterological Association. JAMA 1989;262(21):3031–4.
18. Chopra S, Griffin PH. Laboratory tests and diagnostic procedures in evaluation of liver disease. Am J Med 1985;79(221):230.
19. Aranda-Michel J, Sherman KE. Tests of the liver: use and misuse. Gastroenterologist 1998;6(1):34–43.
20. Giannini EG, Testa R, Savarino V. Liver enzyme alteration: a guide for clinicians. CMAJ 2005;172(3):367–79.
21. Limdi JK, Hyde GM. Evaluation of abnormal liver function tests. Postgrad Med J 2003;79(932):307–12.
22. Rosalki SB, Dooley JS. Liver function profiles and their interpretation. Br J Hosp Med 1994;51(4):181–6.
23. Goldberg DM, Martin JV. Role of gamma-glutamyl transpeptidase activity in the diagnosis of hepatobiliary disease. Digestion 1975;12:232–46.
24. Rochling FA. Evaluation of abnormal liver tests. Clin Cornerstone 2001;3(6):1–12.
25. Johnston DE. Special considerations in interpreting liver function tests. Am Fam Physician 1999;59:2223–30.
26. Neuschwander-Tetri BA. Common blood tests for liver disease. Which ones are most useful? Postgrad Med 1995;98(1):49–56.
27. Olen R, Pickleman J, Freeark RJ. Less is better. The diagnostic workup of the patient with obstructive jaundice. Arch Surg 1989;124(7):791–4.
28. Balfe DM, Ralls PW, Bree RL, et al. Imaging strategies in the initial evaluation of the jaundiced patient. American College of Radiology. ACR Appropriateness Criteria. Radiology 2000;215(Suppl):125–33.
29. Corsetti JP, Arvan DA. Obstructive Jaundice. In: Pranzer RJ, Black ER, Griner PF, editors. Diagnostic Strategies for Common Clinical Problems. Philadelphia: American College of Physicians; 1991. p. 131–40.
30. Castera L. Non-invasive diagnosis of steatosis and fibrosis. Diabetes Metab 2008;34(6 Pt 2):674–9.
31. Chan YL, Chan AC, Lam WW, et al. Choledocholithiasis: comparison of MR cholangiography and endoscopic retrograde cholangiopancreatography. Radiology 1996;200:85–9.
32. Siddique K, Ali Q, Mirza S, et al. Evaluation of the aetiological spectrum of obstructive jaundice. J Ayub Med Coll Abbottabad 2008;20(4):62–6.
33. Chen WX, Zhang Y, Li YM, et al. Endoscopic retrograde cholangiopancreatography in evaluation of choledochal dilatation in patients with obstructive jaundice. Hepatobiliary Pancreat Dis Int 2002;1(1):111–3.
34. Grant A, Neuberger J. Guidelines on the use of liver biopsy in clinical practice. British Society of Gastroenterology. Gut 1999;45(Suppl 4):1–11.
35. Skelly MM, James PD, Ryder SD. Findings on liver biopsy to investigate abnormal liver function tests in the absence of diagnostic serology. J Hepatol 2001;35(2):195–9.
36. Mason PJ, Bautista JM, Gilsanz F. G6PD deficiency: the genotype-phenotype association. Blood Rev 2007;21(5):267–83.
37. Monaghan G, Ryan M, Seddon R, et al. Genetic variation in bilirubin UDP-glucuronosyltransferase gene promoter and Gilbert's syndrome. Lancet 1996;347:578–81.
38. Schwertner HA, Vitek L. Gilbert syndrome, UGT1A1*28 allele, and cardiovascular disease risk: possible protective effects and therapeutic applications of bilirubin. Atherosclerosis 2008;198(1):1–11.

39. Rudensky AS, Halsall DJ. Genetic testing for Gilbert's syndrome: how useful is it in determining the cause of jaundice? Clin Chem 1998;44:1604–9.
40. Pasha TM, Lindor KD. Diagnosis and therapy of cholestatic liver disease. Med Clin North Am 1996;80(5):995–1019.
41. Tung BY, Carithers RL Jr. Cholestasis and alcoholic liver disease. Clin Liver Dis 1999;3(3):585–601.
42. Sass DA, Shaikh OS. Alcoholic hepatitis. Clin Liver Dis 2006;10(2):219–37.
43. Renault M, Nowicki M. Persistent cholestasis following cholecystectomy: a case of Dubin-Johnson syndrome. J Pediatr 2010;157(1):167.
44. Crum NF. Epstein Barr virus hepatitis: case series and review. South Med J 2006; 99(5):544–7.
45. Maheshwari A, Ray S, Thuluvath PJ. Acute hepatitis C. Lancet 2008;372(9635): 321–32.
46. Koff RS. Clinical manifestations and diagnosis of hepatitis A virus infection. Vaccine 1992;10(Suppl 1):S15–7.
47. Hinedi TB, Koff RS. Cholestatic hepatitis induced by Epstein-Barr virus infection in an adult. Dig Dis Sci 2003;48(3):539–41.
48. Garcia-Tsao G, Lim JK, Members of Veterans Affairs Hepatitis C Resource Center, Program. Management and treatment of patients with cirrhosis and portal hypertension: recommendations from the Department of Veterans Affairs Hepatitis C Resource Center Program and the National Hepatitis C Program. Am J Gastroenterol 2009;104(7):1802–29.
49. Steindl P, Ferenci P, Dienes HP, et al. Wilson's disease in patients presenting with liver disease: a diagnostic challenge. Gastroenterology 1997;113:212–8.
50. Green RM, Flam S. AGA technical review on the evaluation of liver chemistry tests. Gastroenterology 2002;123:1367–84.
51. Fregonese L, Stolk J. Hereditary alpha-1-antitrypsin deficiency and its clinical consequences. Orphanet J Rare Dis 2008;3:16.
52. Bjornsson E. Drug-induced liver injury: Hy's rule revisited. Clin Pharmacol Ther 2006;79(6):521–8.
53. Hirschfield GM, Heathcote EJ, Gershwin ME. Pathogenesis of cholestatic liver disease and therapeutic approaches. Gastroenterology 2010;139(5):1481–96.
54. Bjornsson E. The natural history of drug-induced liver injury. Semin Liver Dis 2009;29(4):357–63.
55. Zimmerman HJ. Hepatotoxicity. The adverse effects of drugs and other chemicals on the liver. Philadelphia: Lippincott, Williams & Wilkins; 1999.
56. Faust TW, Reddy KR. Postoperative jaundice. Clin Liver Dis 2004;8(1):151–66.
57. Mohi-ud-din R, Lewis JH. Drug- and chemical-induced cholestasis. Clin Liver Dis 2004;8(1):95–132.
58. Hirschfield GM, Heathcote EJ. Cholestasis and cholestatic syndromes. Curr Opin Gastroenterol 2009;25(3):175–9.
59. Heathcote EJ. Diagnosis and management of cholestatic liver disease. Clin Gastroenterol Hepatol 2007;5(7):776–82.
60. Mortele KJ, Wiesner W, Cantisani V, et al. Usual and unusual causes of extrahepatic cholestasis: assessment with magnetic resonance cholangiography and fast MRI. Abdom Imaging 2004;29(1):87–99.
61. Veillette G, Castillo CF. Distal biliary malignancy. Surg Clin North Am 2008;88(6): 1429–47.
62. Tajiri T, Yoshida H, Mamada Y, et al. Diagnosis and initial management of cholangiocarcinoma with obstructive jaundice. World J Gastroenterol 2008;14(19): 3000–5.

63. Lai EC, Lau WY. Hepatocellular carcinoma presenting with obstructive jaundice. ANZ J Surg 2006;76(7):631–6.

64. Freelove R, Walling AD. Pancreatic cancer: diagnosis and management. Am Fam Physician 2006;73(3):485–92.

65. Frossard JL, Steer ML, Pastor CM. Acute pancreatitis. Lancet 2008;371(9607): 143–52.

66. Rohrmann CA Jr, Baron RL. Biliary complications of pancreatitis. Radiol Clin North Am 1989;27(1):93–104.

67. Boraschi P, Donati F, Gigoni R, et al. MR cholangiography in orthotopic liver transplantation: sensitivity and specificity in detecting biliary complications. Clin Transplant 2010;24(4):E82–7.

68. Deziel DJ, Millikan KW, Economou SG, et al. Complications of laparoscopic cholecystectomy: a national survey of 4,292 hospitals and an analysis of 77,604 cases. Am J Surg 1993;165(1):9–14.

69. Sanders G, Kingsnorth AN. Gallstones. BMJ 2007;335(7614):295–9.

70. Williams EJ, Green J, Beckingham I, et al. Guidelines on the management of common bile duct stones (CBDS). Gut 2008;57(7):1004–21.

71. Zaliekas J, Munson JL. Complications of gallstones: the Mirizzi syndrome, gallstone ileus, gallstone pancreatitis, complications of "lost" gallstones. Surg Clin North Am 2008;88(6):1345–68.

# Care of Chronic Liver Disease

Dongsheng Jiang, MD

**KEYWORDS**

- Chronic liver disease • Viral hepatitis • Hepatitis B • Hepatitis C
- Cirrhosis • NAFLD • NASH • Hemochromatosis

According to Centers for Disease Control and Prevention 2010 National Vital Statistics Reports, chronic liver disease was the 12th leading cause of death in the United States in 2007. Chronic liver diseases represent a group of common hepatic disorders and many patients can have the disease for life. Primary care physicians see these patients often and make the diagnosis for some but frequently leave treatment-related issues to gastroenterologists. To improve primary care physicians' familiarity with these illnesses, this article focuses on treatment of the most common chronic liver diseases.

## HEPATITIS B

The goal for treatment of chronic hepatitis B virus (HBV) infection is to reduce inflammation of the liver, prevent liver failure and cirrhosis, and reduce the risk of hepatocellular carcinoma (HCC). Because cirrhosis, HCC, and death often do not occur for many years after infection with HBV, a long-term evaluation of therapy to demonstrate benefit from anti-HBV therapy is needed. Most published reports of anti-HBV therapy use changes in short-term virologic, biochemical, and histologic parameters to infer the likelihood of long-term benefit. It is important to understand the limitations of this practice when assessing potential benefit.[1]

### Treatment Indications

Fifteen percent to twenty-five percent of chronic HBV patients are at risk for premature death from cirrhosis and liver cancer, so patients should be evaluated soon after infection is identified. Therapy is indicated with patients who have acute liver failure, cirrhosis and clinical complications, cirrhosis or advanced fibrosis, and HBV DNA in serum or reactivation of chronic HBV after chemotherapy or immunosuppression. Patients with an elevated level of alanine aminotransferase (ALT) are more likely to have potentially durable hepatitis B envelope antigen (HBeAg), biochemical, and histologic responses. Therefore, clinically, treatment is often indicated when ALT is

This article is not under consideration by any other publication and has not been published elsewhere. The author reports no conflicts of interest.

Family and Community Medicine, Hershey Medical College, Penn State University, 1850 East Park Avenue, Suite #312, State College, PA 16801, USA

E-mail address: DJiang@hmc.psu.edu

Prim Care Clin Office Pract 38 (2011) 483–498
doi:10.1016/j.pop.2011.05.005  **primarycare.theclinics.com**

greater than 2 times the upper limit of normal range and HBV DNA greater than 20,000 IU/mL.[2,3] With decompensated cirrhosis, nucleoside or nucleotide analogs are used, because pegylated interferons are contraindicated. For infants born to women who are hepatitis B surface antigen (HBsAg) positive, immunoglobulin and vaccination are indicated. Therapy may be indicated for patients in the immune-active phase who do not have advanced fibrosis or cirrhosis.[1]

According to the National Institutes of Health 2008 hepatitis B consensus, patients for whom immediate therapy is not routinely indicated include

- Patients with chronic hepatitis B in the immune-tolerant phase (with high levels of serum HBV DNA but normal serum ALT levels or little activity on liver biopsy)
- Patients in the inactive carrier or low replicative phase (with low levels of or no detectable HBV DNA in serum and normal serum ALT levels)
- Patients who have latent HBV infection (HBV DNA without HBsAg).

### Treatment Choices

The 7 drugs licensed in the United States include interferons (interferon alfa-2b and peginterferon alfa-2a) and nucleoside or nucleotide analogs (lamivudine, adefovir, entecavir, tenofovir, and telbivudine).[3]

Pegylated interferon alfa-2a is a first-line option for patients who do not have cirrhosis.[4] Its strengths include no resistance, highest seroconversion rate, and finite treatment time (48 weeks), but there are also a few weaknesses, such as being expensive (more than $32,590 a year),[5] not well tolerated, and only available in the injected form. Side effects include bone marrow suppression, depression, and autoimmune disorders, such as thyroiditis. Thus, cytopenias, depression, and thyroid-stimulating hormone should be monitored for during treatment.

For oral agents, first-line therapy is tenofovir or entecavir.[4] Combinations of available antiviral drugs for HBV infection in patients who have not received treatment do not increase efficacy. Adefovir and tenofovir can be nephrotoxic, which requires monitoring creatinine. Oral agents are generally well tolerated, but, if prematurely discontinued, these drugs are associated with resurgence of HBV DNA levels or reactivation of hepatitis. Long-term use is also related to resistance.[1]

### Monitoring Therapy

Serologic endpoints of antiviral therapy are loss of HBeAg, HBeAg seroconversion in persons initially HBeAg positive, suppression of HBV DNA to undetectable levels by sensitive polymerase chain reaction (PCR)-based assays in patients who are HBeAg negative and anti-HBe positive, and loss of HBsAg.[6,7] HBsAg loss and seroconversion are associated with durable suppression of HBV DNA; however, this is uncommonly achieved in the short term with current therapy.[7] Treatment for 1 year generally can often reduce serum HBV DNA levels to undetectable by PCR. Because responses are not always durable, careful post-treatment monitoring is required to identify relapse. Various monitoring practices have been recommended, but no clear evidence exists for an optimal approach.[1] One approach is to measure HBV DNA and ALT levels every 12 weeks and HBeAg or anti-HBe levels every 24 weeks in patients who are HBeAg-positive. Most predictive factors of response are a high ALT level, a low HBV DNA level, and mild-to-moderate histologic activity and stage.[8]

### Important Complications

Fifteen percent to twenty-five percent of chronically infected persons die from cirrhosis, liver failure, or HCC. Adults with chronic HBV infection that was acquired in the perinatal period develop HCC at a rate of approximately 5% per decade, which is approximately 100-fold higher than the rate among uninfected persons.[1] The risk factors for developing HCC include Asian/Pacific Islanders/African races, male gender, age older than 50, alcohol abuse, smoking, co-infection with hepatitis C and D virus, HBV DNA viral load greater than 10,000 IU/mL, HBV genotype C, presence of HBeAg, birth in regions where HBV is endemic, longer duration of infection, cirrhosis, type 2 diabetes mellitus, steatohepatitis, exposure to aflatoxin, and family history of HCC.[2,9–11] Patients with chronic HBV infection need to be monitored every 6 months to 12 months for HCC using α-fetoprotein levels and abdominal ultrasonography.[10,12,13] A Cochrane review found insufficient evidence to demonstrate that HCC surveillance improves survival.[5]

### Prevention

Hepatitis B vaccination is 80% to 95% effective in preventing HBV infection and clinical hepatitis among susceptible children and adults. If a protective antibody response develops after vaccination, vaccine recipients are virtually 100% protected against clinical illness. Persons who are not known to be immune to hepatitis A virus should also receive 2 doses of hepatitis A vaccine 6 to 18 months apart.[6]

## HEPATITIS C

The goal of therapy in patients with hepatitis C infection is to slow or halt progression of fibrosis and prevent the development of cirrhosis.[14] Although viral load does not correlate with the severity of hepatitis or with a poorer prognosis (as in HIV infection), it does correlate with the likelihood of a robust response to antiviral therapy. Treatment responses are characterized by the results of hepatitis C virus (HCV) RNA testing.

### Treatment Indications

Patient selection should not be based on symptoms, the mode of acquisition, the genotype, or serum HCV RNA levels. Therapy is widely accepted for patients age 18 years or older with the following: serum positive for HCV RNA, liver biopsy showing chronic hepatitis with significant fibrosis (bridging fibrosis or higher), compensated liver disease (total serum bilirubin <1.5 g/dL, international normalized ratio <1.5, serum albumin >3.4, platelet count >75,000/mm$^3$ and no evidence of hepatic decompensation [hepatic encephalopathy or ascites], and acceptable hematologic and biochemical indices [hemoglobin 13 g/dL for men and >12 g/dL for women, neutrophil count >1500 /mm$^3$, and serum creatinine <1.5 mg/dL]), a willingness to be treated and to adhere to treatment requirements, and no contraindications.[12,15] Patients with clinically decompensated cirrhosis should be referred for consideration of liver transplantation.

### Treatment Initiation

Regardless of ALT level, the decision to initiate therapy with pegylated interferon and ribavirin should be individualized based on the severity of liver disease by liver biopsy, the potential for serious side effects, the likelihood of response, and the presence of comorbid conditions.[15] Liver biopsy before starting treatment is not necessary but is prudent and provides rationale for whether or not therapy is critical. Nevertheless, the major use of liver biopsy is to help in the decision of whether to initiate treatment or to delay until there are further advances in the field.

### Treatment Choices

Common nonmodifiable indicators for a lower probability of response to therapy are genotype 1, high viral load (>500,000 IU/mL), obesity, black or Latino race, advanced age, and high degree of liver fibrosis.[16,17] For genotypes 1, 2, and 3, treatment should be combination therapy with pegylated interferon and ribavirin. For genotypes 4, 5, and 6, patients should probably be treated as genotype 1.[18,19] Peginterferon alfa-2a plus ribavirin produced a significantly higher sustained virologic response rate than peginterferon alfa-2b plus ribavirin in genotypes 1–4.[20]

### Agents

There are 2 forms of peginterferons—alfa-2a and alfa-2b. The former is given in a fixed dose whereas the latter is weight based. Peginterferon is given weekly and with better efficacy, so it has replaced standard interferon both as monotherapy and as combination therapy. Ribavirin is an oral agent given twice a day. It is also weight based and the optimal dose varies depending on genotype.[19]

### Duration

Treatment duration varies depending on whether interferon monotherapy or combination therapy is used as well as by HCV genotype.[19]

For combined therapy for genotype 1 or peginterferon monotherapy regardless of genotype, treatment is continued for 48 weeks. Combined therapy results in sustained virologic response (defined as undetectable HCV RNA in the patient's blood 24 weeks after the end of treatment) rates of up to 50% for genotype 1. Using combined therapy for genotypes 2 or 3, 24 weeks of therapy can result in sustained response rates up to 80%.

### Monitoring during therapy

Side effects, such as severe fatigue, depression, or irritability, can occur. Check complete blood cell count, ALT, and aspartate transaminase (AST) at weeks 1, 2, and 4 and at 4-week to 8-week intervals thereafter and thyroid-stimulating hormone at 3 and to 6 months.[19]

### After therapy

After therapy, measure aminotransferase levels every 2 months for 6 months. Six months after stopping therapy, test for HCV RNA by PCR (or transcription mediated amplification). If HCV RNA is still negative, the chance for a long-term "cure" is excellent; relapses have rarely been reported after this point.

If a patient did not achieve an systemic vascular resistance (HCV RNA negative 24 weeks after cessation of treatment) after a prior full course of peginterferon plus ribavirin, retreatment with peginterferon plus ribavirin is not recommended.[19]

### Contraindications

Common hepatitis C treatment contraindications are listed in **Table 1**.

### Recommendations for Special Patient Groups

Management of individual patients can be challenging in special situations. Treatment recommendations for special patient groups are listed in **Table 2**.

### Important Complications

Among chronically infected persons with HCV, 60% to 70% develop chronic liver disease. Patients with risk factors, such as male gender, alcoholism, age older than 50, cirrhosis, or infection for 20 to 40 years, have an increased risk for HCC.[19] Chronic HBV and HCV infections account for an estimated 78% of global HCC cases.[11] There is no clear evidence showing that ultrasound surveillance improves morbidity or mortality from HCC[14]; however, those who have cirrhosis or advanced liver fibrosis (bridging fibrosis) should be monitored for HCC every 6 months.[12]

**Table 1**
**Hepatitis C treatment contraindications**

| Type of Therapy | Contraindications |
|---|---|
| Monotherapy or combination therapy | • Severe hypertension<br>• Heart failure<br>• Significant coronary artery disease<br>• Poorly controlled diabetes<br>• Obstructive pulmonary disease<br>• Under 3 years of age |
| Peginterferon therapy | • Decompensated liver disease<br>• Severe depression or other neuropsychiatric syndromes<br>• Active substance abuse or alcohol abuse (6-month abstinence is recommended)<br>• Autoimmune disease (such as rheumatoid arthritis, lupus erythematosus, psoriasis, or hyperthyroidism) that is not well controlled (peginterferon therapy can induce autoantibodies)<br>• Bone marrow compromise<br>• Pregnant or inability to practice birth control<br>• Combination therapy with interferon alfa-2b and ribavirin is also contraindicated in males with pregnant partners and hemoglobinopathies (eg, thalassemia major or sickle cell anemia). |
| Ribavirin therapy | • Marked anemia (ribavirin causes red cell hemolysis)<br>• Renal dysfunction (excreted largely by the kidneys)<br>• Coronary artery or cerebrovascular disease (anemia can trigger ischemia)<br>• Pregnant or inability to practice birth control. |

*Data from* Strader DB, Wright T, Thomas D, et al. AASLD practice guideline: diagnosis, management, and treatment of hepatitis C. Hepatology 2004;39(4):1147–71; and Chronic hepatitis C: current disease management-national digestive diseases information clearinghouse. NIH Publication No. 07–4230; November 2006. Available at: www.digestive.niddk.nih.gov.

Other complications of HCV include diabetes mellitus, glomerulonephritis, mixed cryoglobulinemia, porphyria cutanea tarda, neuropathy, non-Hodgkin lymphoma, thyroid cancer, end-stage renal disease, lichen planus, idiopathic thrombocytopenic purpura, and fibromyalgia.[19,21]

### *Preventive Medicine*

Although no hepatitis C vaccination is available, the need for hepatitis A and B vaccination should be evaluated.

## ALCOHOLIC CIRRHOSIS

Alcoholic cirrhosis usually occurs after years of excessive drinking. Cirrhosis involves replacement of the normal hepatic parenchyma with extensive thick bands of fibrous tissue and regenerative nodules, which results in the clinical manifestations of portal hypertension and liver failure.[22]

### *Patient Selection*

All patients should be screened for alcoholic liver disease (ALD). It has been found that cirrhosis develops more commonly in alcohol abusers with fatty liver changes than in those with normal liver histology.[22] Liver biopsy may be useful to confirm the diagnosis or to rule out other diseases.

| Table 2 |  |
|---|---|
| **Recommendations for special patient groups** | |
| **Special Situations** | **Treatment** |
| • Co-infection with HIV | • Treat early even with mild disease.<br>• Treat if benefit is consider as outweighing the risk of morbidity from the adverse effects of therapy. |
| • Acute hepatitis C | • Treatment can be delayed for 8 to 12 weeks to see whether there is spontaneous resolution.<br>• May consider peginterferon (in usual doses) and ribavirin (800 mg/d) for 24 weeks if HCV RNA is still detected 3 months after onset of infection. |
| • Nonresponder | • If stable viral load or failure to achieve more than 100-fold decrease in viral load at week 12, treatment should be discontinued |
| • Chronic kidney disease | • If mild (glomerular filtration rate >60 mL/min), it can be treated with the same combination antiviral therapy. |
| • Decompensated cirrhosis | • Needs to be referred for liver transplantation. |
| • Active injection drug users | • Can be treated only if they are on a methadone program and are able and willing to maintain close monitoring and practice contraception. |
| • Psychiatric illness | • Treat only with the support of a multidisciplinary team that should include psychiatric counseling services |

*Data from* Ghany M, Strader D, Thomas D, et al. AASLD practice guidelines. Diagnosis, management, and treatment of hepatitis C: an update. Hepatology 2009;49(4):1335–74; and Wilkins T, Malcolm J, Raina D, et al. Hepatitis C: diagnosis and treatment. Am Fam Physician 2010;81(11):1351–7.

### *Treatment Choices*

Abstinence from all alcohol is the cornerstone of therapy for patients with ALD.[23]

If abstinence is achieved, clinical and histologic benefits can be impressive, even if a patient is already cirrhotic. It improves long-term survival, although less so short-term mortality. Unfortunately, a significant proportion of patients with alcoholic cirrhosis only abstain from alcohol when they are too sick to drink.[24]

Assessment for nutritional deficiencies (protein-calorie malnutrition) as well as vitamin and mineral deficiencies plays a valuable role in managing the patient with hepatitis C because almost all patients with alcoholic hepatitis have some degree of malnutrition. Correcting protein-calorie malnutrition with enteral nutrition is preferable over parenteral supplementation, and protein should be supplied to provide positive nitrogen balance.[22]

Disulfiram, naltrexone, and acamprosate have been approved for alcohol dependence. Baclofen seems to reduce alcohol craving particularly in individuals with severe alcohol-induced liver disease.[25] Naltrexone or acamprosate may be considered in combination with counseling to decrease the likelihood of relapse.[26]

Glucocorticoids are the most intensely studied and yet most hotly debated treatment for acute alcoholic hepatitis. Results from trials of glucocorticoids for ALD have been variable.[27]

Anabolic-androgenic steroids have demonstrated no significant beneficial effects on any clinically important outcomes.[28]

Pentoxifylline-treated patients had a significant decrease in mortality. This medication is a good clinical option for the treatment of alcoholic hepatitis but is not Food and

Drug Administration approved for this indication. It is unclear if its benefit extends beyond possibly preventing hepatorenal syndrome (HRS).[27]

Topiramate may be generally effective at improving clinical outcomes and physical and psychosocial well-being in patients from 18 to 65 years who drink 35 or more (men) and 28 or more (women) drinks per week.[29]

Colchicine is anti-inflammatory and antifibrotic, but it should not be used for alcoholic, viral, or cryptogenic liver fibrosis or liver cirrhosis outside randomized clinical trials.[30]

Milk thistle (silymarin) is one of the most researched complementary drugs. It is believed to have protective effects on the liver and improve its function. It is typically used to treat liver cirrhosis, chronic hepatitis (liver inflammation), and gallbladder disorders.[31] One Cochrane review concluded that there was no evidence supporting or refuting milk thistle for ALD or HBV or HCV liver diseases.[32] A more recent review, however, still favors this drug due to its oral effectiveness, good safety profile, and low cost.[33]

There is no clear evidence supporting or refuting the use of S-adenosyl-L-methionine (also termed, sulfo-adenosylmethionine or SAMe) for patients with ALDs.[34]

Other American Association for the Study of Liver Disease recommendations on management of ALD are as shown in **Table 3**.

## Adjunctive Therapies

### Zinc deficiency

Zinc sulfate (220 mg orally twice daily) may improve dysgeusia and can stimulate appetite, and it is effective in the treatment of muscle cramps and is adjunctive therapy for hepatic encephalopathy.[35]

### Pain management in patients with cirrrhosis

Tramadol is safer than opioids. Acetaminophen (up to 2 g) can be used if a patient is not actively drinking alcohol. Fentanyl and methadone are not affected by liver impairment. Agents to avoid include nonsteroidal anti-inflammatory drugs, morphine, oxycodone, and oxymorphone.[36]

---

**Table 3**
**Other recommendations on management of alcoholic liver disease by the American Association for the Study of Liver Disease**

| Condition | Recommendations |
|---|---|
| • MDF <32<br>• Without hepatic encephalopathy<br>• Improvement in serum bilirubin or decline in the MDF during the first week of hospitalization | Monitor closely |
| • MDF >32<br>• With or without hepatic encephalopathy | 4-Week course of prednisolone: 40 mg/d for 28 days, typically followed by discontinuation or a 2-week taper |
| • MDF >32<br>• Contraindications to steroid therapy | Pentoxifylline therapy (400 mg orally 3 times/d for 4 weeks) |

*Abbreviation:* MDF, Maddrey discriminant function.
*Data from* O'Shea R, Dasarathy S, McCullough A, et al. Alcoholic liver disease. AASLD practice guidelines. Hepatology 2010;51(1):307–28.

### Nutrition

Patients with ALD should be provided 1.2 to 1.5 g/kg of protein and 35 to 40 kcal/kg of body weight.[37]

### Liver Transplantation

Transplantation has become the standard of care for end-stage liver disease, with 5-year survival rates approaching 70% to 80%.[38] A UK study suggests, however, that, maybe partly due to a misunderstanding about the relationship between ALD and alcoholism, 95% of patients with life-threatening, alcohol-related liver disease are never formally assessed for liver transplantation.[39] Appropriate patients with end-stage liver disease secondary to alcoholic cirrhosis should be considered for liver transplantation. A formal assessment of the likelihood of long-term abstinence should be performed.[26] Contraindications should include HIV positive status, spontaneous bacterial peritonitis or other active infection, severely advanced cardiopulmonary disease, extrahepatic malignancy that does not meet cure criteria, active alcohol or substance abuse, and inability to comply with immunosuppression protocols because of psychosocial situations.[40] Liver transplantation surgery costs $200,000 to $300,000, with the annual cost of drugs and follow-up medical visits thereafter from $12,000 to $20,000.[41]

### Important Complications

#### Ascites

Ascites is the most common complication of alcoholic cirrhosis, with a 55% prevalence at the time of diagnosis.[42] Management of ascites includes sodium restriction (maximum 2 g/d), spironolactone (100 mg by mouth daily to a maximum 400 mg daily), furosemide (40 mg by mouth daily to a maximum 160 mg daily), albumin (8–10 g intravenously per liter of fluid above 5 L removed by paracenteses), and fluid restriction when serum sodium is less than 120 to 125 mEq/L.[43]

#### Hepatic encephalopathy

Pharmacotherapy includes lactulose (30 to 45 mL syrup orally, titrated up to 3–4 times/d or 300 mL retention enema until 2–4 bowel movements/d and mental status improvement), neomycin (4 to 12 g by mouth daily, divided every 6–8 hours), or rifaximin (400 mg 3 times/d).[44]

#### Bacterial infections

They can include urinary tract infections (12%–29%), spontaneous bacterial peritonitis (7%–23%), respiratory tract infections (6%–10%), and primary bacteremia (4%–11%). For spontaneous bacterial peritonitis, antibiotic prophylaxis regimens in trials included norfloxacin orally (400 mg/d); trimethoprim/sulfamethoxazole (160/800 mg orally 5 d/wk); rufloxacin (400 mg orally 3 times in first week, then weekly); and ciprofloxacin (750 mg orally once weekly or 500 mg/d).[45]

#### Variceal hemorrhage

Pimary prophylaxis of variceal hemorrhage includes β-blockers for patients with medium or large varices not at highest risk of hemorrhage. Endoscopic variceal ligation is recommended for patients with medium or large varices that have not previously bled. For secondary prophylaxis of variceal hemorrhage, nonselective β-blockers plus esophageal variceal ligation is the best option. Adjust nonselective β-blocker to maximum tolerated dose, and repeat esophageal variceal ligation every 1 to 2 weeks until obliteration. Emergency sclerotherapy is still widely used as a first-line therapy for variceal bleeding in patients with cirrhosis, particularly when banding ligation is not available or feasible. Vasoactive drugs may be safe and effective, however, whenever endoscopic therapy is not promptly available and seems to be associated with less adverse events than emergency sclerotherapy.[46] Antibiotic prophylaxis should be given if gastrointestinal bleeding is present. Quinolones were tested in most trials with a median duration of treatment of 7 days.[47]

### Hepatorenal syndrome

The complication, HRS, commonly presents as oliguria. In general, terlipressin plus albumin may prolong short-term survival in type 1 HRS.[48] Terlipressin is the drug of choice for treating type 1 HRS (HRS-1) but is expensive and often not readily available. Noradrenaline may be as effective as terlipressin.[49] Paracentesis with 200 mL of 20% human albumin solution infusion may improve renal function and is safe in the treatment of ICU patients.[50]

### Screening HCC

The clinical utility and cost-effectiveness of this strategy remains controversial. Some people choose to perform abdominal ultrasonography and α-fetoprotein testing twice yearly.[35]

## NONALCOHOLIC FATTY LIVER DISEASE/NONALCOHOLIC STEATOHEPATITIS

Treatment of nonalcoholic fatty liver disease (NAFLD) consists of modification of underlying risk factors (weight gain, dyslipidemia, and insulin resistance), detection of patients that have progressed to cirrhosis, management of cirrhosis-related morbidity, and transplantation in patients with end-stage liver disease.[51] There is currently no therapy that is of proved benefit for nonalcoholic steatohepatitis (NASH) and no universal treatment for NAFLD/NASH. Specific therapeutic interventions include weight reduction, ursodeoxycholic acid, clofibrate, gemfibrozil, atorvastatin, troglitazone, and several antioxidants, such as vitamin E, betaine, and N-acetylcysteine.[52]

### Diet and Exercise

Diet and exercise constitute the central strategies in NAFLD treatment.[53] Monounsaturated fatty acids found in olive oil, peanut butter, nuts, and avocados are thought to be generally beneficial because they decrease total cholesterol, triglycerides, and serum low-density lipoprotein and maintain high-density lipoprotein.[54] High fructose content of nondiet sodas is associated with increased hepatic de novo lipogenesis, hypertriglyceridemia, and hepatic insulin resistance. A small randomized study suggests that omega-3 fatty acids have a beneficial effect on liver fat content in women with polycystic ovary syndrome.[55]

### Antioxidants

There is insufficient data to either support or refute the use of antioxidant supplements for patients with NAFLD.[52] Vitamin E can be used for the treatment of NASH in adults without diabetes.[56] The dose response analysis showed a statistically significant relationship between vitamin E dosage and all-cause mortality, with an increased risk of all-cause mortality for dosages greater than 400 IU/day.[52] It seems most prudent to use vitamin E at the lowest dose possible for improvement in liver function tests and histology.

### Weight Loss

Although some people recommended a target weight loss of greater than 7% for overweight patients, the usual goal is 10%. Rapid weight loss has been associated with worsening liver histology, and most experts, therefore, recommend that weight loss in obese patients with NAFLD should be gradual (<1.6 kg/wk).[57] Currently, only 2 drugs are licensed in the United States for the long-term treatment of obesity: orlistat and sibutramine.[58] Orlistat is a reversible inhibitor of gastric and pancreatic lipase. Sibutramine is a pancreatic lipase inhibitor and appetite-suppressive agent and is related to weight loss rather than direct effects of the agents on liver parenchyma. In patients who fail to lose weight with dietary modification and exercise, these classes of pharmacologic agents represent a safe alternative before recommending bariatric surgery.[51] Bariatric surgery is associated with significant improvements in biochemical and histologic markers of NAFLD.[51] It is not a proved therapeutic approach for patients with NASH, however.[59]

### Insulin-Sensitizing Agents

There is insufficient data to either support or refute the use of drugs (metformin, troglitazone, pioglitazone, and rosiglitazone,) for improving insulin resistance for patients with NAFLD, although current limited information suggests a favorable role for drugs that improve insulin resistance.[60] Although metformin is associated with a reduction in liver function tests, there is no evidence that metformin significantly affects prognosis in NAFLD and/or NASH.[60] The thiazolidinediones are still under study. A randomized trial has shown that there is no benefit of pioglitazone for the primary outcome (histology); however, significant benefits of pioglitazone were observed for some of the secondary outcomes (insulin resistance and liver enzymes), although it causes some weight gain.[56]

### Statins

Modest transaminase elevations (<3 times upper limit) are not a contraindication to initiating, continuing, or advancing statin therapy, as long as patients are carefully monitored.[61] Some studies suggest that biochemical markers can improve with statin treatment. But, until larger studies are performed, there is no strong evidence to support statin use for primary treatment of NAFLD.

### Other Agents

There are insufficient data to support or refute the use of ursodeoxycholic acid.[62] The lack of randomized clinical trials makes it impossible to support or refute probiotics.[63] For acetaminophen use in NASH, dosage is the same as for all other chronic liver disease—not to exceed 2 g per day.

### Complications

Older age, obesity, diabetes mellitus, and AST/ALT ratio greater than 1 are significant predictors of severe liver fibrosis.[64] NASH may progress to cirrhosis and liver-related death in 25% and 10% of patients, respectively, and even to HCC. The majority of "cryptogenic" HCCs in the United States are attributed to NAFLD.[65] NAFLD is associated with increased risk of type 2 diabetes mellitus.[66] NAFLD in children is associated with a significantly shorter lifespan.[67]

## HEMOCHROMATOSIS

Hereditary hemochromatosis (HH) is an autosomally recessive inherited condition with variable penetrance. Excessive iron absorption in the small intestine leads to excessive storage in various organs. Men typically develop symptoms by ages 40 to 60 and women after menopause. Management objectives include early diagnosis to prevent organ damage, adequate treatment with effective removal of iron, and vigilant follow-up and maintenance treatment of all cases of HH with the main goal of preventing cirrhosis.

### Phlebotomy

Patients who start phlebotomy before the onset of irreversible organ damage have a normal life expectancy, although there is poor evidence that early therapeutic phlebotomy improves morbidity and mortality in screening-detected versus clinically detected individuals.[68] Ideally, treatment is initiated before the development of symptoms when serum ferritin is greater than 200 µg/L in premenopausal women or 300 µg/L in men and postmenopausal women. The easiest, cheapest, and most effective way to remove iron is by therapeutic phlebotomy. It has never been subjected to a randomized trial, but the strongest supporting evidence for a beneficial effect of phlebotomy is the improvement of liver fibrosis that has been demonstrated on serial liver biopsies.[69] In HH, phlebotomy is indicated with C282Y homozygosity with both increased transferrin saturation and ferritin.[70] All patients with HH who have evidence of iron overload should be strongly encouraged to undergo lifetime regular phlebotomies with the following regimen[71]:

- Perform one phlebotomy (removal of 500 mL of blood) weekly or biweekly.
- Check hematocrit before each phlebotomy; allow hematocrit to fall by no more than 20% of prior level.
- Check serum ferritin level every 10–12 phlebotomies.
- Stop frequent phlebotomy when ferritin <50 ng/mL.
- Continue phlebotomy at intervals to keep serum ferritin at 25–50 ng/mL.

### Deferoxamine

Chelation therapy with deferoxamine is almost never necessary because of the ease, cost, and efficacy of phlebotomy. In patients with secondary iron overload, however, especially chronic dyserythropoietic syndromes or chronic hemolytic anemia, parenteral chelation therapy with deferoxamine is currently the treatment of choice. Dosage is 20 mg/kg to 40 mg/kg body weight per day. Monitoring of the efficacy of therapy during chelation may require repeat liver biopsies to confirm adequate reduction of hepatic iron concentration.[71]

### Diet Modification

Patients with hemochromatosis should avoid iron or vitamin C supplements, and those who have liver damage should avoid alcohol and raw seafood. Although dietary iron is the source of excess iron in hemochromatosis, a decrease in dietary iron has not been shown to decrease iron stores in hemochromatosis.[69]

### Complications

Cardiac dysrhythmias and cardiomyopathy are the most common causes of sudden death in iron overload states.[71] Despite correct elimination of the iron burden, type 1 diabetes mellitus will not resolve, and the risk for HCC remains if cirrhosis was present before phlebotomy therapy.[70] Close life-long surveillance for HCC seems prudent for HH patients with significant fibrosis or cirrhosis.

### SUMMARY

Chronic liver disease is increasing, especially in the elderly population. Because early signs are often vague, vigilance is key in early diagnosis. General management objectives include recognizing underlying risk factors, early diagnosis to prevent organ damage, detection of patients that have progressed to cirrhosis, adequate treatment of the disease, management of cirrhosis-related complications, and transplantation in patients with end-stage liver disease. Although the treatment is similar once the common pathway, such as cirrhosis and liver failure occur, the early state treatment varies according to etiology. As health care providers strive for better care for patients, being more familiar with managing chronic liver disease in the primary care setting can definitely improve morbidity and mortality.

## FIVE KEY POINTS FOR PRIMARY CARE

Approximately 40 million people suffer from chronic liver diseases in the United States and the most common types of diseases include NAFLD, NASH, chronic hepatitis C, ALD, chronic hepatitis B, and hemochromatosis.

Patients with chronic liver diseases are often asymptomatic. If primary care physicians do not look for risk factors, high-risk populations will unlikely be screened and vaccinated, and treatment for those patients can be delayed.

The key to eliminating HBV transmission is identification of people who are living with chronic HBV infection. And, hepatitis B vaccine works.

Alcoholism and ALD may, but do not necessarily, coexist, and many ALD patients are not alcoholic. For NAFLD/NASH, there is no truly effective therapy, so monitoring and modifying risk factors early in life probably make the biggest difference.

Care quality can be enhanced for patients with chronic liver diseases, especially hepatitis C, when primary care physicians become more familiar with treatment options, indications, side effects, and contraindications.

## ACKNOWLEDGMENTS

The author wishes to thank Dr Michael Flanagan for support and proofreading, and Dr Weihong Kong for the support throughout the preparation of the manuscript.

## REFERENCES

1. Sorrell M, Belongia E, Costa J, et al. National Institutes of Health Consensus evelopment Conference Statement: management of hepatitis B. Ann Intern Med 2009;150(2):104–10.
2. Lok AS, McMahon BJ. Chronic hepatitis B [published correction appears in Hepatology 2007;45(6):1347]. Hepatology 2007;45(2):507–39.
3. Dienstag JL. Hepatitis B virus infection. N Engl J Med 2008;359(14):1486–500.
4. Lok AS, McMahon BJ. Chronic hepatitis B: update 2009. Hepatology 2009;50(3): 661–2.
5. Wilkins T, Zimmerman D, Schade R. Hepatitis B: diagnosis and treatment. Am Fam Physician 2010;81(8):965–72.
6. Weinbaum CM, Williams I, Mast EE, et al. Recommendations for identification and public health management of persons with chronic hepatitis B virus infection. MMWR Recomm Rep 2008;57(RR08):1–20.
7. NIH Consensus Development Conference: Management of Hepatitis B 2008; Available at: http://consensus.nih.gov/2008/hepbstatement.htm. Accessed June 12, 2010.
8. Perrillo RP, Lai CL, Liaw YF, et al. Predictors of HBeAg loss after lamivudine treatment for chronic hepatitis B. Hepatology 2002;36:186–94.

9. Bruix J, Sherman M. Management of hepatocellular carcinoma. Hepatology 2005; 42:1208–36.

10. El-Serag HB, Marrero JA, Rudolph L, et al. Diagnosis and treatment of hepatocellular carcinoma. Gastroenterology 2008;134(6):1752–63.

11. O'Connor S, Ward JW, Watson M, et al. Hepatocellular carcinoma—United States, 2001–2006. MMWR Morb Mortal Wkly Rep 2010;59(17):517–20.

12. HM Colvin and AE Mitchell. Hepatitis and liver cancer: a national strategy for prevention and control of hepatitis B and C. consensus report by institute of medicine of the national adademies. 2010. Available at: http://books.nap.edu/catalog/12793.html. Accessed June 18, 2010.

13. Keeffe EB, Dieterich DT, Han SH, et al. A treatment algorithm for the management of chronic hepatitis B virus infection in the United States: 2008 update. Clin Gastroenterol Hepatol 2008;6(12):1315–41.

14. Wilkins T, Malcolm J, Raina D, et al. Hepatitis C: diagnosis and treatment. Am Fam Physician 2010;81(11):1351–7.

15. Ghany M, Strader D, Thomas D, et al. AASLD practice guidelines. Diagnosis, management, and treatment of hepatitis C: an update. Hepatology 2009;49(4): 1335–74.

16. Backus LI, Boothroyd DB, Phillips BR, et al. Predictors of response of US veterans to treatment for the hepatitis C virus. Hepatology 2007;46(1):37–47.

17. Rodriguez-Torres M, Sulkowski MS, Chung RT, et al. Factors associated with rapid and early virologic response to peginterferon alfa-2a/ribavirin treatment in HCV genotype 1 patients representative of the general chronic hepatitis C population. J Viral Hepat 2010;17(2):139–47.

18. Strader DB, Wright T, Thomas D, et al. AASLD Practice guideline: diagnosis, management, and treatment of hepatitis C. Hepatology 2004;39(4):1147–71.

19. Chronic hepatitis C: current disease management-national digestive diseases information clearinghouse. 2006. NIH Publication No. 07–4230. Available at: www.digestive.niddk.nih.gov. Accessed June 18, 2010.

20. Ascione A, De Luca M, Tartaglione MT, et al. Peginterferon alfa-2a plus ribavirin is more effective than peginterferon alfa-2b plus ribavirin for treating chronic hepatitis C virus infection. Gastroenterology 2010;138(1):116–22.

21. Hepatitis C FAQs for health professionals. Available at: http://www.cdc.gov/hepatitis/HCV/HCVfaq.htm#section3. Accessed June 18, 2010.

22. Fairbanks KD. Alcoholic liver disease. 2009. Available at: http://www.clevelandclinicmeded.com/medicalpubs/diseasemanagement/hepatology/alcoholic-liver-disease/#cesec3. Accessed June 18, 2010.

23. Tilg H, Day CP. Management strategies in alcoholic liver disease. Nat Clin Pract Gastroenterol Hepatol 2007;4:24–34.

24. Kalaitzakis E, Wallskog J, Björnsson E. Abstinence in patients with alcoholic liver cirrhosis: A follow-up study. Hepatol Res 2008;38:869–76.

25. Addolorato G, Russell M, Albano E, et al. Understanding and Treating Patients With Alcoholic Cirrhosis: An Update. Alcohol Clin Exp Res 2009;33(7): 1136–44.

26. O'Shea R, Dasarathy S, McCullough A, et al. Alcoholic liver disease. AASLD practice guidelines. Hepatology 2010;51(1):307–28.

27. Tan H, Virmani S, Martin P. Controversies in the management of alcoholic liver disease. Mt Sinai J Med 2009;76:484–98.

28. Rambaldi A, Gluud C. Anabolic-androgenic steroids for alcoholic liver disease. Cochrane Database Syst Rev 2006;4:CD003045.

29. Johnson B, Rosenthal N, Capece J, et al. Improvement of physical health and quality of life of alcohol-dependent individuals with topiramate treatment US multisite randomized controlled trial. Arch Intern Med 2008;168(11):1188–99.
30. Rambaldi A, Gluud C. Colchicine for alcoholic and non-alcoholic liver fibrosis and cirrhosis. Cochrane Database Syst Rev 2005;2:CD002148.
31. National center for complementary and alternative medicine. Available at: http://nccam.nih.gov/health/milkthistle/ataglance.htm. Accessed May 26, 2010.
32. Rambaldi A, Jacobs BP, Gluud C. Milk thistle for alcoholic and/or hepatitis B or C virus liver diseases. Cochrane Database Syst Rev 2007;4:CD003620.
33. Muriel P, Rivera-Espinoza Y. Beneficial drugs for liver diseases. J Appl Toxicol 2008;28:93–103.
34. Rambaldi A, Gluud C. S-adenosyl-L-methionine for alcoholic liver diseases. Cochrane Database Syst Rev 2006;2:CD002235.
35. Wolf D. Cirrhosis. Available at: http://emedicine.medscape.com/article/185856-overview. Updated: 2009. Accessed May 26, 2010.
36. Dynamed. Available at: http://www.ebscohost.com/dynamed/. Accessed May 31, 2010.
37. McCullough AJ, O'Connor JF. Alcoholic liver disease: proposed recommendations for the American College of Gastroenterology. Am J Gastroenterol 1998;93:2022–36.
38. Sorrell M. Immediate listing for liver transplantation for alcoholic cirrhosis: curbing our enthusiasm. Ann Intern Med 2009;150:216–7.
39. O'Grady JG. Liver transplantation alcohol related liver disease: stirring a hornet's nest! Gut 2006;55:1529–31.
40. Manzarbeitia C. Liver transplantation. Available at: http://emedicine.medscape.com/article/431783-overview. Updated: Sep 24, 2009. Accessed May 26, 2010.
41. American association for the study of liver diseases: top ten facts you should know about liver disease in the United States! Available at: http://publish.aasld.org/patients/Pages/liverfacts.aspx. Accessed June 2, 2010.
42. Jepsen P, Ott P, Andersen P, et al. Clinical course of alcoholic liver cirrhosis: a danish population-based cohort study. Hepatology 2010;51:1675–82.
43. Heidelbaugh JJ, Sherbondy M. Cirrhosis and chronic liver failure: part II. Complications and treatment. Am Fam Physician 2006;74:767–76 781.
44. Lawrence KR, Klee JA. Rifaximin for the treatment of hepatic encephalopathy. Pharmacotherapy 2008;28(8):1019–32.
45. Cohen MJ, Sahar T, Benenson S, et al. Antibiotic prophylaxis for spontaneous bacterial peritonitis in cirrhotic patients with ascites, without gastro-intestinal bleeding. Cochrane Database Syst Rev 2009;2:CD004791.
46. D'Amico G, Pagliaro L, Pietrosi G, et al. Emergency sclerotherapy versus vasoactive drugs for bleeding oesophageal varices in cirrhotic patients. Cochrane Database Syst Rev 2010;3:CD002233.
47. Soares-Weiser K, Brezis M, Tur-Kaspa R, et al. Antibiotic prophylaxis for cirrhotic patients with gastrointestinal bleeding. Cochrane Database Syst Rev 2002;2:CD002907.
48. Gluud LL, Christensen K, Christensen E, et al. Systematic review of randomized trials on vasoconstrictor drugs for hepatorenal syndrome. Hepatology 2010;51(2):576–84.
49. Sharma P, Kumar A, Shrama BC, et al. An open label, pilot, randomized controlled trial of noradrenaline versus terlipressin in the treatment of type 1 hepatorenal syndrome and predictors of response. Am J Gastroenterol 2008;103(7):1689–97.

50. Umgelter A, Reindl W, Wagner K, et al. Effects of plasma expansion with albumin and paracentesis on haemodynamics and kidney function in critically ill cirrhotic patients with tense ascites and hepatorenal syndrome: a prospective uncontrolled trial. Critical Care 2008;12:R4.
51. Lewis JR, Mohanty SR. Nonalcoholic fatty liver disease: a review and update. Dig Dis Sci 2010;55:560–78.
52. Lirussi F, Azzalini L, Orando S, et al. Antioxidant supplements for non-alcoholic fatty liver disease and/or steatohepatitis. Cochrane Database Syst Rev 2007;1: CD004996.
53. Neuschwander-Tetri BA, Caldwell SH. Nonalcoholic steatohepatitis: summary of an AASLD Single Topic Conference. Hepatology 2003;37(5):1202–19.
54. Torres DM, Harrison SA. Diagnosis and therapy of nonalcoholic steatohepatitis. Gastroenterology 2008;134(6):1682–98.
55. Cussons AJ, Watts GF, Mori TA, et al. Omega-3 fatty acid supplementation decreases liver fat content in polycystic ovary syndrome: a randomized controlled trial employing proton magnetic resonance spectroscopy. J Clin Endocrinol Metab 2009;94:3842–8.
56. Sanyal AJ, Chalasani N, Kowdley KV, et al. Pioglitazone, vitamin E, or placebo for nonalcoholic steatohepatitis. N Engl J Med 2010;362(18):1675–85.
57. Nugent C, Younossi Z. Evaluation and management of obesity-related NAFLD: Treatment of NASH. Nat Clin Pract Gastroenterol Hepatol CME 2007;4(8): 432–41.
58. Salem V, Bloom SR. Approaches to the pharmacological treatment of obesity. Expert Rev Clin Pharmacol 2010;3(1):73–88.
59. Chavez-Tapia NC, Tellez-Avila FI, Barrientos-Gutierrez T, et al. Bariatric surgery for non-alcoholic steatohepatitis in obese patients. Cochrane Database Syst Rev 2010;1:CD007340.
60. Angelico F, Burattin M, Alessandri C, et al. Drugs improving insulin resistance for non-alcoholic fatty liver disease and/or non-alcoholic steatohepatitis. Cochrane Database Syst Rev 2007;1:CD005166.
61. Pasternak R, Smith S Jr, Bairey-Merz N, et al. ACC/AHA/NHLBI Clinical Advisory on the Use and Safety of Statins. Stroke 2002;33:2337–41.
62. Orlando R, Azzalini L, Orando S, et al. Bile acids for non-alcoholic fatty liver disease and/or steatohepatitis. Cochrane Database Syst Rev 2007;1:CD005160.
63. Lirussi F, Mastropasqua E, Orando S, et al. Probiotics for non-alcoholic fatty liver disease and/or steatohepatitis. Cochrane Database Syst Rev 2007;1: CD005165.
64. Angulo P, Keach JC, Batts KP, et al. Independent predictors of liver fibrosis in patients with nonalcoholic steatohepatitis. Hepatology 1999;30(6):1356–62.
65. Adams LA, Lindor KD. Nonalcoholic fatty liver disease. Ann Epidemiol 2007;17: 863–9.
66. Fraser A, Harris R, Sattar N, et al. Alanine aminotransferase, gamma-glutamyltransferase, and incident diabetes: the British Women's Heart and Health Study and meta-analysis. Diabetes Care 2009;32(4):741–50.
67. Feldstein A, Charatcharoenwitthaya P, Treeprasertsuk S, et al. The natural history of non-alcoholic fatty liver disease in children: a follow-up study for up to 20 years. Gut 2009;58:1538–44.
68. U.S. Preventive Services Task Force. Screening for hemochromatosis: recommendation statement. Ann Intern Med 2006;145(3):204–8.
69. Beaton M, Adams P. The myths and realities of hemochromatosis. Can J Gastroenterol 2007;21(2):101–4.

70. Brissot P, de Bels F. Current approaches to the management of hemochromatosis. Hematology Am Soc Hematol Educ Program 2006;36–41.
71. Tavill A. Diagnosis and management of hemochromatosis. Hepatology 2001; 33(5):1321–8.

# Primary Care of the Liver Transplant Recipient

Augustine J. Sohn, MD, MPH[a],*, Hoonbae Jeon, MD[b],
Joseph Ahn, MD, MS[c]

## KEYWORDS

- Primary care • Liver transplant • Recipient
- Immunosuppressant • Opportunistic infection
- Insulin resistance

*A case: Mr F. O. is a 53-year-old man who presents to a family physician's office for a physical examination and to establish primary care service with a physician. He had a history of hepatitis C and alcohol-related liver cirrhosis and had undergone a liver transplantation 16 months before the visit. The patient had no specific complaints at the time of visit. He had a marked increase in liver enzymes 6 months before this visit and a liver biopsy showed changes of alcoholic and hepatitis C liver disease. He adamantly denied alcohol recidivism and liver enzymes normalized spontaneously. He takes a multivitamin and states that he feels more energy with multivitamins.*

*Review of systems was within normal limits.*

*Past medical history includes hypertension, obesity, left arm fracture.*

*Medications include tacrolimus (Prograf) 2 mg in the morning and 1 mg in the afternoon, mycophenolate mofetil (CellCept) 1 g twice a day.*

*Metoprolol 100 mg twice a day, amlodipine 10 mg daily.*

*Urosodiol 600 mg in the morning and 300 mg in the afternoon.*

*Social history: smokes tobacco (1 pack per day).*

*Alcohol in the past and status post cirrhosis and has not relapsed since the transplantation.*

*Physical examination: alert and oriented times 3, well nourished, blood pressure 136/88, body mass index 35. Pulse 76, respiration rate 18. Temperature 36.9°C (98.4°F). Eyes: non-icteric sclera, pupils equal, round, reactive to light and*

No acknowledged funding support.

[a] Department of Family Medicine, College of Medicine, University of Illinois at Chicago, 1919 West Taylor Street, Chicago, IL 60612, USA

[b] Liver Transplant and Hepatobiliary Surgery, Transplant Surgery Fellowship Program, Division of Transplant (MC958), Department of Surgery, University of Illinois at Chicago, 840 South Wood Street, CSB 402, Chicago, IL 60612, USA

[c] Liver Transplantation, Loyola University Medical Center, Room 167, Building 54, 2160 South First Avenue, Maywood, IL 60153, USA

* Corresponding author.

*E-mail address:* ajsohn@uic.edu

*accommodation, extraocular muscles intact. Neck: no thyroidmegaly. Lungs: clear on auscultation and percussion. Heart: regular without murmur, point of maximal impulse non-displaced. Abdomen: soft, well-healed subcostal transverse scars. Legs: no pedal edema.*

*The patient was given instruction to continue his medications and to follow up in 3 months. The patient was also educated regarding smoking cessation.*

*He was seen by the psychiatry service a few months later. He was referred because of depression. He mentioned to the psychiatrist that he had onset of drinking alcohol at age 10 years. He stated that he had suffered physical abuse as a boy. He also had history of cocaine, intravenous heroine, and marijuana abuse. He mentioned that the last time he used alcohol or drugs was 6 years before the transplantation surgery. He still smokes. He was diagnosed with major depression and started on sertraline.*

Liver transplantation outcomes have evolved significantly since the development of the surgical procedure in the 1960s. Survival after liver transplantation has improved significantly, with the 1-year survival rate more than 85%, and liver transplantation has become the treatment of choice for chronic liver failure, acute liver failure, and selected patients with early stage, unresectable hepatocellular carcinoma.[1] This improved survival was caused by the introduction of potent immunosuppression for the treatment and prevention of cellular rejection. However, potent immunosuppression has led to increased incidence and prevalence of immunosuppression-associated complications. Immunosuppression is a double-edged sword, with a need to carefully consider the risk/benefit ratio in titrating the doses for the optimal benefit of the liver transplant recipients. With an increasing number of long-term survivors, primary care physicians are expected to see larger numbers of these patients. This article provides a guideline for the care of liver transplant recipients in the office of primary care physicians. It is also important to have close communication and collaboration with the patient's transplantation center for optimal care.

## ORGAN REJECTION
### Late-onset Organ Rejection

Late-onset organ rejection of the liver transplant graft by the host immune system can be divided into acute and chronic rejection. Advances in immunosuppressive medications have allowed liver transplantation to move from a theory to a viable life-saving procedure by decreasing the risk of rejection. However, despite improvements in immunosuppression, patients still remain at risk of developing acute cellular rejection within 3 months of liver transplantation in up to 20% to 40% of cases.[2] These cases are eminently treatable with corticosteroid therapy, and long-term graft survival is not significantly impaired by these early cases of acute cellular rejection.[3]

By the time patients present for post follow-up to the primary care physician, they are usually at least 6 to 12 months after liver transplantation. The primary care physician needs to be able to recognize late-onset organ rejection and collaborate with the patient's transplant center to effectively manage these cases. Two major types of late-onset rejection exist: late acute cellular rejection and chronic rejection.

### Late acute cellular rejection

Acute cellular rejection is a process characterized by inflammation of the liver graft caused by immunologic injury occurring as a consequence of immunologic disparities between the donor and recipient immune systems. Late acute rejection occurs in up to 10% to 20% of cases, and is a risk factor for the subsequent development of chronic rejection, which has an impact on long-term survival.[4]

Acute rejection is mediated by the cellular arm of the immune system, mainly T cells that develop against donor antigens in the liver graft leading to an inflammatory response directed at hepatocytes and biliary epithelium. Risk factors include a history of autoimmune hepatitis, primary biliary cirrhosis, primary sclerosing cholangitis, and autoimmune cholangiopathy in the recipient. Medication and clinical follow-up noncompliance is also a well-recognized risk factor for developing acute rejection.[5]

Most commonly, acute rejection is detected through asymptomatic increase in liver chemistries including alkaline phosphatase, γ-glutamyl transferase, transaminases, and total bilirubin. Clinical symptoms are found in more severe cases that manifest later in their course after significant inflammatory injury to the graft has already occurred. Nonspecific complaints include nausea, fever, malaise, pruritus, jaundice, and abdominal discomfort. Thus, a high index of suspicion must be maintained to diagnose late acute rejection because the nonspecific nature of symptoms and findings can lead to a delay in diagnosis. Liver biopsy with histologic examination is mandatory to diagnose acute rejection. Histologic findings include lymphocytic infiltration localized to the portal tracts and central vein with progressive damage to the bile ducts in time.[6] However, histologic changes may be subtle, especially early in acute rejection, and can easily be confused with recurrent hepatitis C infection. The differential diagnoses include cytomegalovirus (CMV) infection, drug hepatotoxicity, hepatitis C or B, and recurrence of underlying liver disease.[7]

A delay in recognition and diagnosis can lead to progression of acute rejection leading to a decrease in response to treatment. Treatment is based on pulse corticosteroid therapy along with an increase in baseline maintenance calcineurin inhibitor levels.[8] There is no consensus for optimal corticosteroid therapy, although most transplant centers admit patients for intravenous corticosteroids for the first 3 days to allow close monitoring of response to therapy. In addition, adjuvant agents such as mycophenolate mofetil or rapamycin are often added. Prognosis in late acute rejection remains similar to early acute rejection except that patients may have a lower response to therapy because of a delay in diagnosis.

### Chronic rejection

Chronic rejection is an insidious process characterized histologically by diffuse bile duct loss, or ductopenia.[9] Chronic rejection is observed usually at least 3 months after liver transplantation and occurs in up to 3% to 4% of liver transplant recipients.[10]

The pathophysiology of chronic rejection is incompletely understood but is postulated to be multifactorial. Risk factors for chronic rejection include a previous history of acute cellular rejection, history of autoimmune hepatitis, primary biliary cirrhosis, and CMV infection.[11,12] The mechanism is attributed to the cellular arm of the immune system directed against antigens in the vascular endothelium and biliary tract. Vascular insufficiency leading to hypoxia is hypothesized to predispose the graft to immunologic-mediated injury. Noncompliance with immunosuppression medications may be an important risk factor for developing chronic rejection.[5]

Symptoms of chronic rejection are insidious, with an initial lack of symptoms or nonspecific malaise, fatigue, and abdominal discomfort. With development of significant cholestasis, patients may develop pruritus and jaundice. Chronic rejection is suspected in the setting of abnormal liver enzymes, notably alkaline phosphate and bilirubin and, to a lesser extent, aspartate aminotransferase (AST) and alanine aminotransferase (ALT). Diagnosis can only be made based on histology. Hallmark histologic findings include ductopenia, leading to the term vanishing bile duct syndrome for chronic rejection. Other less common findings include bile duct atrophy, obliterative arteriopathy and venulitis, lymphoid infiltrates, and centrilobular degeneration.[13] The differential diagnoses for chronic rejection include acute cellular rejection, CMV hepatitis, and recurrence of the original liver disease that necessitated the liver transplantation.

Treatment is directed at increasing the baseline immunosuppressive medications and ensuring compliance with prescribed immunosuppression. The use of pulse corticosteroids is not accepted as a treatment option for chronic rejection because of inefficacy and risk of significant adverse events. Patients on cyclosporine-based immunosuppression may respond to conversion of cyclosporine to tacrolimus-based therapy. However, patients with chronic rejection may continue to progress despite these treatment adjustments, requiring reevaluation for liver transplantation. Chronic rejection remains a well-recognized and feared complication of liver transplantation despite improvements in immunosuppression.

### Common Immunosuppression Medications

In 1994, the US multicenter FK506 Liver Study Group published a seminal paper comparing cyclosporine and tacrolimus for immunosuppression after liver transplantation.[14] This study is a landmark in the evolution of liver transplantation. With the introduction of newer immunosuppressive medications, acute rejection rates have decreased and many now believe that excess immunosuppression is the greater concern. More than half of the deaths in liver transplantation are related to complications attributable to immunosuppressive medications, including cardiovascular diseases, renal failure, infection, and malignancy.[15] To prevent acute rejection and manage potential adverse effects, there is a general strategy of using multiple immunosuppressive medications at high doses early after liver transplantation and fewer immunosuppressive medications at lower doses later.

Early after liver transplantation, most centers use a combination of 2 to 4 immunosuppressive medications, including a calcineurin inhibitor, an antimetabolite such as mycophenolate mofetil, and/or corticosteroids. Later, most centers taper doses of immunosuppressive medications and eliminate all but the calcineurin inhibitors and antimetabolites. When the primary care physicians see the patient, they usually are on a calcineurin inhibitor alone or a calcineurin inhibitor with the addition of mycophenolate. Small differences in doses or levels can lead to adverse effects or inefficacy of immunosuppression. **Tables 1** and **2** show the mechanisms, dosing, trough level goals, and side effects of the major immunosuppressive medications.

## CALCINEURIN INHIBITORS: CYCLOSPORINE AND TACROLIMUS

All forms of cyclosporine (Sandimumune, Neoral, Gengraf) and tacrolimus (Prograf) suppress the immune system through the inhibition of calcineurin, a protein that drives production of cytokines, such as interleukin (IL)-2, and is involved in the activation of T cells, the immune cells that attack the liver allograft. Collectively, cyclosporine and tacrolimus are called calcineurin inhibitors. Most patients are maintained on one or the other calcineurin inhibitors lifelong after transplantation. Both are oral agents usually taken every 12 hours. The dosage is adjusted based on trough levels of the drugs and is highly individualized. Higher trough levels are sought initially after liver transplantation when the risk of rejection is high, and lower levels are sought later when concerns about adverse effects start to predominate.

The early challenges of successful transplantation included surgical technique, organ preservation, and immunosuppression. As surgical technique improved, the need for improvements in immunosuppression became more obvious. A report

| Table 1 | | | |
|---------|--|--|--|
| Immunosuppression medication dose and monitoring and adverse events | | | |
| Agent | Daily Dose | Monitoring | Adverse Event |
| Tacrolimus | 1–5 mg twice a day | 5–15 ng/mL | Hypertension<br>Hypercholesterolemia<br>Neurotoxicity<br>Diabetes<br>Renal insufficiency<br>Osteoporosis |
| Cyclosporine | 100–200 mg twice a day | 50–300 ng/mL | Hypertension<br>Hypercholesterolemia<br>Neurotoxicity<br>Diabetes<br>Renal insufficiency<br>Osteoporosis |
| Mycophenolate mofetil | 750–1.5 g twice a day | None | Bone marrow suppression<br>GI side effects |
| Sirolimus | 2–5 mg every day | 5–15 ng/mL | Hyperlipidemia<br>Hypertension<br>Bone marrow suppression<br>Hepatic artery thrombosis |
| Azathioprine | 1–3 mg/kg every day | None | Bone marrow suppression<br>Pancreatitis |
| Corticosteroids | 5–10 mg every day | None | Hypertension<br>Hyperlipidemia<br>Diabetes<br>Osteoporosis<br>Psychiatric disorders |

*Abbreviation:* GI, gastrointestinal.

published in 1980 described a 1-year survival of only 26%.[16] The introduction of cyclosporine the following year signaled a turning point in liver transplantation.[17]

In an update on liver transplantation in 1988, the Pittsburgh Group reported that phase 1 trials of FK506 (tacrolimus) had recently begun.[18] A year later, the same group described use of FK506 as salvage therapy in patients who had failed with cyclosporine.[19] Within about 5 years, tacrolimus would overtake cyclosporine as the mainstay in liver transplantation. By the mid-1990s, most centers agreed that tacrolimus was associated with superior graft and patient survival. In a landmark study,[20] investigators compared the efficiency of tacrolimus versus microemulsified cyclosporine in 606 patients undergoing first orthotopic liver transplant using a composite primary endpoint of death, retransplantation, or treatment failure for immunologic reasons. Both treatment regimens were effective, but tacrolimus was superior for both the composite end point and for patient and graft survival. In addition, more patients in the tacrolimus group survived without an episode of significant rejection. The results of the study were updated with a 2-year extension of the randomized protocol: tacrolimus remained superior.

Multiple subsequent studies have been performed, and the superiority of tacrolimus compared with cyclosporine was confirmed in a meta-analysis of 16 randomized trials.[21] Tacrolimus was superior when analyzed for survival, graft loss, acute rejection, and steroid-resistant rejection in the first year. The incidence of lymphoproliferative disease was similar for the two groups, although de novo diabetes mellitus was

**Table 2**
Side effects of major immunosuppression medications

| | Hypertension | Hypercholesterolemia | Diabetes | Neurotoxicity | Renal Insufficiency | Osteoporosis | Bone Marrow Suppression | GI Side Effects |
|---|---|---|---|---|---|---|---|---|
| Tacrolimus | xxx | x | xx | xx | xx | x | xx | — |
| Cyclosporine | xxxx | xx | x | — | xxx | xx | xxx | — |
| Mycophenolate mofetil | — | — | — | — | — | — | — | x |
| Sirolimus | x | xxx | — | — | — | — | — | — |
| Azathioprine | — | — | — | — | — | — | — | — |
| Corticosteroids | xx | x | xxx | xx | x | xxx | xxxx | — |

Number of ×'s indicates degree of severity; × = mild to ×××× = severe.

more common in the tacrolimus group. More patients stopped cyclosporine than tacrolimus. The investigators estimated that treating 100 patients with tacrolimus versus cyclosporine would avoid rejection and steroid-resistant rejection in 9 and 7 patients respectively, graft loss and death in 5 and 2 patients respectively, but that 4 additional patients would develop diabetes after liver transplantation.

There are several side effects common to both calcineurin inhibitors, including hyperkalemia, hypertension, neurotoxicity (headaches, tremors, neuropathy, and seizures), and nephrotoxicity. Renal insufficiency remains a major cause of morbidity and mortality after liver transplantation. Cyclosporine is more commonly associated with dyslipidemia and gingival hyperplasia, whereas tacrolimus is more commonly associated with diabetes.

## ANTIMETABOLITES

Azathioprine (Immuran, Azasan), mycophenolate mofetil (CellCept) and mycophenolic acid (Myfortic) are antimetabolites. Antimetabolites are a group of medications that interfere with purine nucleotide synthesis, which leads to preferential inhibition of T and B cell lymphocytes. The antimetabolites are generally not potent enough to be used alone, but are important as adjunctive agents. Mycophenolate mofetil or myco-phenolic acid may be discontinued within a year after transplant. However, there is evidence that if mycophenolate mofetil or mycophenolic acid is continued, lower doses of calcineurin inhibitors can be used with a resulting improvement in renal function.[22] Azathioprine was used in the early years of liver transplantation but, in recent years, mycophenolate mofetil and mycophenolic acid have replaced azathioprine because it can be associated with the development of cholestatic hepatitis. Known side effects of mycophenolate mofetil and mycophenolic acid include bone marrow suppression and gastrointestinal (GI) side effects including gastritis, diarrhea, and abdominal pain.

## SIROLIMUS/RAPAMYCIN

Sirolimus (Rapamune) is a newer immunosuppressive agent that inhibits T cell prolif-eration through cell cycle inhibition. It is regarded as an agent that is potent enough to be used as a primary immunosuppressive agent but without the nephrotoxicity of cal-cineurin inhibitors. Sirolimus is therefore considered as an alternative to calcineurin inhibitors or, in some instances, in combination with lower doses of one of the calci-neurin inhibitors. However, sirolimus has been associated with an increased risk for hepatic artery thrombosis and, as a result, had received a black-box warning for liver transplant recipients, which has led to avoidance of its use in the early months after transplantation. Other side effects include rash, dyslipidemia, cytopenia, poor wound healing, and oral ulcerations. There is also an association with an unusual but poten-tially fatal interstitial pneumonitis. Because of these side effects, 20% to 30% of those patients who receive the drug are not able to tolerate it.

## CORTICOSTEROIDS

Corticosteroids (prednisone or prednisolone) are generally given in large doses during the first week after liver transplantation and tapered rapidly to lower levels or completely eliminated within weeks or months following liver transplantation. Given the substantial long-term side effects of corticosteroids, most transplant centers are trying to eliminate or minimize corticosteroids use in transplant recipients. However, in patients with autoimmune liver diseases or history of recurrent rejection, steroids are frequently continued indefinitely.

## DRUG INTERACTIONS OF IMMUNOSUPPRESSANTS

Tacrolimus, cyclosporin, and sirolimus have dose-related toxicity and narrow therapeutic windows. The 2 pathways that are important for calcineurin inhibitor metabolism are cytochrome P-450 3A4 and P-glycoprotein. Certain drugs can induce, inhibit, or slow metabolism of calcineurin inhibitors. For example, use of azithromycin for a simple case of bacterial infection may result in significant increase of calcineurin inhibitors and cause nephrotoxicity. On the other hand, other drugs such as phenobarbital or phenytoin may lower the calcineurin inhibitor serum levels and cause rejection. Whenever any new medications are started, it is important to check for possible interactions between the new medicine and calcineurin inhibitors, or consult with the transplant center. **Boxes 1** and **2** provide a list of substances that can increase or decrease levels of immunosuppressants.

Transplant recipients have a high prevalence of insulin resistance syndromes including hypertension, type 2 diabetes, obesity, and dyslipidemia. Drugs that are generally well tolerated include amlodipine, nifedipine, clonidine, angiotensin-converting enzyme (ACE) inhibitors, angiotensin receptor blockers, and β-blockers (except carvedilol) for hypertension; oral hypoglycemics, metformin, sulfonylureas, and thiazolidinediones for diabetes. Statin drugs, ezetimibe, niacin, and intestinal binders of bile acids have been used for dyslipidemia. Because of interaction between calcineurin inhibitors and statins or ezetimibe, these lipid-lowering drugs should be given at lower dosages and monitored for side effects and serum trough levels of calcineurin inhibitors.[23] Intestinal binders of bile acids should be given 2 hours before or after calcineurin inhibitors and should not be used in patients also taking mycophenolate mofetil or mycophenolic acid.[24] Narcotics are usually safe outside their addictive potential, and antidepressants are usually well tolerated. Up to 2 g/d of acetaminophen can be given to liver transplant recipients with functioning livers without reservation.

Selected antibiotics including any of the penicillins, cephalosporins, quinolones, sulfonamides, and topical (not oral) antifungal agents are generally well tolerated.

### Opportunistic Infections

Despite improvements in surgical techniques, immunosuppressants, and antibiotics in the last 20 years, infections continue to pose the greatest mortality risk after liver transplantation.[25] The risk of infection is dependent on the patient's epidemiologic infectious risk factors as well as the net state of immunosuppression. These epidemiologic risk factors include procedures, surgeries, vaccination history, previous infectious exposures, travel history, location, and antimicrobial use history. The net state or level of immunosuppression is dependent on the type, dose, and duration of

---

**Box 1**
**Drugs and substances that may increase levels of cyclosporine and tacrolimus and sirolimus (this list is not all inclusive)**

Antifungals: fluconazole, ketoconazole, itraconazole, voriconazole, caspofungin

Antibiotics: azithromycin, erythromycin, clarithromycin

Calcium channel blockers: diltiazem, verapamil, nicardipine, nifedipine

Others: danazol

Protease inhibitors for hepatitis B virus or human immunodeficiency virus (HIV)

Grapefruit products

> **Box 2**
> **Drugs and substance that may decrease levels of cyclosporine, tacrolimus, and sirolimus (this list is not all inclusive)**
>
> Anticonvulsants: carbamazepine, phenobarbital, phenytoin
>
> Antibiotics: rifampin, isoniazid
>
> Others: St John's wort

immunosuppressant use; underlying medical diseases and comorbidities; presence of fluid collections, catheters, or mechanical devices; as well as immune-modulating diseases such as HIV or cytomegalovirus (CMV) infection.

In addition, the astute clinician must be cognizant of the impact of immunosuppression on the liver transplant recipient presenting with infection. Immunosuppression attenuates inflammatory responses and may mute clinical and radiographic signs of infection in the liver transplant recipient, leading to advanced presentations and delays in diagnosis. Because of more advanced presentation of infection and associated delays in diagnosis, the course of infections may be more aggressive and rapid with a significant risk of morbidity and mortality. Thus, early and accurate diagnosis must be pursued with a low threshold for obtaining imaging studies, removal of foreign bodies and catheters, and tissue diagnosis along with broad empiric treatment while awaiting data to narrow and taper antimicrobial treatment. Clinicians must also be aware of the complexity of antibiotic choices in the setting of drug interactions with immunosuppression as well as the increased risk of underlying and potential antimicrobial resistance.

Infections after liver transplantation can be divided based on time from liver transplantation as well as the type of infection.[26,27] Immediately following liver transplantation and for up to 4 to 6 weeks, the patient remains at the greatest risk for nosocomial or hospital-acquired infections associated with surgical procedures, mechanical ventilation, catheter placement, or prolonged antibiotic use. Coupling these risks with the high-intensity immunosuppression immediately following liver transplantation, the patient is at increased infectious risk of *Pseudomonas aeruginosa*, methicillin-resistant *Staphylococcus aureus*, (MRSA), vancomycin-resistant enterococcus (VRE), legionella, non-albicans candida, as well as *Clostridium difficile*. Donor-derived infections also pose a rare, but significant, risk to the liver transplant recipient.

Up to 6 months after liver transplantation, the patient remains at greatest risk of opportunistic infection because of the high level of immunosuppression. After 6 months, most patients' immunosuppression levels have been titrated to a maintenance level with a lower net level of immunosuppression, attenuating the risk of opportunistic infections. At this point, patients present with community-acquired infections such as urinary tract infections, pneumonias, and influenza similar to patients without a history of transplantation.

Atypical infectious organisms causing opportunistic infections include CMV, *Pneumocystis jiroveci*, human herpes virus-6, and *Aspergillus*. Less common viruses include varicella zoster virus (VZV), herpes simplex virus (HSV), Epstein-Barr virus (EBV), adenoviruses, parvovirus B19, and respiratory syncytial virus. Fungal infections such as non-albicans candida can occur as well as *Histoplasma capsulatum* (Midwest), *Coccidioides immitis* (Southwest), and *Blastomyces dermatitidis* (Mississippi and Ohio Rivers) depending on the location of patients' domicile and travel history.[28] Mycobacterium infection, although not as common as the organisms listed earlier, is a feared opportunistic infection that can be seen in this time period.

CMV is a human herpesvirus, and has a unique impact on liver transplant recipients because it has not only a direct effect on tissues but immune-modulating effects. The immune-modulating effects of CMV lead to an increased risk of bacterial infections, fungal infections, accelerated hepatitis C recurrence, and chronic rejection.[29] CMV infection (viremia without symptoms) occurs up to 60% of patients after liver transplantation, with up to 20% developing CMV disease in the liver, lungs, GI tract, and retina.[30] Evidence of CMV seropositivity is found in 40% to 60% of healthy adults, leaving them at risk of reactivation of endogenous latent CMV with immunosuppression. However, the greatest risk of CMV infection is in patients without history of CMV exposure who receive a CMV-seropositive liver graft. Presentation of CMV disease can be variable with fever, malaise, bone marrow suppression, and arthralgias with less frequent presentation including a tissue-specific hepatitis, pneumonitis, gastroenteritis, or retinitis.[31]

Universal CMV prophylaxis is recommended for CMV-seronegative patients receiving a CMV-seropositive donor organ. Patients who are CMV seropositive can receive CMV prophylaxis or be treated with preemptive therapy (monitoring for CMV infection and treatment if the patient becomes CMV positive). Treatment regimens vary among transplant centers, although most centers provide CMV prophylaxis for up to 6 months with ganciclovir or valganciclovir.[32] A benefit of universal CMV prophylaxis is that antiviral therapy directed toward CMV has protective activity against other human herpesviruses such as HSV and VZV as well as EBV. Without prophylaxis, patients may have up to 50% recurrence risk of HSV and an increased risk of other viral infections.[33,34] Although valganciclovir is not approved by the US Food and Drug Administration for liver transplant patients because of an increased incidence of CMV disease compared with ganciclovir,[35] many transplant programs are using valganciclovir because of its greater bioavailability compared with ganciclovir as well as its easier dosing regimen.

*P jiroveci* is a yeast like fungus that poses unique risk for immunosuppressed patients. Pneumocystis was previously misclassified as a protozoan and historically called *Pneumocystis carinii*, although that name is now designated only for *Pneumocystis* variants occurring in animals.[36] PCP continues to be used as the acronym for pneumocystis pneumonia given its familiarity and extended history of use. Prophylaxis with daily single-strength trimethoprim-sulfamethoxazole or 3 times a week double-strength trimethoprim-sulfamethoxazole is recommended up to 6 to 12 months after liver transplantation. Patients who cannot tolerate trimethoprim-sulfamethoxazole because of sulfonamide allergy can be treated with atovaquone, inhaled pentamidine, or dapsone. However, these second-line agents do not provide the added benefit of trimethoprim-sulfamethoxazole activity against *Toxoplasma gondii*, nocardiosis, and *Listeria monocytogenes*.

Vaccination is recommended after liver transplantation for hepatitis A and B as well as pneumococcal and inactivated influenza. However, active, live vaccines are not recommended, including measles, mumps, and varicella.

### Noninfectious Complication of Liver Transplantation

#### Hypertension

Hypertension is a common complication in liver transplant recipients.[37] Corticosteroids and calcineurin inhibitors increase the risk of blood pressure increase in transplant recipients. Calcineurin inhibitors cause sympathetic stimulation with resultant vasoconstrictions and sodium retention.[38] Cyclosporine is associated with a higher incidence of hypertension following liver transplantation compared with tacrolimus.[39]

The goal of antihypertensive therapy should be adequate blood pressure control. Treatment of hypertension may include diuretics, especially in patients with peripheral edema. However, those diuretics must be used with caution because thiazides may cause gout. The calcium channel blockers, particularly the dihydropyridine class, are particularly attractive because their vasodilatory effects may overcome the vasoconstriction caused by the calcineurin inhibitors. Representative dihydropyridine calcium channel blockers include amlodipine, felodipine, and nifedipine. Among other calcium channel blockers, diltiazem, verapamil, and nicardipine should be avoided because they increase serum levels of the calcineurin inhibitors.

α-Blockers such as clonidine and doxazosin are frequently used for posttransplantation hypertension. β-Blockers can be used and do not affect calcineurin inhibitor levels, except carvedilol, which can cause increased levels of calcineurin inhibitors and usually requires reduction in calcineurin inhibitor dosage to maintain therapeutic serum level.[40] ACE inhibitors and angiotensin II receptor blockers are not used initially for hypertension because of the increased risk of renal insufficiency and hyperkalemia in early transplant recipients. However, after the immediate posttransplant period, these medications may be helpful in preventing diabetic nephropathy.

### Diabetes mellitus

Prevalence of diabetes mellitus is higher in liver transplant recipients than in the general population. The prevalence of diabetes is as high as 33%.[41] Risk factors of diabetes in liver transplant recipients include use of corticosteroids, high-dose calcineurin inhibitors, hepatitis C seropositivity, ethnicity, pretransplantation diabetes, and obesity. Although liver transplantation may cure hepatogenous diabetes, many pretransplant type 1 diabetic patients remain on insulin after liver transplantation.

Management of posttransplant diabetes is similar to that of patients without liver diseases, with the same treatment goals to prevent complications such as coronary artery diseases, renal failure, neuropathy, and retinopathy. Education for diet and exercise are important in managing diabetes. Insulin therapy may be needed in the early stages after transplantation. Oral hypoglycemic agents can be used with minimal concern of interaction with immunosuppressive medications or damage to the transplanted liver.[42] Early withdrawal or dose reduction of corticosteroid may improve glycemic control. Because tacrolimus is associated with diabetes, another therapeutic maneuver may be necessary to lower the dosage of tacrolimus.

### Dyslipidemia

Because most patients with end-stage liver disease have low serum cholesterols because of impaired hepatic synthesis and esterification of cholesterols, they have increased plasma cholesterol after liver transplantation. Risk factors for posttransplant dyslipidemia include cholestatic liver disease, pretransplant cholesterol increase, diabetes, obesity, and use of immunosuppressive agents.[43] Cyclosporine, steroids, and sirolimus have significant effects on serum lipid levels. Tacrolimus has a minor effect on serum lipids, and mycophenolate mofetil and azathiprine have no significant effects on serum lipids. Cyclosporine increases serum total cholesterol, low-density lipoprotein (LDL) cholesterol, and triglyceride.[44]

Treatment of posttransplant dyslipidemia is similar to the treatment without liver disease. The first step of treatment is lifestyle modification including low-fat diet and exercise. If the lifestyle modification is not successful after approximately 6 months, the next step is switching medications that are associated with dyslipidemia. The transplantation center should be contacted to consider reducing or eliminating steroids and substituting tacrolimus for cyclosporine.

All agents reducing cholesterol have been used in liver transplant recipients successfully, but all have potential side effects. Bile acid sequestrants (cholestyramine, colestipol, and colesevelam) can decrease plasma mycophenolate mofetil and myco-phenolic acid levels by 35%.[24] In addition, bile acid sequestrants decrease absorption of calcineurin inhibitors. Thus, bile acid sequestrants should not be used in patients taking mycophenolate mofetil or mycophenolic acid and should be given greater than 2 hours before or after calcineurin inhibitor dosing. Fibric acid (gemfibrozil fenofibrate and clofibrate) can cause biliary sludge, dyspepsia, or myopathy. Statins can cause myopathy or increase in liver enzymes. If a statin is used, hydrophilic statins (pravastatin or fluvestatin) are preferred because they are not metabolized by the same cytochrome P-450 3A4 metabolic pathway that metabolizes calcineurin inhibitors and sirolimus.

### Obesity

The obesity rate in the United States has been rising steadily in the past 3 decades. However, 22% of nonobese liver transplant recipients became obese in a 2-year follow-up.[45] Liver transplant recipient who were overweight before surgery tend to gain more weight. Corticosteroids contribute to weight gain, and one study suggests that cyclosporine is associated with more weight gain compared with tacrolimus.[46]

Treatment of obesity in liver transplant recipients is not different from patients without liver diseases. Lifestyle modification, including portion control and aerobic exercise should be considered first. Also, lowering or discontinuing corticosteroids or switching from cyclosporine to tacrolimus should be considered. Orlistat is not rec-ommended for patients who are also receiving cyclosporine, because this combina-tion may decrease cyclosporine absorption. Orlistat has been safely used with tacrolimus-based immunosuppression, but efficacy has not been verified.[47]

### Psychological Aspects of Care for Liver Transplant Recipient

Relapse of alcohol use after liver transplantation often affects not only the quality of life but also adherence to immunosuppressive medications. Problematic and harmful drinking after liver transplantation occurs in up to 20% of liver transplant recipients. Some deaths in this group are related to death caused by poor compliance with immu-nosuppressive agents.[48] One study showed potential predictors of return to harmful drinking: diagnosis of depression, the lack of stable partner, grams per day consumed in the years before assessment for transplant, reliance on family and friends for post-transplant support, tobacco consumption at time of assessment, and lack of insight into the alcoholic cause of liver disease.[49] Alcoholic disease is a chronic illness requiring a continuous management, before and after transplantation.

Neuropsychiatric complications, especially depression, are frequent in liver trans-plant recipients. According to a study, the type of immunosuppression did not alter the frequency of complications. However, depression is significantly more common in patients transplanted for hepatitis C.[50] Underlying depression in patients with hepa-titis C should be identified and treated before liver transplantation and special atten-tion should be given to patients with hepatitis C who received liver transplantation for posttransplantation depression.

As liver transplant recipients live longer, their quality of life is an important aspect of care by primary care physicians. A meta-analysis of health-related quality of life after liver transplantation showed significant improvements in posttransplantation physical health, sexual functioning, general health-related quality of health and social func-tioning, but not psychological health. Investigators of the study recommended that transplantation treatment programs expand the psychological and social support available to patients both before and after transplantation.[51]

The purpose of liver transplantation includes not only the extension of survival and improvement of quality of life but also the return of the liver transplant recipient as a contributing member of society. Employment is one measure of the ability to return to society. A recent study of 308 adult liver transplant recipients showed that pretransplant variables that were independently associated with posttransplantation employment included lack of disability benefit, the absence of diabetes mellitus, the number of jobs before transplantation, high physical functioning before transplantation, and possession of private medical insurance.[52]

---

**Key Points**

1. Chronic rejection of liver graft is an insidious process. Primary care physicians should have a high index of suspicion when patients show any sign of malaise, fever, or jaundice. Chronic rejection should be suspected in the setting of abnormal liver enzymes, notably alkaline phosphate and bilirubin and, to a lesser extent, AST and ALT. Diagnosis can be made based on histology.

2. Major immunosuppression medications such as tacrolimus, cyclosporin, and sirolimus have dose-related toxicity and narrow therapeutic windows. Certain drugs can induce, inhibit, or slow metabolism of calcineurin inhibitors. Whenever any new medications are started, it is imperative to check possible interaction between the new medicine and calcineurin inhibitors, or consult with the transplant center.

3. Up to 6 months after liver transplantation, the patient remains at greatest risk of opportunistic infection caused by the high level of immunosuppression. After 6 months, most patients' immunosuppression medication levels have been titrated to a maintenance level with a lower net level of immunosuppression, attenuating the risk of opportunistic infections. At this point, patients present with community-acquired infections such as urinary tract infections, pneumonias, and influenza, similar to patients without a history of transplantation. However, primary care physicians should be vigilant for any unusual opportunistic infection in liver transplant recipients.

4. Long-term use of immunosuppression with calcineurin inhibitors may lead to conditions associated with insulin resistance: hypertension, type 2 diabetes mellitus, dyslipidemia, and obesity. Lifestyle modification, especially exercise and diet, should be encouraged at every visit. When medications are started, they should be used with care, paying careful attention to possible interaction with calcineurin inhibitors.

5. As liver transplant recipients live longer, their quality of life is an important aspect of care by primary care physicians. Health-related quality of life after liver transplantation showed significant improvement in posttransplantation physical health, sexual functioning, general health-related quality of health, and social functioning, but psychological health has only minor improvement. Alcohol relapse and possibility of depression in liver transplant recipients should be a continuous concern for primary care physicians. Depression is common among those who have had hepatitis C.

---

**REFERENCES**

1. McGuire BM, Rosenthal P, Brown CC, et al. Long-term management of the liver transplant patient: recommendation for the primary care doctor. Am J Transplant 2009;9:1988–2003.
2. Fisher LR, Henley KS, Lucey MR. Acute cellular rejection after liver transplantation: variability, morbidity, and mortality. Liver Transpl Surg 1995;1(1):10–5.
3. Meier-Kriesche HU, Li S, Gruessner RW, et al. Immunosuppression: evolution in practice and trends, 1994–2004. Am J Transplant 2006;6(5):1111–31.
4. Uemura T, Ikegami T, Sanchez EQ, et al. Late acute rejection after liver transplantation impacts patient survival. Clin Transplant 2008;22(3):316–23.

5. Mor E, Gonwa TA, Husberg BS. Late onset acute rejection in orthotopic liver transplantation - associated risk factors and outcome. Transplantation 1992; 54(5):821–4.

6. Banff schema for grading liver allograft rejection: an international consensus document. Hepatology 1997;25(3):658–63.

7. Demetrius AJ, Qian SC, Sun H, et al. Liver allograft rejection: an overview of morphologic findings. Am J Surg Pathol 1990;14(Suppl 1):49–63.

8. Volpin R, Angeli P, Galioto A, et al. Comparison between two high-dose methyl-prednisolone schedules in the treatment of acute hepatic rejection in liver transplant recipients: a controlled clinical trial. Liver Transpl 2002;8(6):527–34.

9. Demetris AJ, Adeyi O, Bellamy CO, et al. Liver biopsy interpretation for causes of late liver allograft dysfunction. Hepatology 2006;44(2):489–501.

10. Wiesner RH, Menon KV. Late hepatic allograft dysfunction. Liver Transpl 2001; 7(11):S60–73.

11. O'Grady JG, Alexander GJ, Sutherland S, et al. Cytomegalovirus infection and donor/recipient HLA antigens: interdependent co-factors in pathogenesis of vanishing bile-duct syndrome after liver transplantation. Lancet 1988;2:302–5.

12. Soin AS, Rasmussen A, Jamieson NV, et al. CsA levels in the early posttransplant period - predictive of chronic rejection in liver transplantation? Transplantation 1995;59(8):1119–23.

13. Demetris AJ, Adams D, Bellamy C, et al. Update of the international Banff schema for liver allograft rejection: working recommendations for the histopathologic staging and reporting of chronic rejection. An international panel. Hepatology 2000;31(3):792–9.

14. The U.S. Multicenter FK506 Liver Study Group. A comparison of tacrolimus (FK 506) and cyclosporine for immunosuppression in liver transplantation. N Engl J Med 1994;331(17):1110–5.

15. Abbasoglu O, Levy MF, Brkic F, et al. Ten years after liver transplantation: an evolving understanding of late graft loss. Transplantation 1997;64:1801–7.

16. Starzl TE, Koep L, Porter KA, et al. Decline in survival after liver transplantation. Arch Surg 1980;115(7):815–9.

17. Starzl TE, Klintmalm GB, Porter KA, et al. Liver transplantation with use of cyclosporin a and prednisone. N Engl J Med 1981;305(5):266–9.

18. Gordon RD, Starzl TE. Changing perspectives on liver transplantation in 1988. Clin Transplant 1988;5–27.

19. Starzl TE, Todo S, Fung J, et al. FK 506 for liver, kidney, and pancreas transplantation. Lancet 1989;2(8670):1000–4.

20. O'Grady JG, Hardy P, Burroughs AK, et al. Tacrolimus versus microemulsified ciclosporin in liver transplantation: the TMC randomized controlled trial. Lancet 2002;360(9340):1119–25.

21. McAlister VC, Haddad E, Renouf E, et al. Cyclosporine verses tacrolimus as primary immunosuppressant after liver transplantation: a meta-analysis. Am J Transplant 2006;6(7):1578–85.

22. Pageaux GP, Rostaing L, Calmus Y, et al. Mycophenolate mofetil in combination with reduction of calcineurin inhibitors for chronic renal dysfunction after liver transplantation. Liver Transpl 2006;12:1755–60.

23. Ucar M, Mjorndal T, Dahlqvist R. HMG-CoA reductase inhibitors and myotoxicity. Drug Saf 2000;22:441–57.

24. Bullingham RE, Nicholls AJ, Kamm BR. Clinical pharmacokinetics of mycophenolate mofetil. Clin Pharmacokinet 1998;34:429–55.

25. Rubin RH. The direct and indirect effects of infection in liver transplantation: pathogenesis, impact, and clinical management. Curr Clin Top Infect Dis 2002;22:125–54.
26. Barkholt L, Ericzon BG, Tollemar J, et al. Infections in human liver recipients: different patterns early and late after transplantation. Transpl Int 1993;6:77–84.
27. Blair JE, Kusne S. Bacterial, mycobacterial, and protozoal infections after liver transplantation - part I. Liver Transpl 2006;11(12):1452–9.
28. Kusne S, Blair JE. Viral and fungal infections after liver transplantation - part II. Liver Transpl 2006;12(1):2–11.
29. Razonable RR. Cytomegalovirus infection after liver transplantation: current concepts and challenges. World J Gastroenterol 2008;14:4849.
30. Winston DJ, Emmanouilides C, Busuttil RW. Infections in liver transplant recipients. Clin Infect Dis 1995;21(5):1077–89.
31. Ljungman P, Plotkin SA. Workshop on CMV disease: definitions, clinical severity, scores, and new syndromes. Scand J Infect Dis 1995;99:S87–9.
32. Cytomegalovirus. Am J Transplant 2004;4(Suppl 10):51–8.
33. Singh N, Dummer JS, Kusne S, et al. Infections with cytomegalovirus and other herpesviruses in 121 liver transplant recipients: transmission by donated organ and the effect of OKT3 antibodies. J Infect Dis 1988;158:124–31.
34. Kalil AC, Levitsky J, Lyden E, et al. Meta-analysis: the efficacy of strategies to prevent organ disease by cytomegalovirus in sold organ transplant recipients. Ann Intern Med 2005;143:870–80.
35. Paya C, Human A, Dominguez E, et al. Efficacy and safety of valganciclovir vs. oral ganciclovir for prevention of cytomegalovirus disease in solid organ transplant recipients. Am J Transplant 2004;4:611–20.
36. Aliouat-Denis CM, Chabe M, Demanche C, et al. Pneumocystis species, coevolution and pathogenic power. Infect Genet Evol 2008;8(5):708–26.
37. Gonwa TA. Hypertension and renal dysfunction in long-term liver transplant recipients. Liver Transpl 2001;7(Suppl 1):S22–6.
38. Moss NG, Powell SL, Falk RJ. Intravenous cyclosporine activates afferent and efferent renal nerves and causes sodium retention in innervated kidneys in rats. Proc Natl Acad Sci U S A 1985;82:8222–6.
39. Canzanello VJ, Textar SC, Taler SJ, et al. Late hypertension after liver transplantation: a comparison of cyclosporine and tacrolimus (FK 506). Liver Transpl Surg 1998;4:328–34.
40. Galioto A, Semplicini A, Zanus G, et al. Nifedipine versus carvedilol in the treatment of de novo arterial hypertension after liver transplantation: results of a controlled clinical trial. Liver Transpl 2008;14:1020–8.
41. Reuben A. Long-term management of the liver transplant patient: diabetes, hyperlipidemia, and obesity. Liver Transpl 2001;7(Suppl 1):S13–21.
42. Marchetti P. New-onset diabetes after liver transplantation: from pathogenesis to management. Liver Transpl 2005;11:612–20.
43. Gisbert C, Prieto M, Berenguer M, et al. Hyperlipidemia in liver transplant recipients: prevalence and risk factors. Liver Transpl Surg 1997;3:416–22.
44. Kobashigawa JA, Kasiske BL. Hyperlipidemia in solid organ transplantation. Transplantation 1997;63:331–8.
45. Everhart JE, Lombardero M, Lake JR, et al. Weight change and obesity after liver transplantation. Incidence and risk factors. Liver Transpl Surg 1998;4:285–96.
46. Contos MJ, Cales W, Sterling RK, et al. Development of nonalcoholic fatty liver disease after orthotopic liver transplantation for cryptogenic cirrhosis. Liver Transpl 2001;7:363–73.

47. Cassiman D, Roelants M, Vandenplas G, et al. Orlistat treatment is safe in overweight and obese liver transplant recipients: a prospective open label trial. Transpl Int 2006;19:1000–15.
48. Pageaux GP, Bismuth M, Perney P, et al. Alcohol relapse after liver transplantation for alcoholic liver disease: does it matter? J Hepatol 2003;38(5):629–34.
49. Kelly M, Chick J, Cribble R, et al. Predictors of relapse to harmful alcohol after orthotopic liver transplantation. Alcohol Alcohol 2006;41(3):278–83.
50. Tombazzi CR, Waters B, Shokouh-Amiri MH, et al. Neuropsychiatric complications after liver transplantation: role of immunosuppression and hepatitis C. Dig Dis Sci 2006;51(6):1079–81.
51. Bravata DM, Olkin I, Barnato AE, et al. Health-related quality of life after liver transplantation: a meta-analysis. Liver Transpl Surg 1999;5:318–31.
52. Saab S, Wiese C, Ibrahim AB, et al. Employment and quality of life in liver transplant recipients. Liver Transpl 2007;13:1330–8.

# Chronic Pancreatitis and Exocrine Insufficiency

John Affronti, MS, MD

**KEYWORDS**

- Pancreatic insufficiency • Pancreas enzymes • Epidemiology
- Diagnosis • Management • Complications

It is common to describe patients with chronic pancreatitis (CP) as a group that is separate from those with acute pancreatitis (AP). However there is abundant evidence documenting the evolution from acute to CP in many patients.[1] It is probably most accurate to think of the 2 conditions as separate ends of the same continuum. Patients with repeated bouts of pancreatitis or acute recurrent pancreatitis without the sequelae of CP may be somewhere in between these 2 ends of the continuum.

The traditional definition of CP has been permanent and irreversible damage to the pancreas, with histologic evidence of chronic inflammation and fibrosis along with destruction of the parenchyma of the gland. However, it is rare that pancreatic tissue is available for evaluation. Moreover, some histologic findings associated with CP are not specific. For example, some may be similar to those found in normal aging. In addition, sampling errors and small tissue volumes may lead to misleading interpretations. Therefore, even when histologic information is available, the diagnosis of CP may be imprecise.

Alternative methods of defining CP have included the combination of clinical features such as pain and pancreatic insufficiency with findings on various imaging studies such as ultrasonography (US), computed tomography (CT), endoscopic US (EUS), magnetic resonance imaging (MRI), and endoscopic retrograde cholangiopancreatography (ERCP). Again, the ability to make a diagnosis of CP may be imperfect because of subtle or intermittent clinical findings. It may also take years for findings on imaging studies to develop. The early diagnosis of CP, at a time when some effective therapy might be given, is therefore often impossible.

Given these shortcomings, when communicating with colleagues about pancreatitis it is helpful to describe how a diagnosis of CP has been made for a particular patient. For example to say that Mr Smith has a diagnosis of CP based on his history of alcohol

The author has nothing to disclose.

Division of Gastroenterology, Hepatology and Nutrition, Stritch School of Medicine, Loyola University of Chicago, 2160 South First Avenue, Maywood, IL 60153, USA

*E-mail address:* jaffronti@lumc.edu

use, recurrent pain, and CT findings of pancreatic calcifications as well as a dilated main pancreatic duct communicates both the level of certainty about the diagnosis as well as the severity of the disease.

## EPIDEMIOLOGY

It has been estimated that in the United States there are 210,000 admissions for AP each year.[2] CP in the United States results in more than 122,000 outpatient visits and more than 56,000 hospitalizations per year.[3] The incidence of CP ranges from 1.6 to 23 cases per 100,000 per year worldwide. The gradual increase in incidence observed in some countries may be attributed to increasing alcohol consumption and earlier diagnosis.[3]

Despite decades of research, the epidemiology of CP remains vague. As in other parts of the digestive tract, it is reasonable to assume that CP develops after numerous antecedent bouts of AP. Although this is generally accepted, it is difficult to document this logical sequence of events.[4] Epidemiologic research on CP has been substantially hindered by several factors. Classifications have been based on morphology and clinical findings rather than on cause; the diagnostic differences between acute and CP are sometimes vague and confusing; and coding by the International Classification of Diseases (ICD) has mostly not been useful for research projects that seek epidemiologic information.

Of the approximately 2.4 million deaths in the United States in 1999, pancreatitis was listed as the underlying cause for 3289 deaths, making it the 235th leading cause of death.[5] AP accounted for 84% of these deaths, and CP the remaining 16%. Alcohol is a primary cause of both acute and CP in most developed countries. About one-third of AP in the United States is alcohol induced. In the United States and other developed countries, 60% to 90% of CP is alcohol induced. Both forms are more common in men.[5] The development of CP is proportional to the dose and duration of alcohol consumption (minimum, 6–12 years of approximately 80 g of alcohol per day).[5] Autopsy studies reveal subclinical CP in another 10% of alcohol abusers. However, because less than 10% of chronic alcoholics develop CP, it is apparent that other predisposing factors in addition to alcohol are involved. Such factors as genetic variability and environmental exposures, like diet, have been suggested as probable disease promoters.[5] The most common presenting complaint for patients with CP is exacerbation of abdominal pain. Hospital admissions average 10 days for these exacerbations.[6]

Additional epidemiologic studies would be beneficial in improving the quality of existing baseline epidemiologic data and allow better assessment of risk. Moreover, many believe that improved diagnostic precision, more complete and specific coding, and greater understanding of covariables and mechanisms would also advance the field.[5]

## PATHOPHYSIOLOGY AND PHYSIOLOGY

The pathophysiology of pancreatitis is less of a mystery than in the past but still not completely understood. There are probably many different mechanisms and combinations of mechanisms that can contribute to pancreatitis. Several protective systems probably exist in the healthy human that overlap and are redundant that prevent the activation of inflammatory and/or enzymatic activity in the pancreas leading to pancreatitis.

Ground-breaking research by Whitcomb[7] and others has elucidated one defective protective mechanism in a family plagued with a hereditary form of CP. They found that there was a mutation in the cationic trypsinogen gene that predisposes this family to recurrent pancreatitis. This mutation prevented the inhibition of trypsinogen activation in the pancreas, which causes cell damage and inflammation. It is conceivable that many additional protective mechanisms of varying importance exist that have not yet been discovered. Moreover, some people may silently possess more defective protective mechanisms than others because of their genetic makeup. Perhaps a combination of many less important defective protective mechanisms, or just a few important defective mechanisms, causes these individuals to develop CP. It is also possible that such patients only develop pancreatitis when they are exposed to certain coexisting factors such as repeated alcohol use; this would explain why some individuals can drink alcohol heavily without developing pancreatitis, whereas others go on to develop a crippling pancreatic disease.

The function of activated pancreatic enzymes in the intestinal lumen is important to consider when treating patients with pancreatitis for at least 2 reasons. Most importantly, steatorrhea can occur in patients who have decreased luminal pancreatic enzyme activity because of a damaged gland, which is believed to occur when more than 90% of the capacity of the pancreas to produce lipase has been lost.[8] Providing exogenous pancreatic enzymes to patients with each meal and snack is an effective way to treat steatorrhea after it has been properly diagnosed.[9]

Another function of active pancreatic enzymes in the intestinal lumen seems to be the stimulation of pancreatic exocrine function through various feedback mechanisms.[10] The inhibitory effects of exogenous pancreas enzyme administration on endogenous pancreatic enzyme concentrations in healthy humans have been shown.[11] It has been proposed that supplementing the duodenal activity of endogenous pancreatic enzymes with exogenous pancreatic enzymes may decrease the stimulation of the pancreas in the early stages of CP or recurrent AP, thereby reducing the frequency and severity of the painful episodes in these patients.[10]

The feedback mechanisms mentioned earlier are probably no longer functional in those individuals who have had CP for many years. Therefore, exogenous pancreatic enzymes are probably not going to be effective for pain control in these patients. However, in those individuals without evidence of long-standing disease, such as those without ectatic pancreatic ducts or calcification, exogenous enzymes may be of benefit.[10] Gupta and Toskes[10] and others have categorized these patients as having small duct disease as opposed to those patients with long-standing CP with dilated pancreatic ducts who are categorized as having big duct disease.

For patients with small duct CP to have the best chance of pain reduction, the exogenous pancreatic enzyme should be given in a nonencapsulated form so it can act in the proximal duodenum. An antacid should be administered to the patient to prevent the degradation of the nonencapsulated enzyme preparation as it passes through the stomach.

### Causes and Associated Conditions

Although the exact pathophysiology leading to CP is not always clear, several conditions are known to be associated with an increased risk for this disease. These conditions have been sorted into categories of the TIGAR-O (toxic-metabolic, idiopathic, genetic, autoimmune, recurrent, obstructive) classification system.[12] The classification is based on the prevalence of each cause, and each class has implications for possible treatments. Each letter in the acronym for the TIGAR-O system corresponds to the first letter of a category. **Box 1** is a list of these categories and conditions that are associated with the development of pancreatitis. Some clinical highlights regarding these items and additional conditions associated with recurrent AP are outlined later.

**Box 1**
**Causal risk factors associated with CP: TIGAR-O classification system (version 1.0)**

- Toxic-metabolic
  - Alcoholic
  - Tobacco smoking
  - Hypercalcemia
  - Hyperparathyroidism
  - Hyperlipidemia (rare and controversial)
  - Chronic renal failure
  - Medications
    - Phenacetin abuse (possibly from chronic renal insufficiency)
  - Toxins
- Idiopathic
  - Early onset
  - Late onset
  - Tropical
    - Tropical calcific pancreatitis
    - Fibrocalculous pancreatic diabetes
  - Other
- Genetic
  - Autosomal dominant
    - Cationic trypsinogen (codon 29 and 122 mutations)
  - Autosomal recessive/modifier genes
    - CFTR mutations
    - SPINK1 mutations
    - Cationic trypsinogen (codon 16, 22, 23 mutations)
    - a1-Antitrypsin deficiency (possible)
- Autoimmune
  - Isolated autoimmune CP
  - Syndromic autoimmune CP
    - Sjögren syndrome–associated CP
    - Inflammatory bowel disease–associated CP
    - Primary biliary cirrhosis–associated CP
- Recurrent and severe AP
  - Postnecrotic (severe AP)
  - Recurrent AP
  - Vascular diseases/ischemic
  - After irradiation

- Obstructive
  - Pancreatic divisum
  - Sphincter of Oddi disorders (controversial)
  - Duct obstruction (eg, tumor)
  - Preampullary duodenal wall cysts
  - Posttraumatic pancreatic duct scars

### Alcohol and Tobacco Use

Sometimes a history of alcohol use is difficult to elicit and the erroneous diagnosis of idiopathic pancreatitis is made. Although several surveys[13] can be helpful in detecting this syndrome, the social and psychological stigma that can result from being labeled with this condition may drive the patient to conceal information and intentionally fill out surveys incorrectly. Including a concerned family member in the interview process with the patient's permission can sometimes be helpful in detecting this behavior. Asking about convictions for driving under the influence (DUI) or past alcohol-related accidents can be revealing as well. If alcoholism is persistent, psychiatric and/or rehabilitation consultation should be strongly encouraged. Abstinence from alcohol has been shown to reduce pain and recurrent attacks, especially in those who have not developed the long-term findings of CP.[14]

The odds ratio for smokers developing CP compared with nonsmokers ranges from 7.8 to 17.3,[15,16] and the risk increases with the amount of smoking.[16] Smoking and alcohol seem to be independent risk factors for CP.[16]

### Hypercalcemia and Hyperparathyroidism

The relationship between hypercalcemia, familial hyperparathyroidism, and CP has been accepted by most clinicians,[6,17] and therefore calcium levels should be checked in patients in whom the cause of CP is in question.

### Hypertriglyceridemia

Although hypertriglyceridemia is associated with recurrent AP, the relationship between hypertriglyceridemia or other hyperlipidemias and CP remains controversial. It seems that in the most severe, prolonged, and poorly controlled cases of hyperlipidemia (eg, genetic lipoprotein lipase deficiencies) dominated by recurrent AP, CP can develop. However, this seems to be rare.[6]

### Chronic Renal Failure

Renal failure is associated with increased rates of both AP[18,19] and CP.[20–22] Even though many of these patients have findings on imaging suggestive of CP, few such patients had clinical CP. Nonetheless, it is appropriate to include pancreatitis in the differential diagnosis when patients with renal failure have abdominal pain, nausea, vomiting, or diarrhea.

### Medications and Toxins

Although there is 1 report of phenacetin being associated with CP,[23] little has been published beyond this, and the questionable influence of renal failure in this situation has been raised.[6] Because the concept of CP being a result of persistent and relapsing AP has become more evident, it seems plausible that medications known to be associated with AP may also cause CP. However, this is only speculation at this point. Nonetheless, the reader is referred to an evidenced-based review of medications associated with AP[24] if this concern arises in the evaluation of a patient with CP.

As with medications, few, if any, toxins have been shown to be conclusively associated with CP. However, 1 report does describe chronic relapsing pancreatitis from a scorpion sting in Trinidad, even though this is believed to be rare.[25]

### Idiopathic Pancreatitis

Idiopathic pancreatitis accounts for 10% to 30% of all cases of CP.[8] There seems to be a bimodal distribution of age onset for patients with idiopathic CP.[23,26] Patients with early age onset idiopathic CP are commonly diagnosed in their 20s and almost always present with abdominal pain. The coexistent findings of pancreatic calcification, exocrine insufficiency, and endocrine insufficiency are usually not present.[23] Most patients with late-onset idiopathic CP still have abdominal pain as their predominant symptom but it is less often seen on presentation than in the patients with early onset CP.[23] Also, the coexistent findings of pancreatic calcification, exocrine insufficiency, and endocrine insufficiency are more commonly found on initial presentation in late-onset idiopathic CP. Many believe that some groups of patients with idiopathic CP contain some patients with covert alcohol use as well as undiagnosed autoimmune CP, especially in earlier studies when testing for autoimmune CP was less common.

Tropical pancreatitis is more commonly found in certain areas of southwest India. It also has been reported from several other areas, including Africa, southeast Asia, and Brazil.[8] One form, tropical calcific pancreatitis, is characterized by multiple episodes of severe abdominal pain in childhood, and is associated with extensive pancreatic calcifications, as well as pancreatic dysfunction, but no diabetes mellitus. In fibrocalculous pancreatic diabetes, diabetes mellitus is the first clinical finding leading to the diagnosis.[27]

### Genetic (Familial) CP

It is important to inquire about a family history of pancreatitis or undiagnosed abdominal pain in patients with CP. At the time of this writing, there is only one autosomal dominant mutation known to cause CP.[6] Other mutations are believed to be autosomal recessive or genetic mutations that result in modification of CP when other causes of pancreatitis are present. The ramifications of being tested for a genetic cause of CP should be carefully considered before this is suggested.[6] Consultation with a pancreatitis expert and/or genetic counselor should occur before this is done.

### Autoimmune CP

In this form of CP, there is a characteristic dense infiltration of the pancreas, and often other organs, with lymphocytes and plasma cells.[28] Autoimmune pancreatitis may be isolated or observed in association with the Sjögren syndrome, primary biliary cirrhosis, primary sclerosing cholangitis, Crohn disease, and ulcerative colitis, or other immune-mediated disorders.[6] It is important to make this diagnosis, when present, because it characteristically responds well to steroids. Also, autoimmune CP can sometimes mimic pancreas cancer. Therefore, a proper diagnosis in this situation can possibly avoid surgical intervention and substantially change management plans. Details regarding the diagnosis of autoimmune CP are given later.

### Severe and Recurrent AP

As mentioned earlier, it is becoming more apparent that persistence of inflammatory activity after acute episodes of pancreatitis may cause CP in some patients.[6,8,29]

With this in mind, it is appropriate to inquire about prior episodes of AP or undiagnosed abdominal pain, along with risk factors that have been traditionally associated with AP,[1,30] when the cause of CP is in question.

### Gallbladder Stones and Microlithiasis

It is uncommon for patients with known gallstones to have a prolonged course of repeated pancreatitis episodes before a cholecystectomy is performed, so cholelithiasis has not been commonly associated with CP. However, severe gallstone pancreatitis has been reported to cause CP.[31] Microlithiasis can be present when gallbladder US is normal, and has been reported to be associated with recurrent pancreatitis.[32] Cholesterol granules and crystals can be seen in bile aspirated from the duodenum during endoscopy after *cholecystokinin* has been given. Some believe that this is a common cause of undiagnosed biliary pain and idiopathic pancreatitis.[32] Given the information discussed earlier regarding severe and recurrent AP leading to CP, it is plausible that undetected microlithiasis could be the cause of idiopathic CP in some patients.

### Pancreatic Ischemia

Ischemia of the pancreas rarely causes AP but can result from several conditions, including vasculitis (systemic lupus erythematosus and polyarteritis nodosa), and ergotamine use.[1] As in the situations mentioned earlier, it is conceivable that severe AP or relapsing AP resulting from these conditions could progress to CP.

### Radiation-associated CP

There are reports that suggest radiotherapy as a cause of CP, but these seem to be rare events.[33,34]

### Pancreas Divisum

Pancreas divisum occurs when the ventral and dorsal ducts of the pancreas fail to fuse during organogenesis. It is the most common congenital variant of pancreatic ductal development, occurring in approximately 10% of individuals.[35] In most patients with pancreatitis and pancreas divisum, it is debatable whether pancreas divisum is a causal factor, but, in those who have recurrent episodes of AP, a subset of patients may benefit from a minor duct sphincterotomy.[36] Its role in CP remains controversial.

### Sphincter of Oddi Disorders

Sphincter of Oddi disorders can impede the outflow of pancreatic fluid and/or bile in some patients in the absence of tumor or stone disease. It remains a controversial cause for CP.[6,8,37] It is not clear whether the manometric findings of a hypertensive sphincter are a result or a causal factor in these cases.

### Pancreas and Ampullary Cancer

Obstruction of the main pancreatic duct or ampulla by tumors can produce CP in the parenchyma upstream of the obstruction.[8] A strong suspicion for cancer should accompany new signs or symptoms of CP or AP in individuals without another known cause; this is especially true in elderly individuals who develop diabetes, steatorrhea, or nausea, vomiting, and abdominal pain along with laboratory or radiologic findings indicating pancreatitis. It is often difficult to clearly show a tumor in the setting of CP because the findings can be similar.[8]

### Duodenal and Choledochal Cysts

Duodenal duplication cysts are rare congenital anomalies that usually present in infancy and childhood. Acute presentation in adults is even rarer. An association between recurrent pancreatitis and duodenal duplication cysts has been reported.[38] Cystic changes of the bile duct are also uncommon.[39] Nonetheless, these have also been associated with CP.[40,41]

### Trauma

Blunt and penetrating trauma to the pancreas can also lead to pancreatic duct strictures, most commonly in the midbody of the gland where the duct crosses the spine.[8] As with tumors, pancreatitis can occur upstream from the injury. In a patient with pancreatitis from an unknown cause, a careful history may uncover a motor vehicle accident or other traumatic event resulting in blunt force to the epigastrium or back.[42] Information such as this could indicate an undiagnosed traumatic pancreatic duct injury in the past that resulted in a subclinical pancreatitis.

## CLINICAL MANIFESTATIONS (HISTORY AND PHYSICAL FINDINGS)

Box 2 lists items that should be considered when obtaining a history and physical examination from a patient with suspected or known CP.

Pain is often the overriding symptom in patients with CP. It is usually described as boring, deep, and penetrating through to the back. It is often associated with nausea and vomiting. The pain may be relieved by sitting or leaning forward as well as the knee-chest position. It may worsen with eating and is often perceived to be worse at night.

Episodes of AP in the setting of CP can occur, leading to findings that correspond with the complications associated with AP as well as CP. With this in mind, other symptoms that may be present include abdominal distension from abdominal fluid collections or ileus. Shortness of breath can also be seen with abdominal fluid collections or pleural effusions. Jaundice may occur from compression of the common bile duct (CBD) as it courses through the diseased pancreas. Fever may indicate cholangitis, infection of fluid collections, or necrosis as well as coexisting acute inflammation. During episodes of AP, inflammatory processes involving the splenic vein can result in gastric varices and hematemesis or melena.

Exocrine insufficiency in CP can result in steatorrhea described as large-volume, foul-smelling, oily bowel movements. Endocrine insufficiency resulting in diabetes has been observed to occur in more than 80% of patients who were followed for 25 years.[43]

Findings on physical examination can include varying degrees of abdominal tenderness including guarding. Decreased bowel sounds may be caused by narcotic medication use as well as the underlying pancreatitis. Palpable abdominal masses may rarely be present and can be caused by pseudocyst formation and/or splenomegaly in the event of splenic vein thrombosis. In some patients with autoimmune pancreatitis, evidence of a coexistent autoimmune feature, such as salivary gland enlargement or lymphadenopathy, may be found.[8] Signs of malnutrition, such as temporal wasting, may also be found. However, no single physical finding is highly specific for CP.

## DIAGNOSIS

The diagnosis of CP can be made easily if the disease has progressed to the point at which imaging and laboratory studies reveal a constellation of findings commonly seen with the disease. However, early in the course of CP (and perhaps at the point

---

**Box 2**
**Items to consider when obtaining a history from a patient with suspected or known CP**

- Symptoms
  - Abdominal pain, flank pain, back pain
  - Nausea, vomiting, hematemesis, melena
  - Diarrhea with foul-smelling, oily bowel movements
  - Abdominal distension
  - Shortness of breath
  - Jaundice
  - Weight loss and fever
- Historical information to suggest a cause or increased risk for CP and recurring AP
  - Prior pancreatitis,
  - Alcohol use, alcoholism, DUI, counseling because of alcohol use
  - Tobacco smoking
  - Gallbladder stones, gallbladder surgery
  - Family history of pancreatitis or cystic fibrosis
  - Abdominal or back trauma
  - Hypertriglyceridemia, hypercalcemia
  - CMV, Coxsackie, mumps, ascaris, clonorchis, or mycoplasma infection
  - Ischemic diseases including PVD, CAD, and diabetes
  - Scorpion stings
  - Autoimmune diseases including PBC, IBD, and Sjögren syndrome
  - Exposure to organophosphates
  - Obstruction of the ampullary region, ampullary neoplasm, diverticula, sphincter of Oddi dysfunction, choledochal cyst pancreas divisum
  - History of surgery
  - Renal failure
  - History of radiotherapy to the abdomen or back
  - Use of medications associated with pancreatitis[24]
- Historical information suggesting endocrine insufficiency
  - Diabetes
- Possible findings on physical examination
  - Jaundice
  - Fever
  - Temporal wasting and muscle wasting
  - Salivary gland enlargement or lymphadenopathy
  - Decreased bowel sounds
  - Varying degrees of abdominal tenderness including guarding
  - Palpable abdominal mass

at which interventions would be the most effective), the classic findings are not always present. A conclusive diagnosis may be impossible if the only abnormalities present are subtle histologic changes in small locations scattered throughout a pancreas gland that still seems to be functioning properly. In these situations, laboratory and imaging studies can result in normal or ambiguous findings. However, there is no single laboratory or imaging test that can conclusively rule in or rule out CP in all situations.

When the presenting symptoms and clinical information suggest an exocrine insufficiency (ie, malnutrition and/or steatorrhea) or endocrine insufficiency (diabetes), the disease process is usually far enough along that simple diagnostic tests discussed later, such as serum trypsinogen, fecal elastase, and/or abdominal CT, will reveal results that are consistent with CP. However, when the presenting primary complaint is only abdominal pain, a diagnostic evaluation may be more challenging.

**Box 3** presents a list of diagnostic tests that can be used in the evaluation of a patient suspected of having CP. Each of these tests is discussed later. Suggestions for an initial diagnostic strategy are also provided, with the understanding that it is common practice for such evaluations to be done in collaboration and consultation with a subspecialist who has expertise in this field.

Information regarding the sensitivity and specificity of these tests is often not available for the wide variety of clinical scenarios with which a patient may present. In general, all of these tests are less accurate in less advanced or early CP.

### Amylase and Lipase

Although commonly used to detect AP, these tests are of little use in the diagnosis of CP. They are sometimes increased and can be used in detecting acute relapsing AP or episodes of AP in the setting of CP but, even in these situations, they may not be

---

**Box 3**
**Diagnostic tests to consider in a patient suspected of having CP**

- Laboratory tests
  - Serum trypsinogen (trypsin)
  - Fecal chymotrypsin and elastase
  - Quantitative 72-hour fecal fat collection
  - Sudan stain
  - Serum IgG$_4$ antinuclear antibodies, antilactoferrin antibodies, anticarbonic anhydrase II antibodies, anti–smooth muscle antibodies, rheumatoid factor and antimitochondrial antibodies (for suspected autoimmune pancreatitis)
- Imaging tests
  - Plain abdominal radiography
  - US
  - CT
  - MRI
  - ERCP
  - EUS
  - Direct pancreatic function testing

abnormal, especially when much of the pancreas is affected by CP. With this in mind, normal amylase and lipase levels should not be used to rule out CP.

### Serum Trypsinogen

Serum trypsinogen (also called serum trypsin) can be used as a rough estimation of pancreatic function. In patients with advanced CP associated with steatorrhea, low levels of serum trypsinogen (<20 ng/mL) can be measured in the blood.[44] The test is specific but can also be seen in patients with a neoplasm obstructing the pancreatic duct.[8] However, the sensitivity is low, especially in early CP.

### Fecal Chymotrypsin and Elastase

Both of these pancreatic enzymes can be measured in random stool samples, and low concentrations can indicate that decreased amounts of the enzymes are being delivered from the pancreas into the duodenum. Fecal chymotrypsin has been shown to be low in patients with CP who have steatorrhea.[45] However, low levels have also been reported in other malabsorptive conditions such as celiac disease and Crohn's disease.[8] Again, the sensitivity is low and it is usually normal in patients who do not have steatorrhea. Likewise, fecal elastase seems to be an accurate method for detecting patients with advanced CP,[46] but it can also be low in other diseases causing diarrhea, such as small bowel overgrowth and short bowel syndrome.[8] Fecal elastase has been reported to be superior to chymotrypsin for the detection of pancreas involvement in a group of pediatric patients with cystic fibrosis with mild steatorrhea.[47]

### Fecal Fat Detection

The measurement of fecal fat excretion during a 72-hour collection of stool is the simplest evaluation of pancreatic lipase action. However, the test is difficult to perform in practice. It is imperative that the patient follow a diet containing 100 g/d fat for at least 3 days before the test. Normally, less than 7 g of fat should be present in stool in these conditions. Patients outside tightly controlled environments such as clinical research wards often stray from required dietary and collection activities, often making the results unreliable. Qualitative analysis of fecal fat can also be performed with a Sudan III stain of a random specimen of stool, but this is positive only in patients with substantial steatorrhea. However, it is generally agreed that the accuracy of the qualitative study is less than that of the quantitative 72-hour collection. More than 6 globules per high-power field is considered a positive result but, once again, the patient must be on a diet with adequate fat intake for positive results to be detected. These tests can also be positive in other disorders such as small bowel overgrowth, so the specificity for CP is limited. Therefore, they are mostly used in a supportive role when making a diagnosis of CP.

### Serum IgG₄ and Autoimmune Antibodies (for Suspected Autoimmune Pancreatitis)

A large United States study found a sensitivity of 76% and a specificity of 93% when patients suspected of having autoimmune pancreatitis had $IgG_4$ levels higher than 140 mg/dL.[48] This study also points out that patients with histologically proved autoimmune pancreatitis can have a normal serum level of $IgG_4$. Even more concerning is the finding that up to 10% of patients with adenocarcinoma of the pancreas may have increases in $IgG_4$ levels. A variety of autoimmune antibodies can also be found in these patients, including antinuclear antibodies, antilactoferrin antibodies, anticarbonic anhydrase II antibodies, anti–smooth muscle antibodies, rheumatoid factor, and antimitochondrial antibodies. These autoimmune antibodies are less specific than $IgG_4$ and therefore less useful in making a diagnosis.

### Plain Abdominal Radiography

The finding of diffuse pancreatic calcifications on plain abdominal films is specific for CP. Other calcifications can be seen but they are usually not diffuse. Focal calcifications may be seen in cystic and islet cell tumors of the pancreas, and in peripancreatic vascular calcifications. As with most other findings in CP, calcifications are more likely to be present in patients with CP with long-standing disease and may not be seen in early CP.

### Abdominal US

US is not always a useful diagnostic tool for CP. This modality is sometimes limited in its ability to image the pancreas because of overlying bowel gas. This limitation can often be minimized by simply having the patient drink large quantities of water before attempts to visualize the pancreas (personal observations). One of the findings that indicate pancreatitis is a dilated main pancreatic duct. Other findings include ductal stones, gland atrophy or enlargement, irregular gland margins, pseudocysts, and changes in the parenchymal texture.

### CT

The findings described earlier for US are also seen on CT. The sensitivity of CT for CP is between 75% and 90%, and the specificity is 85% or higher.[49,50] Here again, the accuracy can be less in early stages of the disease. CT is able to image the pancreas in all patients, which is an advantage compared with US. Pancreatic calcifications can be more apparent on CT than plain abdominal radiography and, although CT is more expensive than US and exposes the patient to ionizing radiation, it is more sensitive and more specific.

### MRI

For diagnostic purposes, MRI is probably as accurate as CT. However, calcifications are not as easily seen with MRI as with CT.[49] MRI with magnetic resonance cholangiopancreatography can better show the ductal anatomy and evaluate for beading or ectasia of duct side branches along with the parenchyma, which may provide advantages in certain situations. Variations in MRI examination quality have been known to exist in different imaging centers, which may also affect accuracy in certain situations.[35]

It is common practice to pursue certain diagnostic testing modalities via consultation with a subspecialist.

### ERCP

In situations in which there is a strong clinical suspicion for CP but the imaging studies described earlier are not confirmatory, ERCP is sometimes used to explore for objective findings that support the diagnosis. Magnetic resonance cholangiopancreatography seems to have more difficulty visualizing small side branches than ERCP in some settings.[49] However, operator variability in technique as well as interobserver variability when interpreting ERCP findings can be substantial. Nonetheless, other information can be gained during ERCP, such as sphincter of Oddi manometry measurements to determine whether a hypertensive sphincter is present. Moreover, therapeutic interventions such as stone removal or stricture dilation can be accomplished during the same procedure. These benefits come with a trade-off for the possibility of complications including exacerbation of pancreatitis. This risk is increased when an ERCP is done in patients with AP, CP, or sphincter of Oddi dysfunction.[51]

## EUS

EUS has the advantage of imaging both the pancreas parenchyma as well as duct structures in high resolution without the risk of pancreatitis that accompanies ERCP. Here again, operator variability in technique, as well as interobserver variability when interpreting EUS findings, can be substantial. An added benefit of EUS is the ability to obtain directed fine-needle aspiration specimens of suspicious lesions. As with other testing, the accuracy seems to be less in early CP. The accuracy of EUS in patients with suspected pancreatitis who had no findings on other imaging has been studied.[52] Diagnostic certainty was only 50% (positive predictive value 0.5) when at least 6 EUS features for pancreatitis were needed to make a diagnosis of CP. CP was excluded with greater than 70% certainty when less than 3 criteria were present.

### Direct Pancreatic Function Testing

These tests require hormone stimulation and duodenal tube collection of pancreatic fluid. They were used as a reference standard in the study that determined the accuracy of EUS (discussed earlier).[52] They have been used as a reference standard for detecting CP in its earliest form and the results of these tests correlate well with histologic findings.[53] However, even though they directly measure pancreatic function, they cannot be diagnostic in the same manner as a histologic diagnosis. The sensitivity and specificity is believed to be the best of any test, but it is still not perfect, and these can vary depending on the technique used and the type of patients being evaluated.[52] The method of performing the test is not standardized and it is available in only a few centers in the United States.

### Initial Diagnostic Strategy

The suspicion of CP can arise in the evaluation of patients with abdominal pain, especially when some of the symptoms outlined in **Box 3** are present and one or more risk factors found in **Box 2** are detected. It is important to consider possible causes other than CP in these situations. For comprehensive reviews of the differential diagnosis and evaluation of various abdominal pain syndromes, the reader may find References[54,55] helpful.

For the initial diagnostic work-up specifically for CP in these situations, if the risk factors are obvious and there are signs/symptoms of exocrine and endocrine insufficiency, simple plain abdominal radiography showing calcifications, along with a positive Sudan stain or fecal elastase, may be sufficient to confirm the diagnosis. However, a more commonly used initial imaging modality is CT or MRI, because it provides more information that may be helpful in eliminating other diagnostic possibilities than plain abdominal radiography. If these initial laboratory and imaging studies are unrevealing or ambiguous, especially in the setting of limited clinical findings, continued evaluation with a higher quality CT, EUS, or direct pancreatic functioning should be pursued with the consultation of a subspecialist. In rare situations, ERCP may be suggested by the consultant for diagnostic purposes but it is more commonly used when therapeutic options are being considered for management.

## MANAGEMENT

The long-term management of a patient with CP can often be simply a matter of refilling medications as needed and monitoring for new symptoms. However, patients with CP can also be challenging in terms of management; for example, if symptoms persist despite therapy, or it is early in the course of CP, the decision process can be complicated, especially if the diagnosis is not certain. Although subspecialists should be consulted for assistance in managing the conditions that are problematic in CP, it is important for the primary care provider to have an appreciation for what these conditions are, as well as an understanding of the evidence-based literature supporting the ways that they are managed. To this end, the major clinical issues that accompany the management of patients with CP are reviewed here.

### Pain Management

The management of abdominal pain is the most common problem encountered in patients with CP. In some patients, the severity and frequency of exacerbations decrease in time.[56] However, approximately half of patients with CP continue to report significant pain after 10 years of follow-up. The initial management of the pain and the management of recurrent exacerbations should include the search for conditions that have effective therapeutic remedies, such as pancreatic pseudocysts and bile duct obstruction. The clinical examination and/or an imaging study such as CT or MRI usually reveal these conditions during the initial evaluation. Beyond this, the evaluation and management may include ERCP, EUS, or surgical options and should be done with a subspecialist.

Once overt treatable causes have been excluded or addressed, medical management of long-term pain is appropriate. Ideally, consultation with subspecialists in a pain clinic that has experience treating patients with CP seems the best approach. In practice, however, these resources may not be available. Moreover, if a pain clinic is being considered, good communication with the primary care physician as well as other consultants is essential. Also, the ideal pain clinic should actively pursue a variety of nonnarcotic alternatives in addition to the appropriate use of narcotics in an attempt to minimize narcotic addiction in these patients. A common practice in these situations is to have 1 provider (often the primary care provider) designated as the prescriber of pain medications. This practice is usually with the understanding that if the prescribed medications are inadequate, the patient will be promptly reevaluated by the pain clinic. The medical management of pain in these patients can include many modalities. A review of the clinical highlights for each of these modalities is presented below.

### Lifestyle Changes

As mentioned earlier, the cessation of alcohol can reduce painful relapses.[14] As many as three-quarters of patients with CP caused by alcohol report cessation of pain with abstinence.[57] This, and the reduction of mortality[58] in these patients, supports the aggressive treatment of this behavior with use of psychiatric and/or rehabilitation resources if necessary.

Many patients reduce oral intake on their own at home, along with bed rest, to avoid hospitalization during exacerbations of their pain. Although this may be effective and practical on a limited short-term basis, this practice, if overused, can lead to substantial malnutrition and be substantially disruptive to both work and lifestyle. Therefore, the patient should be encouraged seek medical attention rather than resorting to this alternative on a frequent basis.

### Medications

Some patients have mild chronic pain that responds to over-the-counter pain medications; however, most require more potent pain control, resulting in the use of narcotics. As many as 10% to 30% of patients may become addicted to these medications.[8] Therefore, a reasonable strategy is to start with a dose that is as low as possible. It is also important to explain to the patient that the goal is to make the pain tolerable, not to completely eliminate it. With its limited effects on gastrointestinal motility, tramadol should be considered when choosing a medication regimen in these situations.

It is also important to consider supplemental medications that can reduce the need for narcotics. Many patients with CP have a coexisting depression and benefit from antidepressant medications such as serotonin reuptake inhibitors or tricyclic antidepressants. These medications can be helpful in treating depression but also can potentially alter central pain perception and reduce narcotic use. Other nonnarcotic medications used for chronic pain syndromes, such as gabapentin and pregabalin, may also be of benefit.

### Antioxidants

It has been suggested that activation of oxygen derived free radical products might have a role in the pathogenesis of CP.[59] At least 1 study has shown a modest reduction in the pain of patients with CP when they were given the following antioxidants on a daily basis: 75 mg of selenium, 3 mg β-carotene, 47 mg D-α-tocopherol acetate (vitamin E), 150 mg ascorbic acid (vitamin C), and 400 mg methionone.[60,61] Incorporating these in the treatment plan of patients with CP seems reasonable and has little, if any, risk of untoward effects.

### Pancreatic Enzymes

As mentioned earlier, the use of unencapsulated exogenous pancreatic enzymes for the treatment of pain can be effective in select patients.[10] A meta-analysis of studies using pancreatic enzymes for the treatment of pain in CP concluded that there was no benefit.[62] Without understanding the details, this may seem confusing at first. However, this combined analysis did not take into account the use of enteric coated enzymes and study populations with long-standing CP in some studies. For the reasons explained earlier, selections of patients with early CP or small duct disease have a better chance of pain reduction.[10]

### Nerve Blocks

Celiac plexus neurolysis via EUS-guided or CT-guided alcohol injections are used rarely in patients with pain from CP because of their short duration.[8] They are more often used in patients who have pancreas cancer.

### Endoscopic Therapy

Endoscopic therapy for pain control also includes its use in the treatment of the complications of CP, which is explained later. In addition, the use of endoscopic therapies to treat pain may also be helpful in select groups of patients. More specifically, some subsets of patients with CP in the obstructive category of the TIGAR-O classification system (see **Box 1**) might benefit from endoscopic intervention. Some patients with CP with pancreas divisum may benefit from an endoscopic sphincterotomy of the minor papilla and temporary stent placement but the reliable selection of those who will respond remains a challenge.[35,36,63] Stent placement for a dominant stricture can be an effective treatment of pain in highly selected patients with CP[64] but, again, can be difficult to predict whether it will be effective in individual patients. The measurement of pancreatic duct pressures[65] or changes in duct diameter[66] also are not helpful in determining who will experience a reduction in pain. Therefore, it is necessary to counsel patients undergoing these procedures about the possibility of persistent pain in addition to the chance of complications when considering such a procedure. Pancreatic duct stones can sometimes be removed endoscopically after a sphincterotomy and may require extracorporeal shockwave lithotripsy if they are large or impacted.[67,68] Not all stones can be removed because many calcifications are in side branches or the pancreatic parenchyma. Again, relief of pain can be seen in highly selected patients but is not always achieved.

### Surgical Therapy

As was the case with endoscopic therapy, surgical therapy for pain control also includes its use in the treatment of the complications of CP, which is explained later. Surgical therapy for pain relief has generally involved 3 concepts: improving duct drainage, removing diseased pancreatic tissue, and interrupting nerve transmission of pain by sectioning the greater splanchnic nerve.

The pancreatic fluids in a poorly draining dilated main pancreatic duct can be redirected into the intestinal lumen by a lateral pancreaticojejunostomy (also called a Puestow procedure). Here, a longitudinal incision is made in the pancreatic duct and it is anastomosed to a limb of small bowel. In the Partington-Rochelle modification of the Puestow procedure, the pancreatic duct is opened longitudinally and anastomosed to a defunctionalized limb of small bowel, which is connected with a Roux-en-Y anastomosis. The morbidity and mortality with these procedures is low and, in some circumstances, they can be performed laparoscopically.[8] Long-term pain control is less than 60 % in some studies.[69]

Surgical procedures involving the removal of diseased pancreatic tissue include Whipple and duodenal preserving Whipple procedures. The long-term results for pain control may be similar to the drainage procedures described earlier,[70] but the morbidity and mortality is generally higher than for drainage procedures. However, those patients undergoing Whipple procedures usually have severe disease in the head of the pancreas, possibly including bile duct obstruction, findings suspicious for a mass or vascular involvement. The Frey procedure is a combination of a partial pancreatic head resection and lateral pancreaticojejunostomy where less of the head of the pancreas is cored out, leaving the bile duct and peripancreatic vessels undisturbed.[71] Results, morbidity, and mortality for all these procedures vary depending on the characteristics of the patient and the expertise of the surgeon. Careful follow-up after the procedure should include evaluation or empiric treatment of exocrine insufficiency, which can be present with minimal symptoms.

Sectioning the greater splanchnic nerve on 1 or both sides can provide pain relief in some patients who have failed other attempts at pain control. In one long-term follow-up study, pain relief was reported in about half of the patients at 1 year and one-quarter of the patients at 4 years.[72] The procedure can be done thoracoscopically in some centers and is associated with few complications.

Total pancreatectomy and islet cell autotransplantation has rarely been used in patients with CP.[73] Many patients still experience pain, requiring narcotics after the procedure, although the severity of pain is decreased. In theory, this should reduce the risk of pancreas cancer in these patients, especially in those with genetically linked CP. However, using this as an indication to do the procedure is without evidence-based support at this time.

### Management of Steatorrhea

The cumbersome and often unreliable 72-hour fecal fat collection is not always necessary for the diagnosis of steatorrhea in patients with other findings consistent with CP and the clinical manifestations of steatorrhea described earlier. A qualitative analysis of fecal fat in a random stool sample can be helpful to confirm suspicions of steatorrhea if needed. Pancreatic enzymes can reduce the frequency of bowel movements in normal individuals, so a change in bowel habits while on exogenous pancreas enzymes is not always conclusively diagnostic for steatorrhea. Moreover, it is proper to check for other causes of diarrhea, including infectious causes, such as *Clostridium difficile* colitis and small bowel overgrowth, when there are sudden changes in bowel habits in a patient who has an otherwise slowly progressive course of CP.

Administering exogenous pancreatic enzymes with each meal is an effective method of treating steatorrhea that is associated with the exocrine insufficiency of CP. Dosages should be adjusted according to the description of bowel habits provided by the patient. Based on the estimated amount needed to treat steatorrhea in most patients, the initial dose usually involves preparations that provide 30,000 IU (90,000 USP units) of lipase per meal.[8] This commonly involves taking multiple pills immediately before, during, and after each meal. It is important to routinely evaluate for deficiencies of fat-soluble vitamins (vitamins A, D, E, and K), in these patients. It is also appropriate to check for osteopenia or osteoporosis with a bone density test.

## COMPLICATIONS
### Pseudocyst

The most common symptom signaling the presence of a pseudocyst is abdominal pain, so searching for a pseudocyst should be a part of evaluating the patient with CP who reports increased or new abdominal pain. Other presenting symptoms include increased nausea or jaundice (from compression of the stomach, duodenum, or bile duct by the enlarging cyst) or bleeding from vessels disrupted by the cyst wall. Pseudocysts are easily found with US, CT, or MRI. Not all cysts require treatment,[74,75] but those that are associated with symptoms should be reviewed by a subspecialist to determine whether they are mature enough for therapeutic interventions to be considered. Those cysts more than 4 weeks of age and/or having a capsule that is seen on CT are usually amenable to percutaneous, endoscopic, or surgical drainage. Imaging of the pancreatic duct system and treating any strictures that are found via ERCP may help quicken the resolution of the cyst following the drainage procedure. EUS-guided cystgastrostomy with the placement of 1 or more pigtail stents has become the preferred option in many centers,[76] thereby avoiding the chance of percutaneous fistula formation with percutaneous drainage procedures. Surgical options including drainage of the cyst into small bowel can be considered if other options are unsuccessful or if other surgical interventions, as described earlier, are being considered.

### Compression of the Bile Duct and/or Duodenum

The progression of fibrosis and/or an inflammatory mass in the pancreatic head of patients can distort the surrounding anatomy, resulting in the compression of the bile duct and/or duodenum. Duodenal obstruction is usually discovered with CT using oral contrast to evaluate increased nausea, vomiting, and abdominal pain. Although improvement with medical therapy is possible, usually surgical therapy in the form of a gastrojejunostomy is required for long-term treatment. The CBD can also be compressed by progression of fibrosis or enlargement of an inflammatory mass. ERCP usually reveals a smooth, tapered stricture in the CBD where it passes through the head of the pancreas. Long-term resolution of the CBD obstruction has been achieved with multiple stents being placed endoscopically[77] to avoid surgical intervention. It is important to evaluate for the possibility of malignancy in these situations, as is discussed later.

### Gastrointestinal Bleeding

Patients with CP can have gastrointestinal bleeding from the more common causes such as peptic ulcers, esophagitis, and Mallory-Weiss tear, as well as causes that are more closely associated with CP. Pseudoaneurysms[78] can form when the walls of an artery, such as the splenic artery, are damaged by inflammatory changes, and possibly from enzymatic action as well. The artery can rupture into the retroperitoneum, peritoneal cavity pancreatic duct system, or into a nearby gastrointestinal lumen. On noncontrast CT, they can mimic pseudocysts and they can also rupture into pseudocysts to make things more confusing. They may present with pain as these structures fill with blood or a sudden drop in hemoglobin without overt bleeding, or a small self-limiting sentinel bleed as a small amount of blood escapes into the gastrointestinal tract before tamponade from the filled structure can occur. A massive hemorrhage can follow if the tamponade effect is no longer able to contain the bleeding. If a pseudoaneurysm is suspected, CT with IV contrast (and preferably without oral contrast) should be urgently done. Once a pseudoaneurysm is discovered, angiography with consideration of therapeutic intervention, such as embolization, should be arranged even when there is no evidence of active bleeding.

### Malignancy

The risk of pancreas malignancy in patients with CP is approximately 5%.[79] However, it can be as high as 40% in those with genetic (familial) pancreatitis.[80] Screening for pancreas cancer with imaging studies such as EUS has been studied in select CP with a high risk for cancer.[81] This screening program has discovered numerous premalignant lesions in this highly select group of patients. However, there is no evidence to support screening in other populations of patients with CP at this time. Moreover, the detection of cancer can be difficult when changes consistent with CP are already present on imaging studies because there are no distinct findings on US, EUS, CT, or MRI to distinguish between cancer and CP, except perhaps metastatic lesions when they are present. The tumor marker CA 19-9 is also not usually used for detection of cancer in patients with CP because it can be increased in patients without cancer, especially those with biliary obstruction and/or cholangitis.

### Fistula Formation

Fistula formation can result in internal drainage into nearby structures, or externally to the skin. This condition may occur after instrumentation from drainage procedures as well as spontaneously from inflammation or a pseudocyst eroding into a nearby structure. In some cases, a fistulous tract is desirable; in most cases, the goal of an endoscopic procedure to treat a pseudocyst is to create a fistulous tract between the stomach and the pseudocyst and to keep it patent with stents so the pseudocyst can drain. Unwanted fistulas can be treated with complete bowel rest and hyperalimentation. Some have advocated the use of octreotide to hasten the healing process[8]; however, depending on the size of the fistula, this can take weeks to heal. If a fistula can be identified that is connected to the pancreatic duct at ERCP, placing a stent across the leak can be effective in promoting healing.[82]

### Dysmotility

When patients with small duct CP were identified with direct pancreatic function testing they were also evaluated with a gastric emptying study, and a substantial proportion of them (44%) were found to have gastroparesis.[83] The gastroparesis may have also prevented adequate delivery of the exogenous enzymes to the duodenum, perhaps explaining why their pain was not reduced with enzyme administration. Most of these patients were women and all had no findings suggestive of CP on imaging studies. One wonders how many of the patients with unexplained abdominal pain associated with nausea and vomiting or painful idiopathic gastroparesis may have this form of CP.

## GUIDELINES FOR REFERRAL AND HOSPITAL ADMISSION OF PATIENTS WITH CP

Hospital admission and consultation should generally be considered for patients with pain that cannot be managed with oral medication, or vomiting that prevents adequate oral intake. Also, hospitalization may be required following any therapeutic interventions for pain control or complications of CP.

Referral to an appropriate subspecialist is appropriate for all but the most straightforward evaluation and management activities described earlier.

## FIVE KEY POINTS FOR PRIMARY CARE PROVIDERS

1. The evaluation, management, and follow-up of patients with CP can be simple in many cases.
2. The evaluation, management, and follow-up of patients with CP can be complex in many cases, so having a good referral network of subspecialists experienced in this field is essential.
3. Identifying the cause of CP, if possible, is important and requires a systematic review of the many potential causes when the cause is not obvious.
4. The identification of patients with autoimmune CP is particularly important because treatment with steroids may be effective in this form of CP.
5. Alterations in pain or other symptoms in patients with CP should not be attributed to worsening disease before evaluations for complications including malignancy are done.

## REFERENCES

1. Tenner S, Steinberg WM. Acute pancreatitis. In: Feldman M, Friedman LS, Brand LJ, editors. Sleisenger and Fordtran's gastrointestinal and liver disease. 9th edition. Philadelphia: Saunders Elsevier; 2010. p. 959.
2. Swaroop VS, Chari ST, Clain JE. Severe acute pancreatitis. JAMA 2004;291(23): 2865–8.
3. Stevens T, Conwell DL. Chronic pancreatitis. In: Carey W, editor. Current clinical medicine. 2nd edition. Philadelphia: Saunders Elsevier; 2009. p. 451–6.
4. Lowenfels AB, Maisonneuve P. Epidemiology of chronic pancreatitis. In: Forsmark CE, editor. Pancreatitis and its complications. Totowa (NJ): Humana Press; 2005. p. 137.
5. Dufour MC, Adamson MD. The epidemiology of alcohol-induced pancreatitis. Pancreas 2003;27(4):286–90.
6. Etemad B, Whitcomb DC. Chronic pancreatitis: diagnosis, classification, and new genetic developments. Gastroenterology 2001;120(3):682–707.
7. Whitcomb DC, Gorry MC, Preston RA, et al. Hereditary pancreatitis is caused by a mutation in the cationic trypsinogen gene. Nat Genet 1996;14(2):141–5.
8. Forsmark CE. Chronic pancreatitis. In: Feldman M, Friedman LS, Brand LJ, editors. Sleisenger and Fordtran's gastrointestinal and liver disease. 9th edition. Philadelphia: Saunders Elsevier; 2010. p. 985.
9. Safdi M, Bekal PK, Martin S, et al. The effects of oral pancreatic enzymes (creon 10 capsule) on steatorrhea: a multicenter, placebo-controlled, parallel group trial in subjects with chronic pancreatitis. Pancreas 2006;33(2):156–62.
10. Gupta V, Toskes PP. Diagnosis and management of chronic pancreatitis. Postgrad Med J 2005;81(958):491–7.

11. Walkowiak J, Witmanowski H, Strzykala K, et al. Inhibition of endogenous pancreatic enzyme secretion by oral pancreatic enzyme treatment. Eur J Clin Invest 2003;33(1):65–9.
12. Chari ST, Singer MV. The problem of classification and staging of chronic pancreatitis. Proposals based on current knowledge of its natural history. Scand J Gastroenterol 1994;29(10):949–60.
13. Maisto SA, Connors GJ, Allen JP. Contrasting self-report screens for alcohol problems: a review. Alcohol Clin Exp Res 1995;19(6):1510–6.
14. Pelli H, Lappalainen-Lehto R, Piironen A, et al. Risk factors for recurrent acute alcohol-associated pancreatitis: a prospective analysis. Scand J Gastroenterol 2008;43(5):614–21.
15. Talamini G, Bassi C, Falconi M, et al. Alcohol and smoking as risk factors in chronic pancreatitis and pancreatic cancer. Dig Dis Sci 1999;44(7):1303–11.
16. Lin Y, Tamakoshi A, Hayakawa T, et al. Cigarette smoking as a risk factor for chronic pancreatitis: a case-control study in Japan. Research Committee on Intractable Pancreatic Diseases. Pancreas 2000;21(2):109–14.
17. Prinz RA, Aranha GV. The association of primary hyperparathyroidism and pancreatitis. Am Surg 1985;51(6):325–9.
18. Pitchumoni CS, Arguello P, Agarwal N, et al. Acute pancreatitis in chronic renal failure. Am J Gastroenterol 1996;91(12):2477–82.
19. Rutsky EA, Robards M, Van Dyke JA, et al. Acute pancreatitis in patients with end-stage renal disease without transplantation. Arch Intern Med 1986;146(9):1741–5.
20. Lerch MM, Riehl J, Mann H, et al. Sonographic changes of the pancreas in chronic renal failure. Gastrointest Radiol 1989;14(4):311–4.
21. Araki T, Ueda M, Ogawa K, et al. Histological pancreatitis in end-stage renal disease. Int J Pancreatol 1992;12(3):263–9.
22. Avram MM. High prevalence of pancreatic disease in chronic renal failure. Nephron 1977;18(1):68–71.
23. Ammann RW, Buehler H, Muench R, et al. Differences in the natural history of idiopathic (nonalcoholic) and alcoholic chronic pancreatitis. A comparative long-term study of 287 patients. Pancreas 1987;2(4):368–77.
24. Badalov N, Baradarian R, Iswara K, et al. Drug-induced acute pancreatitis: an evidence-based review. Clin Gastroenterol Hepatol 2007;5(6):648–61.
25. George Angus LD, Salzman S, Fritz K, et al. Chronic relapsing pancreatitis from a scorpion sting in Trinidad. Ann Trop Paediatr 1995;15(4):285–9.
26. Layer P, Yamamoto H, Kalthoff L, et al. The different courses of early- and late-onset idiopathic and alcoholic chronic pancreatitis. Gastroenterology 1994;107(5):1481–7.
27. Rossi L, Whitcomb DC, Ehrlich GD, et al. Lack of R117H mutation in the cationic trypsinogen gene in patients with tropical pancreatitis from Bangladesh. Pancreas 1998;17(3):278–80.
28. Gardner TB, Chari ST. Autoimmune pancreatitis. Gastroenterol Clin North Am 2008; 37(2):439–60, vii.
29. Seidensticker F, Otto J, Lankisch PG. Recovery of the pancreas after acute pancreatitis is not necessarily complete. Int J Pancreatol 1995;17(3):225–9.
30. Somogyi L, Martin SP, Venkatesan T, et al. Recurrent acute pancreatitis: an algorithmic approach to identification and elimination of inciting factors. Gastroenterology 2001;120(3):708–17.
31. Boreham B, Ammori BJ. A prospective evaluation of pancreatic exocrine function in patients with acute pancreatitis: correlation with extent of necrosis and pancreatic endocrine insufficiency. Pancreatology 2003;3(4):303–8.

32. Saraswat VA, Sharma BC, Agarwal DK, et al. Biliary microlithiasis in patients with idiopathic acute pancreatitis and unexplained biliary pain: response to therapy. J Gastroenterol Hepatol 2004;19(10):1206–11.
33. Mitchell CJ, Simpson FG, Davison AM, et al. Radiation pancreatitis: a clinical entity? Digestion 1979;19(2):134–6.
34. Levy P, Menzelxhiu A, Paillot B, et al. Abdominal radiotherapy is a cause for chronic pancreatitis. Gastroenterology 1993;105(3):905–9.
35. Klein SD, Affronti JP. Pancreas divisum, an evidence-based review: part I, pathophysiology. Gastrointest Endosc 2004;60(3):419–25.
36. Klein SD, Affronti JP. Pancreas divisum, an evidence-based review: part II, patient selection and treatment. Gastrointest Endosc 2004;60(4):585–9.
37. Tarnasky PR, Hoffman B, Aabakken L, et al. Sphincter of Oddi dysfunction is associated with chronic pancreatitis. Am J Gastroenterol 1997;92(7):1125–9.
38. Bong JJ, Spalding D. Duodenal duplication cyst (DDC) communicating with the pancreatobiliary duct–a rare cause of recurrent acute pancreatitis in adults. J Gastrointest Surg 2010;14(1):199–202.
39. Vallera R, Affronti J. Caroli's disease and choledochal cysts. In: Benjamin S, Dimarino AJ, editors. Endoscopy: an endoscopic approach to gastrointestinal disease. 2nd edition. Thorofare (NJ): Slack; 2002. p. 1233–44.
40. Saluja SS, Mishra PK, Nayeem M, et al. Choledochal cyst with chronic pancreatitis: presentation and management. JOP 2010;11(6):601–3.
41. Gouda BP, Desai DC, Abraham P, et al. Choledochal cysts with chronic pancreatitis in adults: report of two cases with a review of the literature. JOP 2010;11(4):373–6.
42. Newby LK, Affronti J, Baillie J, et al. Post-traumatic pancreatitis. Gastrointest Endosc 1990;36(1):79.
43. Malka D, Hammel P, Sauvanet A, et al. Risk factors for diabetes mellitus in chronic pancreatitis. Gastroenterology 2000;119(5):1324–32.
44. Jacobson DG, Curington C, Connery K, et al. Trypsin-like immunoreactivity as a test for pancreatic insufficiency. N Engl J Med 1984;310(20):1307–9.
45. Niederau C, Grendell JH. Diagnosis of chronic pancreatitis. Gastroenterology 1985;88(6):1973–95.
46. Naruse S, Ishiguro H, Ko SB, et al. Fecal pancreatic elastase: a reproducible marker for severe exocrine pancreatic insufficiency. J Gastroenterol 2006;41(9):901–8.
47. Walkowiak J, Herzig KH, Strzykala K, et al. Fecal elastase-1 is superior to fecal chymotrypsin in the assessment of pancreatic involvement in cystic fibrosis. Pediatrics 2002;110(1 Pt 1):e7.
48. Ghazale A, Chari ST, Smyrk TC, et al. Value of serum IgG4 in the diagnosis of autoimmune pancreatitis and in distinguishing it from pancreatic cancer. Am J Gastroenterol 2007;102(8):1646–53.
49. Kim DH, Pickhardt PJ. Radiologic assessment of acute and chronic pancreatitis. Surg Clin North Am 2007;87(6):1341–58, viii.
50. Siddiqi AJ, Miller F. Chronic pancreatitis: ultrasound, computed tomography, and magnetic resonance imaging features. Semin Ultrasound CT MR 2007;28(5):384–94.
51. Cotton PB, Garrow DA, Gallagher J, et al. Risk factors for complications after ERCP: a multivariate analysis of 11,497 procedures over 12 years. Gastrointest Endosc 2009;70(1):80–8.
52. Chowdhury R, Bhutani MS, Mishra G, et al. Comparative analysis of direct pancreatic function testing versus morphological assessment by endoscopic

ultrasonography for the evaluation of chronic unexplained abdominal pain of presumed pancreatic origin. Pancreas 2005;31(1):63–8.

53. Hayakawa T, Kondo T, Shibata T, et al. Relationship between pancreatic exocrine function and histological changes in chronic pancreatitis. Am J Gastroenterol 1992;87(9):1170–4.

54. Milham FH. Acute abdominal pain. In: Feldman M, Friedman LS, Brand LJ, editors. Sleisenger and Fordtran's gastrointestinal and liver disease. 9th edition. Philadelphia: Saunders Elsevier; 2010. p. 151.

55. Yarze JC, Friedman LS. Chronic abdominal pain. In: Feldman M, Friedman LS, Brand LJ, editors. Sleisenger and Fordtran's gastrointestinal and liver disease. 9th edition. Philadelphia: Saunders Elsevier; 2010. p. 163.

56. Lankisch PG, Seidensticker F, Lohr-Happe A, et al. The course of pain is the same in alcohol- and nonalcohol-induced chronic pancreatitis. Pancreas 1995;10(4):338–41.

57. Strum WB. Abstinence in alcoholic chronic pancreatitis. Effect on pain and outcome. J Clin Gastroenterol 1995;20(1):37–41.

58. Prognosis of chronic pancreatitis: an international multicenter study. International Pancreatitis Study Group [Internet]. Valhalla (NY): United States: Department of Surgery, New York Medical College; 1994.

59. Basso D, Panozzo MP, Fabris C, et al. Oxygen derived free radicals in patients with chronic pancreatic and other digestive diseases. J Clin Pathol 1990;43(5):403–5.

60. Kirk GR, White JS, McKie L, et al. Combined antioxidant therapy reduces pain and improves quality of life in chronic pancreatitis. J Gastrointest Surg 2006;10(4):499–503.

61. Sateesh J, Bhardwaj P, Singh N, et al. Effect of antioxidant therapy on hospital stay and complications in patients with early acute pancreatitis: a randomised controlled trial. Trop Gastroenterol 2009;30(4):201–6.

62. Brown A, Hughes M, Tenner S, et al. Does pancreatic enzyme supplementation reduce pain in patients with chronic pancreatitis: a meta-analysis. Am J Gastroenterol 1997;92(11):2032–5.

63. Chacko LN, Chen YK, Shah RJ. Clinical outcomes and nonendoscopic interventions after minor papilla endotherapy in patients with symptomatic pancreas divisum. Gastrointest Endosc 2008;68(4):667–73.

64. Rosch T, Daniel S, Scholz M, et al. Endoscopic treatment of chronic pancreatitis: a multicenter study of 1000 patients with long-term follow-up. Endoscopy 2002;34(10):765–71.

65. Renou C, Grandval P, Ville E, et al. Endoscopic treatment of the main pancreatic duct: correlations among morphology, manometry, and clinical follow-up. Int J Pancreatol 2000;27(2):143–9.

66. Morgan DE, Smith JK, Hawkins K, et al. Endoscopic stent therapy in advanced chronic pancreatitis: relationships between ductal changes, clinical response, and stent patency. Am J Gastroenterol 2003;98(4):821–6.

67. Affronti J, Branch M, Jowell P, et al. How often is extracorporeal shockwave lithotripsy needed for the treatment of pancreatic and biliary duct stones? Am J Gastroenterol 1996;91(9):1928.

68. Guda NM, Partington S, Freeman ML. Extracorporeal shock wave lithotripsy in the management of chronic calcific pancreatitis: a meta-analysis. JOP 2005;6(1):6–12.

69. Buchler MW, Warshaw AL. Resection versus drainage in treatment of chronic pancreatitis. Gastroenterology 2008;134(5):1605–7.

70. Strate T, Bachmann K, Busch P, et al. Resection vs drainage in treatment of chronic pancreatitis: long-term results of a randomized trial. Gastroenterology 2008;134(5):1406–11.

71. Frey CF, Reber HA. Local resection of the head of the pancreas with pancreatico-jejunostomy. J Gastrointest Surg 2005;9(6):863–8.

72. Buscher HC, Schipper EE, Wilder-Smith OH, et al. Limited effect of thoracoscopic splanchnicectomy in the treatment of severe chronic pancreatitis pain: a prospective long-term analysis of 75 cases. Surgery 2008;143(6):715–22.

73. Sutton JM, Schmulewitz N, Sussman JJ, et al. Total pancreatectomy and islet cell autotransplantation as a means of treating patients with genetically linked pancreatitis. Surgery 2010;148(4):676–85 [discussion: 685–6].

74. Baillie J. Pancreatic pseudocysts (part I). Gastrointest Endosc 2004;59(7):873–9.

75. Baillie J. Pancreatic pseudocysts (part II). Gastrointest Endosc 2004;60(1):105–13.

76. Baron TH. Endoscopic drainage of pancreatic pseudocysts. J Gastrointest Surg 2008;12(2):369–72.

77. Catalano MF, Linder JD, George S, et al. Treatment of symptomatic distal common bile duct stenosis secondary to chronic pancreatitis: comparison of single vs. multiple simultaneous stents. Gastrointest Endosc 2004;60(6):945–52.

78. Zyromski NJ, Vieira C, Stecker M, et al. Improved outcomes in postoperative and pancreatitis-related visceral pseudoaneurysms. J Gastrointest Surg 2007;11(1):50–5.

79. Dite P, Novotny I, Precechtelova M, et al. Incidence of pancreatic carcinoma in patients with chronic pancreatitis. Hepatogastroenterology 2010;57(101):957–60.

80. Vitone LJ, Greenhalf W, Howes NR, et al. Hereditary pancreatitis and secondary screening for early pancreatic cancer. Rocz Akad Med Bialymst 2005;50:73–84.

81. Canto MI, Goggins M, Hruban RH, et al. Screening for early pancreatic neoplasia in high-risk individuals: a prospective controlled study. Clin Gastroenterol Hepatol 2006;4(6):766–81 [quiz: 665].

82. Cicek B, Parlak E, Oguz D, et al. Endoscopic treatment of pancreatic fistulas. Surg Endosc 2006;20(11):1706–12.

83. Chowdhury RS, Forsmark CE, Davis RH, et al. Prevalence of gastroparesis in patients with small duct chronic pancreatitis. Pancreas 2003;26(3):235–8.

# Acute Infectious Diarrhea

Rebecca L. McClarren, MD*, Brodi Lynch, MD,
Neelima Nyayapati, MD

**KEYWORDS**

• Diarrhea • Infectious • Foodborne • Enteric pathogens

Infectious diarrhea is both a common and a complex entity. In adults and older children, a formal definition of diarrhea includes the passage of three or more loose or liquid stools daily with a cumulative mass greater than 200 gm.[1,2] Organisms responsible for infectious diarrhea include viruses, bacteria, parasites, and fungi.

## DEFINITION AND PATHOPHYSIOLOGY

Approximately 9 L of fluid pass into an adult's intestine each day. This daily fluid load consists of 1 to 2 L of dietary liquid and about 7 L of endogenous gastrointestinal secretions. Roughly 98% to 99% of this liquid is absorbed; 7.5 L are taken up by the duodenum and jejunum and an additional 1 to 2 L are removed by the colon.[2,3] The maximum absorptive capacity of the adult intestinal tract is 12 to 18 L daily.[2] In simplest terms, infectious diarrhea is a result of two basic mechanisms—increased endogenous fluid production or decreased fluid resorption. It often is classified as noninflammatory or inflammatory.

Noninflammatory infectious diarrhea usually originates in the upper intestinal tract. Toxins produced by the offending organisms may cause marked increases in enteric secretions and gut motility resulting in frequent, voluminous, watery stools. Sometimes toxins are generated by the organism before consumption, as in food poisoning due to *Staphylococcus aureus*. This leads to the abrupt onset of symptoms within a few hours of ingestion. In other illnesses, the toxins are formed following colonization of the small intestine and the onset of symptoms is more delayed. In both types of illness, nausea and vomiting often precede diarrhea. Patients are usually afebrile or have low-grade fevers. In severe cases, profound dehydration may occur over the span of several hours. Cholera is the prototypic infection in this group. Other examples include viral gastroenteritis, giardiasis, and food poisoning due to *Clostridium perfringens* and *S aureus*.

The authors have nothing to disclose.
Family Medicine Residency Program, St Luke's Hospital, University of Toledo, 6005 Monclova Road, Maumee, OH 43537, USA
* Corresponding author.
*E-mail address:* rebecca.mcclarren@utoledo.edu

Inflammatory infectious diarrhea typically is due to attacks on the gut by the offending agent. The invasive or cytotoxin-producing organisms trigger an inflammatory response in the bowel mucosa. This inflammation results in increased permeability and/or decreased absorptive area. Patients are usually febrile and often appear toxic. Severe cramps are followed by the passage of frequent, small-volume stools that often contain blood and mucus. Dysentery is the term denoting this disease process. Common inflammatory pathogens include *Shigella, Campylobacter, Salmonella,* and *Clostridium difficile.*

Diarrhea may also be classified by its chronicity. Knowledge of the length of illness gives clues to cause and helps guide both diagnostic work-up and treatment considerations.

Although there are minor variations in classification, in general

1. Acute diarrhea has duration of several hours to 14 days
2. Persistent diarrhea lasts 2 to 4 weeks
3. Chronic diarrhea extends beyond 1 month.

## EPIDEMIOLOGY

Globally, there are approximately 1.5 to 2 billion cases of diarrhea yearly.[4,5] About 375 million of these infections occur in the United States.[5] Internationally, in the year 2000, diarrhea was responsible for the deaths of 1.5 to 2 million children who were under the age of 5 years.[4] In resource-poor countries, diarrhea is second only to pneumonia in lethality in this age group.[4] The annual incidence of infectious diarrhea in the United States is estimated to be 1.4 episodes per person year.[5] Population groups at particular risk for significant morbidity and mortality are the very young, the elderly, the undernourished, and the immunocompromised. Those who live in areas lacking safe food and water supplies, good hygiene practices, basic medical care, and adequate nutrition are especially vulnerable.

## EVALUATION

Most cases of diarrhea are mild and resolve without medical care. When assistance is sought however, the medical history is of prime importance. Specific questions should be asked regarding comorbidities such as diabetes, immunodeficiencies, and conditions or medications resulting in decreased gastric acidity. Inquiries should be made regarding exposure to other ill persons, involvement with daycare and group residential facilities, travel, immunization history, water and food sources, contact with animals, and, when appropriate, sexual practices.

The presence of fever, vomiting, cramping, tenesmus, and abdominal pain should be noted. Questions should be asked regarding oral intake, complaints of thirst or weakness, and frequency, appearance, and relative amounts of both stool and urinary output. Systemic manifestations of illness should not be ignored, as diarrhea may be a symptom of other disease processes such as urinary tract infections and influenza.

In patients with diarrhea, the most important aspect of the physical examination is assessment of hydration status. Weight should be documented. Dry mucus membranes, tachycardia, fever, and hypotension may be indicative of dehydration. Conversely, bradycardia, deep erratic respirations, and hypothermia, may signal severe volume depletion. Abdominal examination should focus on bowel sounds, distension, palpable masses, pain, tenderness, guarding, and rebound.

## LABORATORY STUDIES

Initial laboratory studies for the patient with diarrhea should be limited to tests necessary to assess severity of illness and to deliver appropriate supportive care. Aside from public health concerns, no testing is needed in patients with mild diarrhea of short duration. In the presence of dehydration, dipstick urinalysis, electrolytes, blood urea nitrogen, creatinine, and glucose are useful in evaluating metabolic derangements. If the patient appears toxic or has dysenteric stools, a complete blood count is indicated.

Guidelines regarding stool studies are determined by epidemiologic concerns and severity, and duration of illness. In previously healthy individuals who are not severely ill, some authorities advise not ordering stool studies until diarrhea has persisted for 3 to 7 days.[6] Patients who appear toxic or develop dysentery should have prompt stool examinations. Diarrhea that originates in the upper gut tends to be watery and voluminous and may have a pH less than 5.5; diarrheal stools resulting from lower bowel pathology often contain blood and/or mucus and have a pH above 5.5.[1] The presence of fecal leukocytes as seen with methylene blue staining indicates an inflammatory process, due to either an infectious process or an inflammatory bowel disease. Alternatively, the presence of fecal lactoferrin, a protein made by neutrophils, can be measured. This test is only valid in persons older than 15 years and relies on a latex agglutination method; as such, it is both more user-friendly and more costly.[6]

Testing for *C difficile* toxin should be considered in patients with diarrhea who have been on antibiotics in the preceding 3 months or have other predisposing factors for *C difficile* infections. Rapid ELISAs test for toxin A, toxin B, or both.[7] Sensitivity between 85% and 96% has been reported on the polymerase chain reaction (PCR) assay used by Johns Hopkins' personnel.[8]

Rapid ELISA tests for rotavirus detection provide results within minutes and report specificities between 95.8% and 99.3% and sensitivities between 93.1% and 97.6%.[9,10] A single- step dipstick test for cholera is also available. Sensitivity of 96% and specificity of 92% has been reported.[11] Similar rapid tests are now also available for *Cryptosporidium*, *Giardia*, pathogenic *Escherichia coli*, and *Campylobacter*.

Stool cultures require significant expenditures with a calculated cost of more than $1000 per positive test.[2] In North America, most cases of diarrhea are relatively brief, self-limited, and mild, usually resolving before the results of stool cultures are known. It is generally recommended that cultures be sent if diarrhea has persisted more than 3 to 5 days or if stools are dysenteric or contain leukocytes. Significant fever or toxicity is also an indication for cultures. In addition, outbreaks of illness may require identification of pathogens for epidemiologic purposes. When ordering cultures, it is important to know which organisms are routinely identified in the lab being used. If other bacteria are suspected, they must be specifically requisitioned.

Testing for ova and parasites is generally not advised unless symptoms have persisted for at least 2 weeks. Because of intermittent passage of ova and parasites, three specimens obtained on 3 different days should be obtained.[2]

## GENERAL TREATMENT GUIDELINES

When diarrhea is severe, efforts to replace fluid losses should be of highest priority; rapid deterioration can progress to death in a matter of hours if treatment is delayed. Young children, the elderly, the immunocompromised, and the malnourished are particularly vulnerable. In the past, diarrhea has been classified as mild (3% to 5% fluid deficit), moderate (6% to 9% fluid deficit), and severe ($\geq$10%).[12] Because of difficulty in clinically quantifying fluid losses, mild and moderate levels of dehydration are now grouped together for purposes of treatment planning.[12]

Fortunately, most patients with diarrhea are able to tolerate oral fluids. Breastfed infants should continue to nurse.[13] Commercial rehydration solutions such as Pedialyte are readily available in North America. In many areas, the World Health Organization (WHO) Oral Rehydration Solution (ORS), is supplied in packets to be mixed with clean water. In 2006, WHO published the composition of a new ORS formulation in which the osmolarity was reduced from 311 milliosmole (mOsm)/L to 245 mOsm/L.[14] Concerns have been expressed regarding possible development of hyponatremia with use of the new formula, particularly in cholera patients.[15] A variety of recipes for "homemade" ORS are available on Internet sites.[16–18]

A Cochrane Review of poor-to-moderate quality compared oral rehydration therapy (ORT) to intravenous therapy (IVT) in children with acute gastroenteritis and found "no clinically important differences between ORT and IVT…"[19] It should be noted that 4% of the children failed oral therapy and were then treated with IVT.[19] Detailed fluid and electrolyte management is beyond the scope of this article; however, key concepts are replacement of losses as well as provision of maintenance needs. Daily fluid requirements for cholera patients may be measured in gallons.[20]

When patients with dehydration are unable to consume or retain oral fluids, alternative methods of fluid administration must be used. This may involve intravenous or intraosseous access. Hypodermoclysis is another little-used option for treating mild-to-moderate dehydration, particularly in the frail, elderly, homebound patient.[21–23] Because this method does not require constant nursing care, home administration can be accomplished. Hypodermoclysis is not appropriate for emergency resuscitation because rapid infusion rates cannot be maintained.

Except in rare circumstances, a regular diet is encouraged after the initial correction of dehydration. Although the BRAT (bananas, rice, applesauce, and toast) diet, has been widely used, it is not advised due to nutritional inadequacies. Early re-feeding was shown to decrease stool volume during the recovery period.[24] There does not seem to be a clear consensus regarding avoidance of dairy products due to infection-induced lactase deficiency.[25] In infancy, continuation of breast feeding is uniformly encouraged.[12]

Recent studies have shown a beneficial effect of zinc supplementation in poorly nourished children with diarrhea.[12,26] Supplementation with zinc has led to decreased severity, duration, mortality, and recurrence rate in the subsequent 2 to 3 months.[27–32] Current recommendations are to supplement with 10 mg zinc daily for infants under 6 months of age and 20 mg zinc daily for 10 to 14 days for all children with infectious diarrhea.[27,28] There is contradictory evidence supporting the use of Vitamin A supplementation in the treatment of infectious diarrhea in children.[26]

The possible relationship between infectious diarrhea and zinc in adults is less studied. A decreased frequency of diarrhea and a delay in immune failure was demonstrated in a United States study using zinc supplementation.[33,34] A study performed in rural Kenya among HIV-infected adults showed a beneficial effect only among persons coinfected with both malaria and HIV but not among healthy volunteers or persons infected only with malaria or HIV.[35,36] A single, small study among Peruvian HIV patients with persistent diarrhea failed to show a significant effect on the resolution of diarrhea in those treated with supplemental zinc.[37] No studies were found assessing the role of zinc in treatment of acute infectious diarrhea in previously "healthy" adults.

In adults, symptoms of infectious diarrhea can often be significantly improved by the administration of loperamide (Imodium), or diphenoxylate (combined with atropine in the formulation of Lomotil). Both are antimotility agents and should not be given in the presence of fever, severe pain, or dysenteric stools. Administration to children and the elderly is contraindicated. Central nervous system depression, bloating, constipation, and toxic megacolon have been observed with the use of antimotility agents.[38] Although antibiotics and antimotility agents are sometimes prescribed concurrently, this practice has unknown effectiveness.[39]

Bismuth subsalicylate (Pepto-Bismol and Kaopectate), has been in use for more than a century and is thought to have a multifactorial mechanism of action. According to Epocrates Online, it "possesses topical mucosal effects; reduces secretions; binds bacterial toxins; [and] possesses antimicrobial effects."[40] It also is of some benefit in the prophylaxis of traveler's diarrhea. The use of bismuth subsalicylate is somewhat limited by a host of drug interactions and the recent recommendation against use in the pediatric population due to the relationship between aspirin and Reye syndrome.

Racecadotril is a purely antisecretory drug that has been used successfully in both children and adults. The incidence of adverse side effects is similar to placebo.[41–43] It has been in widespread use internationally for a number of years but cannot be purchased in the United States.

Probiotic use has received attention as both an effective prophylaxis and treatment modality for infectious diarrhea.[44,45] The WHO defines probiotics as "live organisms that, when administered in adequate amounts, confer a health benefit on the host."[46] Preliminary studies support the hypothesis that both the type and quantity of ingested probiotics are factors in the prevention and treatment of some types of infectious diarrhea.[44,47,48]

## TRAVELERS' DIARRHEA

Travelers' diarrhea afflicts an estimated 20% to 50% of international travelers.[49] As such, it is considered the most common illness affecting international travelers.[49,50] Symptoms usually present within the first week of travel[49,51,52] and resolve spontaneously within 1 to 7 days.[49] The likelihood of contracting the malady is inversely related to the socioeconomic status of the destination.

The majority of travelers' diarrhea is due to bacterial infection.[49,51] In a systematic review covering the years from 1973 to 2008, the most frequently identified pathogen was Enterotoxigenic *E coli* (ETEC), which was found in 30.4% of those studied. The second most common organism was enteroaggregative *E coli* (EAEC), which was identified in 19.0% of studied subjects.[50] Predominance of pathogens was dependent upon sites visited.

Host factors also appear to affect susceptibility to travelers' diarrhea. Multiple studies have demonstrated increased susceptibility among persons with decreased gastric acidity.[53] Nonbreastfed infants, young children, the elderly and persons with underlying immunocompromise are at increased risk. In addition, persons traveling from developing countries are at lower risk than those who travel from countries that are more affluent.[52]

The effects of travelers' diarrhea can range from being a mild inconvenience to thwarting the purpose of the trip. Long-advocated preventive recommendations have included efforts to ensure safe food and water supplies: (1) avoidance of salads and fresh fruits and vegetables (unless they can be washed and peeled by the consumer); incompletely cooked meats, seafood, and eggs; raw milk and unpasteurized dairy products and (2) use of only bottled, boiled, or filtered water (including that used in ice and for brushing teeth). Unfortunately, a review of eight studies did not show a correlation between dietary choices and the development of travelers' diarrhea.[54] Daily antibiotic use has been shown to be effective in preventing most travelers' diarrhea. However, there are significant concerns regarding the development of antibiotic resistance and their risks and side effect profiles. Because of these concerns, routine antibiotic prophylaxis is not recommended.[25,49] Antibiotic prophylaxis with daily ciprofloxacin or rifaximin can be considered for high-risk individuals or for persons who cannot "afford to be ill" due to responsibilities inherent in their reason for travel. Prophylactic use of bismuth subsalicylate four times daily can be considered[49]; however, its use is contradicted in pregnancy or when aspirin use is contradicted. Vaccines against ETEC are currently being developed.[55]

In addition to hydration, self-treatment for travelers' diarrhea can include bismuth subsalicylate, ciprofloxacin or norfloxacin, or rifaximin.[53] Antimotility agents may also be considered if fever and dysenteric stools are absent.[49,53]

## SPECIFIC INFECTIONS

Most cases of infectious diarrhea ultimately resolve without a specific diagnosis. From a public health perspective, however, identification of offending organisms is often essential in planning effective prevention and eradication strategies. In severe or prolonged illnesses, such knowledge is also invaluable in guiding individual treatment decisions. Infectious agents will be examined in the following groups: bacteria, viruses, parasites, and fungi.

Although some overlap may occur, infectious diarrhea will be classified here as noninflammatory (primarily due to toxin mediated effects on the upper gut), or inflammatory (characterized by inflammation of the lower intestine with resultant small-volume stools containing white and red blood cells).

## VIRUSES

*Rotavirus* is the most common cause of severe diarrhea among children.[56] Before the reintroduction of rotavirus vaccines in 2006, this diarrheal illness resulted in the hospitalization of approximately 55,000 to 70,000 children in the United States each year.[57] In temperate climates, peak occurrence is during winter months. The highest rate of illness is between the ages of 6 months and 5 years. Globally, rotavirus is responsible for about 40% of pediatric infectious diarrhea and is estimated to cause 352,000 to 592,000 pediatric deaths annually.[58] Rotavirus also causes significant adult morbidity, particularly among caregivers of children, travelers to Central America and the Caribbean, and those residing in long-term care facilities or relatively closed communities (eg, military bases).[59]

Rotaviruses are wheel-shaped, nonenveloped, double-stranded members of the Reoviridae family. Most pediatric infections are due to strains of Group A rotavirus. Groups B and C are also known to be pathogenic, at least in adults. Animal rotavirus strains do not cause human illness.[59] The viruses are hardy, surviving on dry fomites for up to 60 days.[60] Following ingestion of even a very few organisms, the rotaviruses infect the proximal small intestine, where an enterotoxin is elaborated.

The primary mode of transmission of rotavirus infection is fecal-oral. Following an incubation period of 1 to 4 days,[57,61] the typical rotavirus presentation begins abruptly with nausea and vomiting, often accompanied by fever and headache. This is followed by watery diarrhea that may persist for 4 to 5 days.[62] Asymptomatic infection can occur in adults.[59] Reinfection later in life is common.[59]

Rapid ELISA on stool specimens is generally used to diagnose rotavirus infection. Other techniques may be used in research settings.

No specific antidote exists. Treatment is supportive with particular attention to maintaining hydration.

Good hand-washing technique is critical when caring for patients with rotavirus gastroenteritis. Because the virus is resistant to many cleansing agents, a bleach containing disinfectant should be applied to contaminated surfaces.[62] Two live vaccines, Rotarix and RotaTeq, are now in widespread use and have been included in WHO-recommended immunization programs since 2009.[63] A third vaccine, Lanzhou lamb rotavirus (LLR), has been approved for use in China. Rotarix is a monovalent vaccine and is given in two doses at 2 and 4 months of age. RotaTeq is a pentavalent vaccine and is given in three doses at 2, 4, and 6 months of age. Administration of both vaccines must begin between 6 weeks and 14 weeks 6 days. In the United States, there has been a reduction of approximately 85% in the number of rotavirus-related pediatric emergency department visits or hospitalizations since the introduction of widespread rotavirus immunization in 2008.[64] In 2010, the number of rotavirus-confirmed hospitalizations in the United States was approximately 96% less than in 2006.[65] Although seasonal variations continue, both the number of tests performed and the number of positive tests have dramatically declined following routine administration of rotavirus vaccine.[66] For Mexican children under the age of 5, the diarrhea-related mortality rate declined by 35% after the administration of at least one dose of vaccine to infants 11 months old or younger.[67] In a Centers for Disease Control and Prevention (CDC) analysis of laboratory data, a 60% and 64% decline in the percentage of positive rotavirus test results was observed in the first 2 years following widespread rotavirus vaccination in the United States.[68]

*Norovirus* is highly contagious organism responsible for more than half of all foodborne cases of gastroenteritis in the United States. Per CDC estimates, more than 21 million cases of norovirus gastroenteritis occur annually in the United States.[69] Noroviruses are named after the original strain, "Norwalk Virus," which caused an outbreak of gastroenteritis in a school in Norwalk, Ohio in 1968.

Noroviruses are very small, round, nonenveloped, single-stranded RNA viruses belonging to the Calicivirus family. Transmission is thought to be primarily fecal-oral; however, it appears that aerosolization may also lead to infection.[70] Illness may develop after as few as 10 viral particles have been ingested.[69] Numerous outbreaks related to consumption of raw shellfish, particularly oysters, have also been reported.[71–73] Infection with norovirus occurs in the proximal portion of the small intestine. Susceptibility to infection varies among individuals, presumably due to genetic factors.[69]

Often referred to as "the stomach flu," norovirus infection is characterized by an incubation period of 24 to 36 hours followed by the development of nausea, vomiting, abdominal cramps, and watery diarrhea. Low-grade fever and myalgias may also be present. Dehydration may occur in severe cases. Resolution usually occurs within 24 to 48 hours; however, viral shedding may be present for 2 or more weeks.[69] Asymptomatic infections may occur. Reinfection throughout the life cycle is common.

Performed on stool or emesis samples, reverse transcriptase-PCR is used to diagnose norovirus infection, ideally during the acute stage of illness. ELISA techniques are available but less sensitive.[69] Drinking water and shellfish can also be tested for the presence of norovirus.[69,74]

No specific antidote exists. Treatment is supportive with particular attention to maintaining hydration.

No vaccine exists to prevent norovirus infection. Thorough hand-washing with soap and water is of major importance. Because the virus can survive freezing and steaming, provision of a safe food supply is essential. Disinfection of hard surfaces should be done with an approved commercial agent or a solution containing 5 to 25 tablespoons bleach per gallon water.[69]

## Other Viruses

There are several other, less frequent, causes of viral diarrhea to briefly review. Supportive care is the mainstay of treatment for these infections.

Evidence of infection with *Adenoviruses 40* or *41* has been detected primarily among pediatric patients with gastroenteritis. In three non-American studies, 4% to 7.2% of children with diarrhea demonstrated evidence of *Adenovirus* infection.[75–77] Diarrhea, usually lasting 1 to 2 weeks, is the most common symptom of infection due to these strains.[75,78] Vomiting and fever also occur frequently. Asymptomatic infections have been documented.[75] Posttransplantation patients are at increased risk for infection.[78]

*Sapoviruses* are similar to *Noroviruses* and belong to the Calicivirus family. Although *Sapovirus* gastroenteritis is less common than *Norovirus*, its clinical course is very similar. Infection has been documented in both adults and children.[79] Secondary attacks frequently occur.

Gastroenteritis due to *Astrovirus* is generally less severe than that due to other viruses.[80] Its structure is similar to that of the Calicivirus family.

## BACTERIA

*S aureus* gastroenteritis is an extremely common cause of foodborne gastroenteritis.[6,81] It is difficult to estimate the true incidence of the illness due to presumed underdiagnosis and underreporting. As in other types of food poisoning, symptoms usually present simultaneously in groups of individuals who have eaten common foods.

The spherical *S aureus* organism is a gram-positive facultative anaerobe.[82] Episodes of gastroenteritis have been traced to single skin lesions on food handlers.[83,84] The illness is due to ingestion of one of five preformed *S aureus* enterotoxins, (A, B, C, D, or E), which have been elaborated in improperly handled food.[6] Meat and dairy products, (including ham and cheese), are frequently implicated as vehicles of *S aureus* gastroenteritis. The bacteria proliferate at temperatures between 10°C and 48.89°C.[81] Although high temperatures may kill the bacteria, the toxins are heat stable and, therefore, may cause illness from foods that were contaminated before cooking.

Affected individuals develop abrupt onset of nausea, vomiting, abdominal cramps, and watery diarrhea, usually within 1 to 4 hours of ingestion of food containing a *S aureus* enterotoxin. Symptoms generally resolve spontaneously within 1 to 2 days.

The history and epidemiology of an outbreak of *S aureus* gastroenteritis often leads to a presumptive diagnosis. Detection of *S aureus* enterotoxin in suspected foods is confirmatory. Testing can also be performed on patients' stool or emesis, or on skin lesions of food handlers.

Therapy is supportive with complete resolution usually occurring within 1 to 2 days. Complications are exceedingly rare. Safe food-handling practices are the primary means of prevention.

*Bacillus cereus* causes two distinct, food-related, gastrointestinal syndromes—an emetic (or vomiting) form and a diarrheal form. It is not a reportable disease and the actual incidences of illness are unknown. Both syndromes appear to be caused by the same organism.

The gram-positive, rod-shaped *B cereus* is a facultative aerobe that contaminates foods before cooking. The heat-resistant spores of the organism are found in many types of foods.[85,86] If, following cooking, the contaminated foods are allowed to cool slowly, germination can occur.

The emetic form presents with acute onset of vomiting ½ to 6 hours after ingestion of a preformed toxin. Although *B cereus* has been identified in a host of foods, the emetic form is most commonly associated with the consumption of fried rice. The toxin is highly heat-resistant and leads to symptoms in approximately 100% of those who ingest it.[6] The illness resembles *S aureus* food poisoning and is characterized by an acute onset of nausea and vomiting. Approximately one-third of patients also develop diarrhea. Symptoms are self-limited and usually resolve within 8 to 10 hours.[6,86]

The pathogenesis of the diarrhea form of the illness is less clear. Onset of symptoms is 6 to 15 hours after consumption of contaminated food.[6,87] Because of the interval between ingestion and onset of symptoms, it is speculated that the toxin is produced by *B cereus* organisms that have colonized the gut.[86]

Abdominal cramping and watery diarrhea are the predominate symptoms in the diarrhea form of illness. Vomiting occurs in approximately one-fourth of patients.[86] Symptoms mimic infection due to *C perfringens*. Illness resolves spontaneously in 20 to 36 hours.[6,86]

*B cereus* is often present in the stool of well persons.[86] Isolation of the same serotype from implicated food and a patient's stool or emesis is considered confirmatory evidence. In some instances, presumptive diagnosis is made on analysis of only suspect foods or vomit and feces. Supportive therapy generally leads to complete resolution without complications. Safe food-handling practices are the mainstay of prevention.

*Clostridia* are gram-positive, rod-shaped, anaerobic spore producers. The toxins of two of the species, *C difficile* and *C perfringens*, cause significant diarrheal illnesses.

*C perfringens* is frequently implicated in food poisoning involving meats or poultry that has been improperly cooked or stored. A secretory cytotoxin produced during sporulation damages the ileum.[88] Although the toxin can be isolated in stool and the bacteria can be detected in contaminated foods, presumptive diagnosis is often made based on the clinical course. Severe abdominal cramping, often accompanied by vomiting, and watery diarrhea occur 8 to 24 hours after ingestion of contaminated food. Symptoms are self-limited, usually resolving within 24 hours, although patients may not feel well for 1 to 2 weeks.[89] Treatment is supportive and prognosis is generally excellent. A rare variant known as pigbel, or *Enteritis necroticans*, results from consumption of large quantities of improperly cooked pork and primarily afflicts malnourished persons. A pigbel mortality rate of 40% has been reported.[51]

*C difficile* is the major cause of hospital-acquired diarrhea.[51] It is responsible for 15% to 25% of antibiotic-associated diarrhea.[90] Virtually all antibiotics have been implicated in the development of *C difficile* diarrhea; the most common culprits include clindamycin, cephalosporins, fluoroquinolones, and penicillins. Antibiotic-altered gut flora provides an "open" environment for colonization by *C difficile*, which then elaborates two intensely inflammatory exotoxins, toxin A and toxin B. These cytotoxins induce characteristic lesions and a widely variable clinical spectrum of colonic pathology and systemic illness. Asymptomatic colonization has been documented. High levels of antitoxin antibodies are thought to be protective against *C difficile* illness.[91]

The clinical picture of *C difficile* infection is variable but typically includes cramping and tenderness in the lower abdomen, malaise, mild temperature elevation, and diarrhea. Stools may be watery or contain occult blood and mucus. Frank hematochezia or melena is uncommon. Pseudomembranous enterocolitis may be seen on colonoscopy. Toxic megacolon is characterized by fever and marked abdominal distension and tenderness.

Techniques for detecting C difficile disease have evolved significantly and usually include a test for the presence of toxins A and B. A sensitivity range from 85% to 96% has been reported with a PCR assay, which requires a processing time under 3 hours.[92] When interpreting lab results, it is essential that they be viewed in light of the patient's history and medical condition. Because as many as half of infants have tested positive for C difficile by the time they are discharged from the hospital nursery, routine testing of children under the age of 5 years is not recommended.

Factors which predispose to the development of C difficile infection include significant underlying comorbidities, advanced age, the use of a nasogastric tube, immunosuppressive therapy, recent (within 3 months) antibiotic use, and an elevated gastric pH.[51]

Treatment of C difficile diarrhea involves supportive care and discontinuation of antibiotic therapy. Except in very mild cases, oral or intravenous metronidazole should be administered for 10 to 14 days. Oral vancomycin should be reserved for second-line therapy because of emerging drug-resistance and cost concerns.[91] Approximately 20% of patients experience relapses of symptoms.[7] If C difficile diarrhea recurs, a 14-day course of the same antibiotic regimen may be repeated, or dosage may be slowly tapered, in a pulsed manner, over a 5-week period.[91]

Effective programs to decrease the incidence of C difficile focus on decreasing unnecessary use of antibiotics and proton pump inhibitors, and basic infection-control measures. Such efforts have been shown to significantly lower the in-hospital acquisition rate of the infection.[93] Although alcohol cleansers have become readily accessible, it should be noted that they do not eradicate C difficile.

Cholera is the prototype of noninflammatory diarrhea and causes devastating epidemics of illness that ravage areas lacking safe water supplies. In 2009, the WHO reported a grand total of 221,226 cases of cholera with a case-fatality rate of 2.24%.[94] Although North America had seen little cholera activity for many years, the epidemic in postearthquake Haiti complicated an incredibly difficult political and public health crisis. As of February 2011, more than 220,000 Haitians had been diagnosed with cholera in a 4-month period. Early in the course of the epidemic, it was projected that approximately 400,000 persons would develop the infection in the following year.[95]

Vibrio cholera organisms are motile, comma shaped, gram-negative, short rods with single flagellum. They thrive in aerobic, salty, alkaline environments. Multiple pathogenic species of Vibrio exist. The clinical significance of the organism is due to the virulence of the various toxins elaborated by different strains. Contaminated food and water are responsible for most illness.

Although the severity of the illness is variable, the "classic" cholera scenario begins with vomiting and abdominal distension after an incubation period ranging from 6 hours to 5 days.[96] Diarrhea quickly ensues; voluminous stools are described as rice water due to the flecks of mucus that are present in the isotonic liquid stool. Massive quantities of diarrhea can rapidly result in dehydration and shock, in a period of hours. Fever is not a major feature of the illness. Bacteremia is exceedingly rare.[88]

In areas where cholera is endemic, the diagnosis is usually made on clinical grounds. Because mucosal invasion of the gut does not occur, stool examination does not reveal inflammatory cells. Stool dipstick testing can be used if the diagnosis is in question. Stool culture and antibiotic sensitivity testing may be useful in index cases.

Timely aggressive treatment of fluid and electrolyte disturbances is of paramount importance. This may be accomplished by oral rehydration solutions if the patient is able to drink and retain large volumes of fluids. Parenteral replacement is often required. With moderate to severe illness, antibiotic treatment with azithromycin, erythromycin, tetracycline, doxycycline, trimethoprim-sulfamethoxazole, furazolidone, or ciprofloxacin is indicated.[97] Because of emerging resistance, selection should be guided by local sensitivity patterns.

The keys to prevention are the provision of a safe water supply and good hygiene practices. Injectable cholera vaccines used in the past were safe but, according to a Cochrane Review, had an efficacy of 48%, with protection lasting 1 to 3 years.[98] Two oral vaccines have been produced on a limited scale but widespread use has never been implemented. Efficacy rates against V cholera O1 are approximately 85% to 90% at 4 to 6 months for the Dukoral vaccine.[99] A second vaccine, Shanchol, is awaiting WHO approval. It is administered in two doses and confers more sustained protection against two strains—V cholera O1 and O139.[99–101] The limited supply of vaccines coupled with political and social concerns have thwarted the use of the vaccines in Haiti.[102]

*Campylobacter jejuni* are among the leading bacterial causes of infectious diarrhea and, according to some authorities, cause more illness than *Salmonella*.[103,104] In the United States, an estimated 2.4 million persons, or 0.8% of the population, develop the illness each year.[105,106] The case fatality rate is estimated at 0.1%.[104]

The motile, gram-negative, microaerophilic, spiral-shaped rods are fragile and do not tolerate drying, high oxygen concentrations, or high temperatures.[104] The infective dose is below 500 organisms.[104,106] *C jejuni* are part of the normal flora of both wild and domesticated animals. Animal-to-human transmission is common. Improperly cooked chicken is a major source of illness. In 2005, increasing fluoroquinolone resistance prompted a successful effort by the US Food and Drug Administration to ban the use of this class of antibiotics in poultry.[107] Other modes of transmission include person-to-person, fecal-oral, improperly cooked meats, unpasteurized milk, and contaminated water supplies.

After an incubation period of 1 to 10 days,[88] persons may develop abdominal pain and cramps, diarrhea (watery to dysenteric), and fever. Nausea, vomiting, headache, and malaise frequently occur, and bacteremia may be present. Symptoms typically last 2 to 7 days and may be biphasic in nature.

Both white and red cells are seen on examination of feces. Darkfield microscopy may reveal the organism. Stool culture, using a selective antibiotic-containing medium in reduced-oxygen concentrations, is the most reliable method for diagnosing *C jejuni*.

Treatment is primarily supportive with an emphasis on hydration. Among severely ill patients, antibiotic use early in the course of the disease is usually encouraged.[88,108] This appears to decrease the duration of bacterial shedding but has not consistently been shown to alter the clinical course.[88,108] Current treatment recommendations include macrolides or fluoroquinolones. In some areas of the world, quinolone resistance has become a major problem, thereby limiting the usefulness of this antibiotic class.[51,88]

Relapses are quite common, occurring in up to one-fourth of cases.[51,88] Rare complications may include Guillain-Barré syndrome, hemolytic uremic syndrome, toxic megacolon, cholecystitis, meningitis, and reactive arthritis.

*E coli* are facultative anaerobic, gram-negative rods that normally inhabit the guts of all animals. The presence of *E coli* in prepared food is an indication of fecal contamination.[109] Although a host of *E coli* strains abounds in the environment, only a handful is recognized as seriously enteropathogenic in humans. Clinical course, prognosis, and treatment are variable, depending on the strain.

EAEC most frequently afflicts AIDS patients and malnourished children with diarrhea. The organism's name is derived from its characteristic "stacked brick" appearance as they adhere to cultured human epidermoid (HEP)-2 cells in the assay used for diagnosis of the infection.[51] The pathogenesis of EAEC diarrhea is incompletely understood but appears to involve enterotoxin and cytotoxin production.[110] The clinical picture may include low grade fever, vomiting and watery stools containing blood or mucus.[110]

Enterohemorrhagic *E coli* (EHEC) adheres to gut epithelium and produces *Shiga* toxins, (also called verotoxins), which are similar or identical to the toxin elaborated by *Shigella*. The best known EHEC serotype is 0157:H7, which has been responsible for outbreaks related to consumption of undercooked hamburger, alfalfa sprouts, raw milk, spinach, and lettuce.[111–113] A European study has also implicated wild game as a probable significant source of EHEC infections.[114] The incubation period is between 2 and 10 days.[115] The illness is initially characterized by watery diarrhea followed by grossly bloody stools within a few days. Abdominal pain (especially in the right-lower quadrant), cramping, and mild leukocytosis are common. Fever is either absent or low-grade.[51] Symptoms may persist for as long as 2 weeks. Diagnosis relies on clinical picture and stool cultures or ELISA for *Shiga* toxin. As many as 10% of EHEC patients develop hemolytic uremic syndrome (HUS).[116] This complication, which has a case fatality rate of 3% to 5%, is a common cause of renal failure as well as neurologic sequelae, hemolytic anemia, and thrombocytopenia.[116] Children are particularly vulnerable. Treatment is supportive with avoidance of antimotility agents. Antibiotic therapy has shown no benefit and may actually predispose to the development of HUS.[51]

Enteropathogenic *E coli* (EPEC) is most often associated with illness in formula-fed infants[117] but has occasionally been found in older children and adults. It currently is not a major pathogen in North America. The hallmark pathologic findings include "attaching and effacing" lesions in the small and large intestine due to adherence to the entereocytes.[118] Diarrhea may be either watery or bloody and may lead to dehydration. In developing countries, a mortality rate of 50% has been reported.[117] Supportive therapy is essential; treatment with trimethoprim-sulfamethoxazole has appeared beneficial.[51]

ETEC is ranked as the leading cause of travelers' diarrhea.[119] Similar strains also cause devastating disease in livestock and other domesticated animals. Virulence is due to production in the intestine of a heat-labile toxin and a heat-stable toxin, both of which cause watery diarrhea.[51,119] Contact with contaminated water or food is responsible for most illnesses. A relatively high infective dose of the bacteria is necessary for colonization to occur. Symptoms of low-grade fever, nausea, malaise, abdominal cramping, and diarrhea usually occur within 1 to 3 days of ingestion and resolve within 3 to 4 days.[119] The diagnosis is most often based on clinical course because laboratory confirmation may require a week.[117] Hydration is the mainstay of therapy, although fluoroquinolones and rifaximin decrease the length of illness.[51] The use of antibiotics must be weighed against concerns of increasing drug resistance. Vaccine testing is in progress.[120,121]

*Salmonellae* comprise a large division of Enterobacteriaceae. They are hydrogen sulfide-producing, gram-negative bacilli that can survive in a multitude of hosts. They are frequently found in contaminated water and foods. Although optimal growth occurs between 35°C and 37°C and a pH of 7.0 to 7.5, most serotypes are relatively resistant to drying and freezing. Fortunately, temperatures above 70°C and most disinfectants will eradicate the organisms. More than 2400 serotypes of *Salmonellae* have been identified, all of which are considered potentially pathogenic.[122] Most of the *Salmonellae* are flagellated. Typing is antigen-based. From a human medicine perspective, the two groups of primary concern are nontyphoidal and typhoidal (or the closely related paratyphoidal).

Nontyphoidal salmonellosis is culture-confirmed in approximately 40,000 persons in the United States annually. However, it is estimated that the actual number of infections approaches 1.4 million.[123] The annual salmonellosis death toll in the United States is about 400 persons. Acquisition may be related to consumption of contaminated foods, of both plant and animal origin. Fecal-oral transmission from infected animals or persons also occurs. In animals, transmission can be both vertical and horizontal. Poultry are particularly prone to colonization by *Salmonella*; disease transmission has occurred while handling birds, consuming undercooked poultry, and eating inadequately cooked eggs.[124,125] Contamination of eggs occurs before shell formation.[122] Recommendations to reduce salmonellosis include testing and immunization of flocks, refrigeration of eggs and meat at all times, use of pasteurized eggs, and cooking of eggs until both the yolks and whites are firm.[125] Handling of pet reptiles is another well known source of infection.[126] Because of this risk, it is illegal to sell or distribute small turtles in the United States.[127] Manure from colonized livestock is thought to be responsible for contamination of plant-based foods.

Following ingestion of the organism, victims typically develop nausea, vomiting, abdominal cramping, and diarrhea within 6 to 48 hours, although an incubation period of greater than 1 week has been reported.[88] Diarrhea usually persists 4 to 7 days and may be watery or dysenteric. Approximately half of patients are febrile and approximately 1 in 10 develop bacteremia, often leading to involvement of other organs.[88] Pain frequently localizes to the periumbilical area or to the right-lower quadrant.[88] Illness course varies greatly among individuals; severity tends to be greatest among infants, immunocompromised patients, and those with hypochlorhydria or achlorhydria.[51,88] *Salmonella* colitis can present identically to new-onset ulcerative colitis. Because symptoms of *Salmonella* colitis may be worsened by the administration of steroids, stool cultures are advised before beginning therapy if the diagnosis is in question. A carrier state develops in a small percentage of patients. About 2% of patients with salmonellosis develop a postinfection reactive arthritis.[128] Reiter syndrome is a well-documented, long-term sequel affecting approximately 2% to 29% of patients with salmonellosis, especially among persons with the HLA-B27 geno-type.[129–132]

In most instances of salmonellosis, supportive treatment without antibiotics is advised, as antimicrobial therapy has not been shown to alter the clinical course and appears to increase the carrier rate.[88] Exceptions to this recommendation include infants, the elderly, the immunocompromised, persons with implanted prosthetic devices, and patients with signs of sepsis.[51,88] Multidrug resistance has made the selection of antibiotics challenging. Currently ciprofloxacin is considered first-line therapy, followed by trimethoprim-sulfamethoxazole, ceftriaxone, or tetracycline.[88]

### Typhoid and Paratyphoid Fever

Infection with *Salmonella typhi* results in an illness that is distinct from that produced by nontyphoidal strains. Similar, but less severe, pictures occur with infection by *S paratyphi* and related serotypes. These organisms require human hosts and differ antigenically from typhoidal *Salmonellae*. Incidence is greatest in areas lacking high standards of sanitation. Annually only about 400 to 500 cases occur in the United States.[88] A 2010 outbreak was linked to consumption of smoothies containing imported mamey fruit.[133] For persons traveling internationally to endemic areas, there are two typhoid vaccines available, both affording a 50% to 80% protection rate. The oral, live, attenuated vaccine should only be administered to children age 6 years or older and should be repeated every 5 years. The injectable, capsular polysaccharide vaccine may be given to persons age 2 years and older and should be boosted every 2 years.[134] The vaccines offer no protection against S paratyphi.

Following ingestion of the bacilli, the organism enters the bloodstream via the small bowel mucosa. Initially, gastrointestinal symptoms are absent but, after an incubation period of 1 to 2 weeks, waves of bacteremia carry the organism throughout the body. Headache, high fever, abdominal pain, and the eventual appearance of a "rose spots" rash are hallmarks of the first week of illness. The fever then becomes more constant, often with the development of altered mental status. Green, "pea soup" diarrhea, sometimes accompanied by intestinal perforation and hemorrhage, may occur during this stage. Multiorgan system involvement is frequently present. The illness generally lasts about 1 month, but relapse, even after antibiotic therapy, is not uncommon. Early diagnosis, usually through blood cultures, is essential to ensure that appropriate treatment is instituted. Antibiotic therapy options include chloramphenicol; fluoroquinolones; amoxicillin; trimethoprim-sulfamethoxazole; and third-generation, injectable cephalosporins.[88,134] High-dose steroids may be beneficial in severely toxic patients.[88] A prolonged, antibiotic-resistant carrier state usually indicates the presence of the disease in the gallbladder and is an indication for cholecystectomy.[88] Untreated typhoid fever carries a mortality rate of 12% to 30%.[135]

Shigella organisms are nonmotile, gram-negative, non–gas-formers that are morphologically similar to E coli. Their only natural hosts are humans. Shigellae are divided into four main species: S dysenteriae, S flexneri, S boydii, and S sonnei. The relative prevalence of each organism varies relative to time and location. Shigellae are sensitive to heating and drying. As few as 10 to 200 bacteria can cause illness.[51,88,136]

Approximately 14,000 documented cases of shigellosis occur annually in the United States, but it is estimated that this number may only represent the most ill 5% of patients.[137] Between 85 million and 165 million persons are infected globally each year.[138] Young children are especially prone to the illness. In recent years, the number of deaths due to shigellosis appears to have significantly decreased in Asia; the reasons behind this trend have not yet been elucidated.[139]

During infections, large numbers of Shigellae are found in feces. Person-to-person contact, food, water, and fly transmission have been documented. The incubation period is usually 12 to 96 hours.[138] Symptoms may be due both to the production of an enterotoxin and the invasion of the colonic epithelium and mucosa. The illness is marked by lower abdominal pain and small-volume, dysenteric stools containing visible blood and mucus. High fever and rectal burning frequently occur. The length of illness varies from 1 to 7 days and may sometimes be biphasic, with frank hematochezia being observed only in the second phase.[88] Potential complications include seizures, meningitis, appendicitis, hemolytic-uremic syndrome, reactive arthritis, and postinfection irritable bowel syndrome.

Treatment of shigellosis should usually be dictated by severity of symptoms. As with other forms of diarrhea, rehydration is of paramount importance. Because of to widespread resistance, ampicillin and trimethoprim-sulfamethoxazole are no longer considered first-line therapy. Fluoroquinolones are generally recommended as drugs of choice; other agents that may be considered include ceftriaxone, azithromycin, nalidixic acid, and cefixime.[88,136] A 2010 Cochrane Review failed to show superiority of any specific antibiotics in the treatment of shigellosis.[140]

Yersinia enterocolitica is another gram-negative, non–lactose-fermenting bacterium that is responsible for infectious diarrhea. In the United States, approximately 17,000 persons have documented yersiniosis yearly. Y enterocolitica has been found in environmental fresh water sources and has been isolated from a variety of animals and animal-based foods.[141] Transmission occurs primarily by consumption of contaminated foods, particularly inadequately cooked pork.[142] Contaminated water sources, direct fecal-oral transmission, and transfusion related transmission have also been documented.[142]

The incubation period for yersiniosis is 1 to 10 days.[51,141,142] The clinical presentation is variable but usually includes abdominal pain, fever, and diarrhea (which may be frankly bloody). Symptoms typically persist for 1 to 3 weeks. Diagnosis by culture requires specific techniques; serologic testing can also be performed. Because of involvement of the lymphatic system, tonsillitis and mesenteric adenitis may be present.[51] The illness can cause right-lower quadrant pain, mimicking inflammatory bowel disease, and acute appendicitis.[51,141] In a 1999 study from Tripoli, analysis of 70 cases of acute appendicitis revealed bacteria in 25 specimens; 11 of 25 (44%), contained *Y enterocolitica*.[143] Postinfection sequelae may include erythema nodosum, erythema multiforme, and reactive polyarthritis.[88,142]

*Listeria monocytogenes* are very hardy, gram-positive, flagellated bacteria that are found in soil, silage, and a multitude of animals. They have been found in 1% to 10% of asymptomatic persons.[144] According to CDC estimates, approximately 1600 persons in the United States develop listeriosis each year.[145] Following an incubation period of approximately 24 hours, a self-limited, febrile gastroenteritis lasting about 2 days may occur in healthy, nonpregnant adults.[146] In the elderly or immunocompromised patient, systemic illness may prove fatal.[147] Patients with AIDS are nearly 300 times more likely to develop listeriosis than the general population.[145] Listeriosis in pregnancy can lead to placental invasion with resultant miscarriage or stillbirth.[147,148]

Acquisition of *L monocytogenes* has been traced to a variety of foods, especially unpasteurized dairy products, raw fruits and vegetables, and raw or undercooked meats and poultry.[144] Because of this, pregnant women are advised to avoid soft cheeses, cold luncheon and deli meats, and cold-smoked seafood.[148] In low-risk individuals, no specific therapy is necessary. Pregnant women or immunocompromised patients should be treated with ampicillin or trimethoprim-sulfamethoxazole.[146]

## PROTOZOA

Several parasites are important causes of diarrhea. These illnesses are often characterized by insidious onset and persistence of symptoms.

*Entamoeba histolytica* is an extremely common pathogen in tropical countries in which poverty is prevalent. In North America, amebiasis is most frequently seen among institutionalized persons, men who have sex with men, and immigrants or travelers returning from endemic countries.[149] Multiple strains of amoebae may colonize the human gastrointestinal tract; however, most have not been linked to pathology.

The life cycle of *E histolytica* begins with ingestion of hardy, infective cysts, usually in contaminated food or water. Although approximately 80% to 90% of colonized persons may be asymptomatic,[51,150,151] some individuals develop illness 2 to 4 weeks after exposure. In the small bowel, excystation occurs; the resultant trophozoites may invade the colonic mucosa causing significant inflammation. Mild diarrhea may be followed by the development of frank dysentery accompanied by low-grade fever, abdominal cramping, and anemia. In cases of severe pancolitis, symptoms can mimic inflammatory bowel disease. Following mucosal invasion, the trophozoites can travel systemically via the bloodstream. Amebic liver abscess formation is a well-known entity.

As cysts are shed only intermittently, examination of three separate stool specimens should be ordered if the diagnosis of amebic dysentery is being considered. Because of inability to distinguish pathogenic from nonpathogenic species of *Entamoeba* cysts on stool examination, confirmation by other techniques such as ELISA are advised.[152]

Treatment recommendations for asymptomatic colonization include iodoquinol or paromomycin. Persons with symptomatic infection should receive metronidazole or tinidazole, followed by iodoquinol or paromomycin.[150] A 2009 Cochrane Review concluded that tinidazole appeared more effective and caused fewer adverse side effects than metronidazole when treating amebic colitis.[153]

*Giardia lamblia* is a pathologic intestinal flagellate that has worldwide distribution. It is the most common protozoan pathogen in the United States[51] and is frequently detected in children at daycare centers, international travelers, and men who have sex with men. In the United States, more than 19,000 cases were reported each year from 2006 through 2008.[154] Peak incidence was between the ages of 1 and 9 years of age.[154]

*G lamblia* reside in several mammals as well as humans. Very hardy cysts are passed in the stool. They are then ingested via contaminated food or water, or direct fecal-oral contact. The trophozoites are released in the upper gut where they multiply and attach to the intestinal epithelium. Although about half of colonized persons remain asymptomatic,[51] many persons become ill 2 to 4 weeks after ingestion of the organisms.[150] Patients may experience diarrhea with steatorrhea, abdominal pain and cramping, flatulence, and nausea and vomiting. Treatment options include tinidazole, metronidazole, paromomycin, nitazoxanide, furazolidone, and quinicrine.[150] The treatment of choice is based on clinical cure rates and side effect profile in a Cochrane Review article from 2007.[155] Without treatment, symptoms usually resolve within a month. However, postinfection irritable bowel symptoms have been reported in a significant number of patients.[156]

*Cryptosporidium* annually infects approximately 300,000 persons in the United States.[157] The two species most commonly found as pathogens for humans are *C parvum* and *C hominis*. The organism has worldwide distribution and infects a variety of mammalian hosts. It has become particularly problematic among HIV-infected individuals. Although cryptosporidiosis is often associated with waterborne illness,[158,159] infection may also be traced to contaminated food or person-to-person contact.

Following ingestion of thick-walled, chlorine-resistant oocysts, *Cryptosporidium* reproduction occurs in the intestine through both sexual and asexual cycles. Infection may be asymptomatic but often leads to abdominal cramping, malaise, and watery diarrhea. Systemic manifestations occasionally occur. Definitive diagnosis is made by direct fluorescent antibody or PCR techniques.[160] Treatment with a 3-day course of nitazoxanide is usually recommended; however, its efficacy in immunosuppressed patients has not been proven.[51,152] In cryptosporidiosis AIDS patients, effective treatment with antiretroviral therapy is key to decreasing or resolving symptoms. To prevent transmission, persons who have been infected with *Cryptosporidium* should not swim for at least 2 weeks after cessation of diarrhea.[161]

### Other Protozoan Infections

Two other organisms, *Cyclospora cayetanensis* and *Cystoisospora belli* (previously known as *Isospora belli*),[162] also occasionally cause diarrheal disease in North America. Both organisms cause watery diarrhea, occur more frequently in tropical or subtropical regions, and are treated primarily with trimethoprim-sulfamethoxazole.[163,164]

## FUNGI AND/OR PROTOZOA

Microsporidia, a huge group of obligate intracellular parasites, are currently classified as fungi and/or protozoa. They have recently been recognized as human pathogens, particularly in immunocompromised persons.[51,165,166] It has been estimated that the organism causes infection in approximately 15% of AIDS patients.[167] In humans, the most common manifestation is diarrhea, which can become chronic. Ocular manifestations can also occur. Because the organisms are ubiquitous, transmission can occur by a variety of routes.[51] Diagnosis of microsporidia infection previously was dependent upon light or electron microscopy; however, recent advances in molecular diagnostic procedures are simplifying the process.[168] Currently, albendazole is recommended for treatment for most *Enterocytozoon* species[167]; however, fumagillin is used for treatment of *E bieneusi*.[169]

## SUMMARY

Infectious diarrhea is a condition that every clinician encounters. In resource-rich countries, most cases are mild, respond well to hydration, and resolve without sequelae. The offending pathogen is frequently unidentified. The increasing globalization of society requires familiarization with illnesses not endemic to North America. Diagnostic evaluation should be conducted in severely ill patients, those with high risk comorbidities, or those with prolonged or complicated illness. In outbreaks of diarrheal illness, identification of pathogens should be pursued for epidemiologic purposes. Examination of stool for fecal leukocytes is usually helpful in determining whether the infection is due to an invasive or toxin-producing organism. A series of three stools should be examined for ova and parasites before excluding the possibility of a protozoan infection.

Assessment of hydration status and administration of fluids is the cornerstone of therapy in treatment of diarrhea. If it is impossible to achieve adequate oral rehydration, intravenous, intraosseous, or hypodermoclysis routes may be used. Empiric antibiotic or antihelmintic therapy may be instituted at times, particularly when dealing with travelers' diarrhea.

Prevention of infectious diarrhea is a multifaceted, challenging task. Key components include provision of safe food and water supplies, good hygiene principles, optimal nutritional status, treatment of comorbid conditions, and development and appropriate use of vaccines.

## REFERENCES

1. Guandalini S, Frye RE, Tamer MA. Diarrhea. eMedicine 2010:1–31. Available at: http://emedicine.medscape.com/article/928598-print. Accessed October 29, 2010.
2. Greenberger NJ, Blumberg RS, Burakoff R. Current diagnosis and treatment gastroenterology, hepatology, and endoscopy. New York: McGraw-Hill Medical; 2009.
3. Lever DS, Soffer E. Acute diarrhea. 2010. Available at: http://www.clevelandclinicmeded.com/medicalpubs/diseasemanagement/gastroenterology. Accessed October 29, 2010.
4. World Health Organization. Diarrhoeal disease. 2009. Available at: http://www.who.int/mediacentre/factsheets/fs330/en/index.html. Accessed October 23, 2010.
5. Farthing M, Lindberg G, Dite P, et al. World gastroenterology organisation practice guideline: acute diarrhea. 2008. Available at: http://www.worldgastroenterology.org/assets/downloads/en/pdf/guidelines/01_acute_diarrhea.pd. Accessed October 24, 2010.

6. Gianella RA. Infectious enteritis and proctocolitis and bacterial food poisoning. In: Feldman M, Friedman LS, Brandt LJ, editors. Gastrointestinal and liver disease, vol. 2. 8th edition. Philadelphia: Saunders; 2006. p. 2333–91.

7. Wilkins TD, Lyerly DM. Clostridium difficile testing: after 20 years, still challenging. J Clin Microbiol 2003;41(2):531–4.

8. Carroll KC. Ushers in changes to *Clostridium difficile* testing, vol. 2010. Baltimore (MD): Johns Hopkins Pathology Blogs Index; 2010. Available at: http://apps. pathology.jhu.edu/blogs/pathology/2010-ushers-in-changes-to-clostridium-difficile-testing. Accessed May 23, 2011.

9. Ltd. BD. Rotavirus rapid test stick immunochromatographic rapid test strip for qualitative detection of rotavirus antigen in feces. 2008. Available at: http://www. docstoc.com/docs/63467149/Rotavirus-Rapid-Test-Stick. Accessed October 31, 2010.

10. Meridian Bioscience I. Immunocard STAT! Rotavirus. 2010. Available at: http:// www.meridianbioscience.com/diagnostic-products/rotovirus-and-adenovirus/ immunocard/immunocard. Accessed October 31, 2010.

11. Bhuiyan NA, Qadri F, Faruque AS, et al. Use of dipsticks for rapid diagnosis of cholera caused by *Vibrio cholerae* O1 and O139 from rectal swabs. J Clin Microbiol 2003;41(8):3939–41.

12. King CK, Glass R, Bresee JS, et al. Managing acute gastroenteritis among children: oral rehydration, maintenance, and nutritional therapy. MMWR Recommendations and Reports: Morbidity and Mortality Weekly Report. Recommendations and Reports/Centers for Disease Control, 52. 2003. Available at: http://www.cdc.gov/mmwr/pdf/rr/rr5216.pdf. Accessed May 23, 2011.

13. Weinberg N, Weinberg M, Maloney S. Traveling safely with infants and children. Atlanta (GA): Yellow Book; 2010. Available at: cdc.gov. Accessed May 23, 2011.

14. World Health Organization. Oral rehydration salts: production of the new ORS. Geneva: World Health Organization; 2006. Available at: http://www.who.int/ child_adolescent_health/en/. Accessed May 23, 2011.

15. Nalin DR, Hirschhorn N, Greenough W 3rd, et al. Clinical concerns about reduced-osmolarity oral rehydration solution. JAMA 2004;291(21):2632–5.

16. Children AHTAfTHfS. Diarrhea: formula-fed infants. Available at: http://partners. aboutkidshealth.ca/HealthAZ/Elimination-Gallery.aspx?articleID=&categoryID= AZ2f. Accessed October 24, 2010.

17. Brown S. Electrolyte replacement drink—Pedialyte alternative. About.com: toddlers. Available at: http://babyparenting.about.com/od/recipesandcooking/ r/electrolytedrnk.htm. Accessed October 24, 2010.

18. Rib DZ. How to make Pedialyte. How to do just about everything! How to videos & articles. Available at: http://www.ehow.com/how_5735256_make-pedialyte-_ homemade-electrolite-solution_.html. Accessed January 30, 2011.

19. Hartling L, Bellemare S, Wiebe N. Oral versus intravenous rehydration for treating dehydration due to gastroenteritis in children. Evid Based Child Health 2007; 2(1):163–218.

20. Roberts KB. Oral rehydration. Whitehouse Station (NJ): Merck Sharpe and Dohme Corp; 2007. Available at: http://www.merckmanuals.com/professional/ sec19/ch276c.html. Accessed January 30, 2011.

21. Barua P, Bhowmick BK. Hypodermoclysis—a victim of historical prejudice. Age Ageing 2005;34:215–7.

22. Committee CP. Hypodermoclysis (HDC) Administration Protocol for Palliative Care Patients. Alberta (CA): Alberta Health Services Covenant Health Seniors

Health Regional Palliative Care Program; 2005. p. 1–7. Available at: http://www.palliative.org/PC/ClinicalInfo/Clinical%20Practice%20Guidelines/ClinicalPractice GuidelinesIDX.html. Accessed May 23, 2011.

23. Moses S. Hypodermoclysis: family practice notebook. 2010. Available at: http://www.fpnotebook.com/er/procedure/Hypdrmclys.htm.

24. Duro D, Duggan C. The BRAT diet for acute diarrhea in children: should it be used? Pract Gastroenterol 2007;60:65–8.

25. Dupont H. The Practice Parameters Committee of the American College of Gastroenterology. Guidelines on infectious diarrhea in adults. Am J Gastroenterol 1997;92(11):1962–75.

26. Grimwood K, Forbes D. Acute and persistent diarrhea. Pediatr Clin North Am 2009;56:1343–61.

27. Expert Committee on the Selection and Use of Essential Medicines. Application for the inclusion of zinc sulfate in the WHO model list of essential medicines. Expert Committee on the Selection and Use of Essential Medicines. Geneva (Switzerland): World Health Organization Child and Adolescent Health Division Johns Hopkins Bloomberg School of Public Health USAID UNICEF; 2005. p. 1–16.

28. Program MTUM. Diarrhoea treatment guidelines for clinic-based healthcare workers including new recommendations for the use of ORS and zinc supplementation Not yet field-tested. In: USAID, Organization WH, UNICEF, et al, editors. Arlington (VA): World Health Organization; 2005.

29. The Center for Sustainable Development. Zinc & Vitamin A: mitigating diarrhea in children. 2008–2011. Available at: http://www.csdi-i.org/zinc-vitamin-a-mitigating-dia/. Accessed February 1, 2011.

30. Can one pill tame the illness no one wants to talk about? TIME Inc. 2009. Available at: http://www.time.com/time/printout/0,00.html,8816,1914655.

31. INCLEN Childnet Zinc Effectiveness for Diarrhea (IC-ZED) Group. Zinc supplementation in acute diarrhea is acceptable, does not interfere with oral rehydration, and reduces the use of other medications: a randomized trial in five countries. J Pediatr Gastroenterol Nutr 2006;42(3):300–5.

32. Bhutta ZA, Bird SM, Black RE, et al, The Zinc Investigators' Collaborative Group. Therapeutic effects of oral zinc in acute and persistent diarrhea in children in developing countries: pooled analysis of randomized controlled trials. Am J Clin Nutr 2000;72:1516–22, October 24, 2010.

33. Baum MK, Shenghan L, Sales S, et al. Randomized, controlled clinical trial of zinc supplementation to prevent immunological failure in HIV-infected adults. Clin Infect Dis 2010;50(12):1653–60, February 2, 2011.

34. Scrimgeour A. Zinc supplements delayed immune failure, decreased diarrhea in adults with HIV. infectiousdiseasenews.com. 2010. Available at: http://www.infectiousdiseasenews.com/print.aspx?id=64976. Accessed February 1, 2011.

35. Bovill ME, Polhemus ME, Otieno L, et al. Zinc supplementation to reduce diarrhea rates in adults in Western Kenya. Natick (MA): United States Army Research Institute of Environmental Medicined; 2010.

36. Scrimgeour A, Lukaski HC, Polhemus ME, et al. Effect of zinc supplementation on diarrhea and malaria morbidity in adults in rural Kenya. US Army MRMC; 2010.

37. Lukacik M, Thomas RL, Aranda JV. A meta-analysis of the effects of oral zinc in the treatment of acute and persistent diarrhea. Pediatrics 2008;121(2):326–36.

38. Baldi F, Bianco MA, Nardone G, et al. Focus on acute diarrhoeal disease. World J Gastroenterol 2009;15(27):3341–8. Available at: www.wjgnet.com. Accessed October 31, 2011.

39. De Bruyn G. Diarrhea in adults (Acute) Clinical Evidence Concise A publication of BMJ Publishing Group. Am Fam Physician 2008;78(4):503–4.

40. Epocrates Online. Bismuth subsalicylate. San Mateo (CA): Epocrates online; 2011. Available at: https://online.epocrates.com/noFrame/showPage. do?method=drugs&MonographId=1820&ActiveSectionId=10. Accessed May 23, 2011.

41. Adis International Limited. Racecadotril: an antidiarrhoeal suitable for use in infants and young children. Drugs Ther Perspect 2001;17(8):1–5. Available at: www.scribd.com/doc/12190481/Racecadotril.

42. Matheson AJ, Noble S. Racecadotril. Drugs 2000;59(4):829–35.

43. Lecomte JM. An overview of clinical studies with racecadotril in adults. Int J Antimicrob Agents 2000;14(1):81–7.

44. Szymanski H, Pejcz J, Jawien M, et al. Treatment of acute infectious diarrhoea in infants and children with a mixture of three Lactobacillus rhamnosus strains– a randomized, double-blind, placebo-controlled trial. Aliment Pharmacol Ther 2006;23(2):247–53.

45. Allen SJ, Okoko B, Martinez EG, et al. Review: probiotics reduced diarrhoea at 3 days in children and adults with proven or presumed infectious diarrhoea. Evid Based Nurs 2004;7(4):107.

46. Prebiotics ISAfPa. Clarification of the definition of a probiotic. 2009. Available at: www.isapp.net. Accessed January 31, 2011.

47. Fang SB, Lee HC, Hu JJ, et al. Dose-dependent effect of *Lactobacillus rhamnosus* on quantitative reduction of faecal rotavirus shedding in children. J Trop Pediatr 2009;55(5):297–301.

48. McFarland L. Meta-analysis of probiotics for the prevention of antibiotic associated diarrhea and the treatment of *Clostridium difficile* disease. Am J Gastroenterol 2006;101(4):812–22.

49. Prevention CfDCa. Travelers' diarrhea. In: Services DoHaH, editor. Atlanta (GA). Available at: cdc.gov. 2006.

50. Shah N, Dupont H, Ramsey D. Global etiology of travelers' diarrhea: systematic review from 1973 to the present. Am J Trop Med Hyg 2009;804(4):609–14.

51. Trier JS. Acute diarrheal disorders. In: Greenberger NJ, Blumberg RS, Burakoff R, editors. Current diagnosis and treatment gastroenterology, hepatology, and endoscopy. New York: McGraw-Hill Medical; 2009. p. 45–63.

52. Steffen R. Epidemiology of Traveler's Diarrhea. Clin Infect Dis 2005;41(Suppl 8): S536–40.

53. Diemart D. Prevention and self-treatment of traveler's diarrhea. Clin Microbiol Rev 2006;19(3):583–94.

54. Shlim D. Looking for evidence that personal hygiene precautions prevent traveler's diarrhea. Clin Infect Dis 2005;41(Suppl 8):S531–5.

55. Organization WH. Diarrhoeal diseases (Updated February 2009). Geneva: World Health Organization; 2009.

56. Centers for Disease, Control and Prevention. Rotavirus: clinical disease information. In: Centers for Disease, Control and Prevention; 2011. Available at: http://www.cdc.gov/rotavirus/clinical.html. Accessed May 23, 2011.

57. Payne D, Stockman L, Gentsch J, et al. Rotavirus. manual for the surveillance of vaccine-preventable diseases. Chapter 13. 4th edition. Atlanta (GA): CDC; 2008.

58. Parashar U, Hummelman E, Bresee J, et al. Global illness and deaths caused by rotavirus disease in children. Emerg Infect Dis 2003;9(5):565–72.

59. Anderson E, Weber S. Rotavirus infection in adults. Lancet Infect Dis 2004;4: 91–9.

60. Kramer A, Schwebke I, Kampf G. How long do nosocomial pathogens persist on inanimate surfaces? A systematic review. BMC Infect Dis 2006;6:130.

61. DynaMed. Rotavirus gastroenteritis. DynaMed summary. 2011. Available at: http://0-dynaweb.ebscohost.com.carlson.edu/Detail?id=AN+114180&sid=901534. Accessed February 20, 2011.

62. Clash K. Rotavirus. Johns-Hopkins Medicine. Available at: http://www.hopkinsmedicine.org/heic/ID/rotavirus/. Accessed May 23, 2011.

63. Soares-Weiser K, MacLehose H, Ben-Aharon I, et al. Vaccines for preventing rotavirus diarrhoea: vaccines in use. Cochrane Database Syst Rev 2010;5: CD008521.

64. Centers for Disease, Control and Prevention. Statement regarding rotarix and rotateq rotavirus vaccines and intussusception. In: Immunizations Va, editor. Department of Health and Human Services; 2010. Available at: http://www.cdc.gov/vaccines/vpd-vac/rotavirus/intussusception-studies-acip.htm. Accessed May 23, 2011.

65. Cortese M. Estimates of benefits and potential risks of rotavirus vaccination in the United States. Presented at ACIP Meeting. Atlanta, October 28, 2010.

66. Chilton L. Rotavirus vaccine—new information. Presented at ACIP Meeting. Atlanta, October 28, 2010.

67. Richardson V, Hernandez-Pichardo J, Quintanar-Solares M, et al. Effect of rotavirus vaccination on death from childhood diarrhea in Mexico. N Engl J Med 2010;362:299–305.

68. Prevention CfDCa. Reduction in rotavirus after vaccine introduction—United States, 2000–2009. In: Services DoHaH, editor. vol. 58. Atlanta (GA); 2009. p. 1146–9. Available at: USA.gov.

69. Centers for Disease, Control and Prevention. Diseases DoV. Norovirus: technical fact sheet. In: Services DoHaH, editor. National Center for Immunization and Respiratory. Atlanta (GA): CDC; 2010. p. 1–6. Available at: http://www.cdc.gov/ncidod/dvrd/revb/gastro/norovirus-factsheet.htm. Accessed May 23, 2011.

70. Marks P, Vipond I, Regan F, et al. A school outbreak of Norwalk-like virus: evidence for airborne transmission. Epidemiol Infect 2003;131(1):727–36.

71. Administration FUSFaD. FDA, CDC, and states investigating norovirus illnesses linked to oysters consumers advised to avoid oysters harvested from San Antonio Bay. U.S. Food and Drug Administration; 2009.

72. Flynn D. Norovirus linked to oysters in British Columbia. 2010. Available at: http://www.foodsafetynews.com/2010/10/bout-of-bad-oysters-in-bč/. Accessed May 23, 2011.

73. Westrell T, Dusch V, Ethelberg S, et al. Norovirus outbreaks linked to oyster consumption in the United Kingdom, Norway, France, Sweden and Denmark, 2010. Euro Surveill 2010;15(12). pii: 19524. Available at: http://www.eurosurveillance.org/ViewArticle.aspx?ArticleId=19524. Accessed May 23, 2011.

74. Le Guyader F, Parnaudeau S, Schaeffer J, et al. Detection and quantification of noroviruses in shellfish. Appl Environ Microbiol 2009;75(3):618–24.

75. Uhnoo I, Wadell G, Svensson L, et al. Importance of enteric adenoviruses 40 and 41 in acute gastroenteritis in infants and young children. J Clin Microbiol 1984;20(3):365–72.

76. Herrmann J, Blacklow N, Perron-Henry D, et al. Incidence of enteric adenoviruses among children in Thailand and the significance of these viruses in gastroenteritis. J Clin Microbiol 1988;26(9):1783–6.

77. de Jong J. III, 2. Epidemiology of enteric adenoviruses 40 and 41 and other adenoviruses in immunocompetent and immunodeficient individuals. Perspect Med Virol 2003;9:407–45.

78. Gompf S, Kelkar D, Oehler R. Adenoviruses. eMedicine 2010. Available at: http://emedicine.medscape.com/article/211738-print. Accessed October 24, 2010.

79. Johhansson P, Bergentoft K, Larsson P, et al. A nosocomial sapovirus-associated outbreak of gastroenteritis in adults. Scand J Infect Dis 2005;37(3):200–4.

80. Logan C, O'Sullivan N. Detection of viral agents of gastroenteritis: norovirus, sapovirus and astrovirus. Future Virology 2008;3(1):61–70. Available at: www.futuremedicine.com.

81. Stehulak N. Staphylococcus aureus a most common cause. In: Family and Consumer Sciences, editor. Columbus (OH): Ohio State University Extension Fact Sheet, US Department of Agriculture. Available at: http://ohioline.osu.edu/hyg-fact/5000/5564.html. Accessed May 23, 2011.

82. Le Loir Y, Baron F, Gautier M. *Staphylococcus aureus* and food poisoning. Genet Mol Res 2003;2(1):63–76.

83. Schmid D, Gschiedl E, Mann M, et al. Outbreak of acute gastroenteritis in an Austrian boarding school, September 2006. Euro Surveill 2007;12(3):224.

84. La Chapelle N, Joy E, Halverson C. A gastroenteritis outbreak of *Staphylococcus aureus*, Type 29. Am J Public Health Nations Health 1966;56(1):94–6.

85. Todar K. Textbook of Bacteriology 2011. Available at: http://www.textbookofbacteriology.net/B.cereus.html. Accessed February 26, 2011.

86. Section LOoPH-IDE. Bacillus cereus toxi-infection. In: Section IDE, Office of Public Health LDoHH, editors. 2004. Available at: http://www.dhh.louisiana.gov/offices/miscdocs/docs-249/Manual/BacillusCereusManual.pdf. Accessed May 23, 2011.

87. Administration FUSFaD. Bacillus cereus and other Bacillus spp. Bad Bug book: foodborne pathogenic microorganisms and natural toxins handbook: FDA U.S. Food and Drug Administration. Available at: http://www.fda.gov/food/foodsafety/foodborneillness/foodborneillnessfoodbornepathogensnaturaltoxins/badbugbook/ucm070492.htm. Accessed May 04, 2009.

88. Gianella RA. Infectious *Enteritis* and proctocolitis and bacterial food poisoning. In: Feldman M, Friedman L, Brandt L, editors. Sleisenger & Fordtran's Gastrointestinal and liver disease, vol. 2. Philadelphia: Saunders; 2006. p. 2333–91.

89. Adminstration FUSFaD. Clostridium perfringens. Bad bug book: foodborne pathogenic microorganisms and natural toxins handbook: FDA US Food and Drug Administration; 2006.

90. Prevention CfDCa. Frequently Asked Questions about *Clostridium difficile* for Healthcare Providers. In: Diseases NCfEaZI, editor. 2011. Available at: cdc.gov.

91. Kelly C, Lamont J. Antibiotic-associated diarrhea, pseudomembranous enterocolitis, and *Clostridium difficile*-associated diarrhea and colitis. In: Feldman MF, Brandt LJ, editors. Sleisenger and Fordtran's Gastrointestinal and liver disease pathophysiology/diagnosis/management, vol. 2. 8th edition. Philadelphia: Saunders; 2006. p. 2393–412.

92. 2010 ushers in changes to *Clostridium difficile* testing, vol. Index JHPB; 2010. Available at: http://apps.pathology.jhu.edu/blogs/pathology/2010-ushers-in-changes-to-clostridium-difficile-testing. Accessed May 23, 2011.

93. O'Reilly K. Preventive measures shown to cut hospital C.*diff* rates. 2010 amednews.com. Available at: http://www.ama-assn.org/amednews/2010/11/01/prsb1101.htm. Accessed November 15, 2010.

94. Organization WH. Cholera 2009. 2010;85(31):293–308. Available at: http://www. who.int/wer/2010/wer8531.pdf. Accessed October 31, 2010.

95. Pan American Health Organization. Cholera and post-earthquake response in Haiti. In: Bulletin HC, editor. Health Cluster Bulletin. World Health Organization; 2011. Available at: http://reliefweb.int/sites/reliefweb.int/files/resources/Full_Report_209. pdf. Accessed May 23, 2011.

96. Adminstration FUSFaD. Foodborne pathogenic microorganisms and natural toxins handbook vibrio cholerae serogroup 01. Bad bug book. U.S. Food and Drug Adminstration; 2010.

97. Handa S. Cholera. 2010:1–22. Available at: http://emedicine.medscape.com/ article/214911-print. Accessed February 19, 2011.

98. Graves PM, Deeks JJ, Demicheli V, et al. Vaccines for preventing cholera: killed whole cell or other subunit vaccines (injected). Cochrane Database Syst Rev 2010;8:CD000974.

99. Organization WH. Cholera. Fact sheet. 2010(N° 107). Available at: http://www. who.int/mediacentre/factsheets/fs107/en/print.html.

100. International Vaccine Institute. Oral Cholera vaccine: first licensed vaccine developed with Gates Foundation support. Available at: http://www.ivi.org/. Accessed May 23, 2011.

101. Sur D, Lopez AL, Kanungo S, et al. Efficacy and safety of a modified killed-whole-cell oral cholera vaccine in India: an interim analysis of a cluster rando-mised, double-blind, placebo-controlled trial. Lancet 2009;374(9702):1694–702.

102. Cyranoski D. Cholera vaccine splits experts. Opinion is divided over how to tackle the disease in Haiti. Nature 2011;469:273–4.

103. Diseases NCfI. *Campylobacter jejuni*. In: Services DoHaH, editor. Atlanta (GA): Centers for Disease Control and Prevention; 2010. Available at: http://www.cdc. gov/nczved/divisions/dfbmd/diseases/campylobacter/. Accessed May 23, 2011.

104. Administration FUSFaD. *Campylobacter jejuni*. Bad bug book: foodborne path-ogenic microorganisms and natural toxins handbook. U.S. Food & Drug Admin-istration; 2009.

105. Viray M, Lynch M. Other infectious diseases related to travel. 2010 Yellow Book. Atlanta (GA): Centers for Disease Control and Prevention; 2010.

106. Division of Foodborne B, and Mycotic Diseases, National Center for Zoonotic, Vector-Borne, and Enteric Diseases. *Campylobacter*. In: Centers for Disease, Control and Prevention, editor. Atlanta (GA): Centers for Disease Control and Prevention; 2010. p. 1–4. Available at: http://www.cdc.gov/nczved/divisions/ dfbmd/diseases/campylobacter/. Accessed May 23, 2011.

107. Nelson J, Chiller T, Powers J, et al. Fluoroquinolone-resistant *Campylobacter* species and the withdrawal of fluoroquinolones from use in poultry: a public health success story. Clin Infect Dis 2007;44:977–80.

108. Medicine A. *Campylobacter* infection. The McGraw-Hill Companies; 2010. Avail-able at: http://0-www.accessmedicine.com.carlson.utoledo.edu/popup.aspx? aID53411366&;print5. Accessed October 30, 2010.

109. EHA Consulting Group I. Why is the finding of generic E. coli in ready-to-eat food a red flag? Baltimore (MD): EHA Consulting Group, Inc. Environmental & Public Health Consultants Since 1980; 2010. Available at: http://blog.ehagroup.com/ blog/2008/11/why-is-the-finding-of-generic-e-coli-in-ready-to-eat-food-a-red-flag.html#more. Accessed May 23, 2011.

110. Nataro J, Steiner T, Guerrant R. Enteroaggregative *Escherichia coli*. Emerg Infect Dis 1998;4(2):251–61.

111. Administration FUSFaD. Escherichia coli 0157:H7 (EHEC). Bad bug book: FDA U.S. Silver Spring (MD): Food and Drug Administration; 2009. Available at: http://www.fda.gov/Food/FoodSafety/FoodborneIllness/FoodborneIllnessFoodborne PathogensNaturalToxins/BadBugBook/ucm071240.htm. Accessed May 23, 2011.

112. Prevention CfDCa. *Escherichia coli* 0157:H7 infections in children associated with raw milk and raw colostrum from cows—California, 2006. MMWR Morb Mortal Wkly Rep 2008;57(23):625–8.

113. Administration FUSFaD. FDA Statement on foodborne *E. coli* 0157: H7 outbreak in spinach. In: Administration FUSFaD, editor. 2006. Available at: www.fda.gov.

114. Lukassowitz I. Meat from wild-living animals underestimated as source of EHEC infections. In: BfR, editor. Berlin: BfR; 2007. p. 1–2.

115. Service AD. Enterohemorrhagic *E. coli*, Including *E. coli* 0157:H7 and *E. coli* 0111. In: Health OSDo, editor. 2008. Available at: http://www.ok.gov/health/documents/E.%20Coli.2008.pdf. Accessed May 23, 2011.

116. Organization WH. Enterohaemorrhagic *Escherichia coli* (EHEC). Geneva: WHO; 2005.

117. Administration FUSFaD. Enteropathogenic *Escherichia coli*. Bad bug book: foodborne pathogenic microorganisms and natural toxins handbook. 2009. Available at: www.fda.gov.

118. Trabulsi L, Keller R, Tardelli Gomes T. Typical and atypical enteropathogenic *Escherichia coli*. Emerg Infect Dis 2002;8(5):508–13.

119. Prevention CfDCa. Enterotoxigenic *Escherichia coli* (ETEC). In: Services DoHaH, editor. Atlanta (GA); 2005. Available at: cdc.gov.

120. (NIAID) NIoAaID. Phase I Study of ETEC Vaccine. In: Diseases NIoAaI, editor. NIAID; 2011. Available at: http://clinicaltrials.gov/ct2/show/NCT01147445. Accessed May 23, 2011.

121. Marathon Medical Communications I. Navy Medical Researchers Tackle ETEC Vaccine. 2011. usmedicine.com. Available at: http://www.usmedicine.com/infectiousdisease/navy-medical-researchers-tackle-etec-vaccine.html. Accessed March 13, 2011.

122. Health S-PA. The control of Salmonella infections in humans. The Netherlands: Schering-Plough Animal Health; 2008. Available at: http://www.merck-animal-health.com/news-media/news-archive.aspx. Accessed May 23, 2011.

123. Prevention CfDCa. Salmonellosis. In: Prevention CfDCa, editor. Atlanta (GA): 2009. Available at: cdc.gov.

124. Prevention CfDCa. Investigation update: multistate outbreak of human *Salmonella enteritidis* infections associated with shell eggs. In: Services DoHaH, editor. Atlanta (GA): 2010. Available at: cdc.gov.

125. Prevention CfDCa. Multistate outbreaks of *Salmonella* infections associated with live poultry—United States, 2007. MMWR Morb Mortal Wkly Rep 2009;58(2):25–9.

126. Prevention CfDCa. Multistate outbreak of human *Salmonella* typhimurium infections associated with pet turtle exposure—United States, 2008. MMWR Morb Mortal Wkly Rep 2010;59(7):191–6.

127. 21 CoFRT. Turtles intrastate and interstate requirements. In: Adminstration FaD, Services DoHaH, editors. vol. 8. 2010. Available at: www.fda.gov.

128. Administration FUSFaD. Salmonella spp. Bad bug book. Available at: www.fda.gov.

129. Wilson I, Whitehead E. Long-term post-Salmonella reactive arthritis due to Salmonella Blockley. Jpn J Infect Dis 2004;57(5):210–1.

130. Paul I, Mitchell ES, Bell A. Salmonella reactive arthritis in established ankylosing spondylitis. Ulster Med J 1988;57(2):215–7.

131. Leirisalo-Repo M, Helenius P, Hannu T, et al. Long-term prognosis of reactive salmonella arthritis. Ann Rheum Dis 1997;56:516–20.
132. Dworkin M, Shoemaker P, Goldoft M, et al. Reactive arthritis and Reiter's syndrome following an outbreak of gastroenteritis caused by *Salmonella enteritidis*. Clin Infect Dis 2001;33:1010–4.
133. Prevention CfDCa. Investigation update: multistate outbreak of human typhoid fever infections associated with frozen mamey fruit pulp. In: Services DoHaH, editor. Atlanta (GA): Centers for Disease Control and Prevention; 2010. Available at: http://www.cdc.gov/salmonella/typhoidfever/index.html. Accessed August 20, 2010.
134. Mintz E. Typhoid and paratyphoid fever. Yellow book. Atlanta (GA): 2010. Available at: cdc.gov.
135. National Center for Zoonotic, Vector-Borne, Enteric Diseases. Typhoid fever. In: National Center for Zoonotic, Vector-Borne, Enteric Diseases, editors. Division of foodborne b, and mycotic diseases. CDC; 2010. Available at: http://www.cdc. gov/nczved/divisions/dfbmd/diseases/typhoid_fever/. Accessed October 5, 2010.
136. Sureshbabu J, Venugopalan P, Abuhammour W. *Shigella* infection. emedicine 2010. Available at: http://emedicine.medscape.com/article/968773-print. Accessed October 24, 2010.
137. Prevention CfDCa. Shigellosis. Atlanta (GA): 2009. Available at: cdc.gov.
138. Mintz E, Schilling K. Shigellosis. Atlanta (GA): Yellow Book; 2010. Available at: cdc.gov. 2010.
139. Bardhan P, Faruque A, Naheed A, et al. Decreasing shigellosis-related-deaths without *Shigella* spp.-specific interventions, Asia. Emerg Infect Dis 2010; 16(11):1718–23.
140. Prince C, David K, John S. Antibiotic therapy for *Shigella* dysentery. Cochrane Database Syst Rev 2010;8:CD006784.
141. Administration FUSFaD. *Yersinia enterocolitica* (and *Yersinia pseudotuberculosis*). Bad bug book: foodborne pathogenic microorganisms and natural toxins handbook. Available at: http://www.fda.gov/Food/FoodSafety/FoodborneIllness/ FoodborneIllnessFoodbornePathogensNaturalToxins/BadBugBook/ucm070064. htm. Accessed June 18, 2009.
142. Prevention CfDCa. *Yersinia enterocolitica*. In: Services DoHaH, editor. Atlanta (GA): 2005. Available at: cdc.gov.
143. El-Sherbini M, Al-Agili S, El-Jali H, et al. Isolation of *Yersinia enterocolitica* from cases of acute appendicitis and ice-cream. East Mediterr Health J 1999;5(1):130–5.
144. Administration FUSFaD. *Listeria monocytogenes*. Bad bug book: foodborne pathogenic microorganisms and natural toxins handbook. U.S. Food and Drug Administration; 2009.
145. Prevention CfDCa. Listeriosis. In: Prevention CfDCa, editor. Atlanta (GA): 2011. Available at: cdc.gov.
146. Ooi S, Lorber B. Gastroenteritis due to *Listeria monocytogenes*. Clin Infect Dis 2005;40:1327–32.
147. Centers for Disease Control and Prevention (CDC). Outbreak of *Listeria monocytogenes* infections associated with pasteurized milk from a local dairy— Massachusetts, 2007. MMWR Morb Mortal Wkly Rep 2008;57(40):1097–100.
148. Prevention CfDCa. Listeriosis (Listeria) and Pregnancy. Atlanta (GA): Centers for Disease Control and Prevention; 2010.
149. Prevention CfDCa. Amebiasis. 2010. Available at: cdc.gov.
150. Roy S, Herwaldt B, Johnston S. Other infectious diseases related to travel. 2010 Yellow Book. Atlanta (GA): Centers for Disease Control and Prevention; 2010.

151. Administration FUSFaD. *Entamoeba histolytica.* Bad bug book: foodborne pathogenic microorganisms and natural toxins handbook. Silver Spring (MD): U.S. Food and Drug Administration; 2009. Available at: http://www.fda.gov/Food/FoodSafety/FoodborneIllness/FoodborneIllnessFoodbornePathogensNaturalToxins/BadBugBook/ucm070739.htm. Accessed May 23, 2011.

152. Huston C. Intestinal protozoa. In: Feldman M, Friedman L, Brandt L, editors. Sleisenger & Fordtran's Gastrointestinal and liver disease, vol. 2. 8th edition. Philadelphia: Saunders; 2006. p. 2413–33.

153. Gonzales M, Dans L, Martinez E. Antiamoebic drugs for treating amoebic colitis [Review]. Cochrane Database Syst Rev 2009;2:CD006085.

154. Yoder J, Harral C, Beach M. Giardiasis surveillance—United States, 2006–2008. MMWR Surveill Summ 2010;59:15–25.

155. Zaat J, Mank T, Assendelft W. Drugs for treating giardiasis. Cochrane Database Syst Rev 2007;2:CD000217.

156. Hanevik K, Dizdar, Langeland N, et al. Development of functional gastrointestinal disorders after *Giardia lamblia* infection. BMC Gastroenterol 2009;9:27.

157. Prevention CfDCa. Cryptosporidiosis. In: Prevention CfDCa, editor. Atlanta (GA): 2010. Available at: cdc.gov.

158. Centers for Disease Control and Prevention (CDC). Outbreak of cryptosporidiosis associated with a splash park—Idaho, 2007. MMWR Morb Mortal Wkly Rep 2009;58(22):615–8.

159. Centers for Disease Control and Prevention (CDC). Communitywide cryptosporidiosis outbreak—Utah, 2007. MMWR Morb Mortal Wkly Rep 2008;57(36): 989–93.

160. Prevention CfDCa. Cryptosporidiosis (*Cryptosporidium* spp.) 2011 case definition. In: Services USDoHaH, editor. 2011. Available at: cdc.gov.

161. Prevention CfDCa. Prevention & control of cryptosporidiosis. In: Prevention CfDCa, editor. Atlanta (GA): 2010. Available at: cdc.gov.

162. Prevention CfDCa. Cystoisosporiasis. In: Prevention CfDCa, editor. Atlanta (GA): 2010. Available at: cdc.gov.

163. Prevention CfDCa. Cystoisosporiasis FAQs. In: Prevention CfDCa, editor. Atlanta (GA): 2010. Available at: cdc.gov.

164. Prevention CfDCa. Cyclosporiasis FAQs for health professionals. In: Prevention CfDCa, editor. Atlanta (GA): 2010. Available at: cdc.gov.

165. Lee S, Corradi N, Bymes E, et al. Microsporidia evolved from ancestral sexual fungi. Curr Biol 2008;18(21):1675–9.

166. Cheng L. Microsporidia. Stanford (CA): 2006. p. 5. Available at: http://www.stanford.edu/class/humbio103/ParaSites2006/Microsporidiosis/microsporidia1.html. Accessed May 23, 2011.

167. Center TNPR. Microsporidiosis. Diseases we investigate. 2006. Available at: http://www.tnprc.tulane.edu/public_micro.html. Accessed March 10, 2011.

168. Ghosh K, Weiss L. Molecular diagnostic tests for microsporidia. Interdiscip Perspect Infect Dis 2009;2009:13.

169. Molina J, Tourneur M, Sarfati C, et al. Fumagillin treatment of intestinal microsporidiosis. N Engl J Med 2002;346(25):1963–9.

# Index

*Note:* Page numbers of article titles are in **boldface** type.

# Moving?

## Make sure your subscription moves with you!

To notify us of your new address, find your **Clinics Account Number** (located on your mailing label above your name), and contact customer service at:

**Email: journalscustomerservice-usa@elsevier.com**

**800-654-2452** (subscribers in the U.S. & Canada)
**314-447-8871** (subscribers outside of the U.S. & Canada)

**Fax number: 314-447-8029**

**Elsevier Health Sciences Division
Subscription Customer Service
3251 Riverport Lane
Maryland Heights, MO 63043**

*To ensure uninterrupted delivery of your subscription, please notify us at least 4 weeks in advance of move.

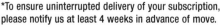
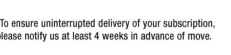

ELSEVIER

Printed and bound by CPI Group (UK) Ltd, Croydon, CR0 4YY

03/10/2024

01040447-0018